HUMAN PAPILLOMAVIRUSES
CLINICAL AND SCIENTIFIC ADVANCES

Edited by

Jane C. Sterling MB BChir MA PhD FRCP

Department of Dermatology
University of Cambridge
Addenbrooke's Hospital
Cambridge, UK

and

Stephen K. Tyring MD PhD

Departments of Dermatology, Microbiology/Immunology and Internal Medicine
The University of Texas Medical Branch at Galveston
Galveston
Texas, USA

A member of the Hodder Headline Group
LONDON • NEW YORK • NEW DELHI

First published in Great Britain in 2001 by
Arnold, a member of the Hodder Headline Goup,
338 Euston Road, London NW1 3BH

http://www.arnoldpublishers.com

Distributed in the United States of America by Oxford University Press Inc.,
198 Madison Avenue, New York, NY10016
Oxford is a registered trademark of Oxford University Press

Whilst the advice and information in this book are believed to be true and
accurate at the date of going to press, neither the authors nor the publisher
can accept any legal responsibility or liability for any errors or omissions
that may be made. In particular (but without limiting the generality of the
preceding disclaimer) every effort has been made to check drug dosages;
however it is still possible that errors have been missed. Furthermore,
dosage schedules are constantly being revised and new side-effects
recognized. For these reasons the reader is strongly urged to consult the
drug companies' printed instructions before administering any of the drugs
recommend in this book.

British Library Cataloguing in Publication Data
A catalogue record for this book is available from the British Library

Library of Congress Cataloging-in-Publication Data
A catalog record for this book is available from the Library of Congress

ISBN 0 340 74215 1

1 2 3 4 5 6 7 8 9 10

Commissioning Editor: Joanna Koster
Production Editor: James Rabson
Production Controller: Iain McWilliams

Typeset in 10.5pt Garamond by J&L Composition Ltd, Filey, North Yorkshire
Printed and bound in Italy by Giunti

Contents

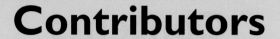

Contributors

Humphrey Birley
Department of Medical Microbiology and Genito-
urinary Medicine
Royal Liverpool University Hospital
Liverpool
UK

Scott Cuthill
Roche Discovery Welwyn
Welwyn Garden City
UK

John Doorbar
National Institute of Medical Research
London
UK

Catherine M Flaitz
Department of Stomatology
The University of Texas Health Science Center at
Houston
Houston
Texas
USA

Isobel Greenfield
Roche Global Department
Roche Products Ltd
Welwyn Garden City
UK

Catherine A Harwood
Centre for Cutaneous Research
St Bartholomew's and the Royal London School of
Medicine and Dentistry
Queen Mary and Westfield College
London
UK

Stephen C Inglis
Cantab Pharmaceuticals
Cambridge
UK

Stefania Jablonska
Department of Dermatology
Warsaw School of Medicine
Warsaw
Poland

Charles J N Lacey
Department of Genitourinary Medicine and
Communicable Diseases
St Mary's Hospital
London
UK

Slawomir Majewski
Department of Dermatology
Warsaw School of Medicine
Warsaw
Poland

Claire P Mansur
Department of Dermatology
New England Medical Center
Boston
Massachusetts
USA

Terence O'Neill
Cantab Pharmaceuticals
Cambridge
UK

Charlotte M Proby
Centre for Cutaneous Research
St Bartholomew's and the Royal London School of
Medicine and Dentistry
Queen Mary and Westfield College
London
UK

Margaret A Stanley
Department of Pathology
University of Cambridge
Cambridge
UK

Jane C Sterling
Department of Dermatology
University of Cambridge
Addenbrooke's Hospital
Cambridge
UK

Zoltan Trizna
Department of Dermatology
Texas Tech University Health Science Center
Lubbock
Texas
USA

Stephen K Tyring
Departments of Dermatology,
Microbiology/Immunology and Internal Medicine
University of Texas Medical Branch
Galveston
Texas
USA

Angela Yen Moore
Department of Dermatology
University of Texas Southwest Medical Center
Dallas
Texas
USA

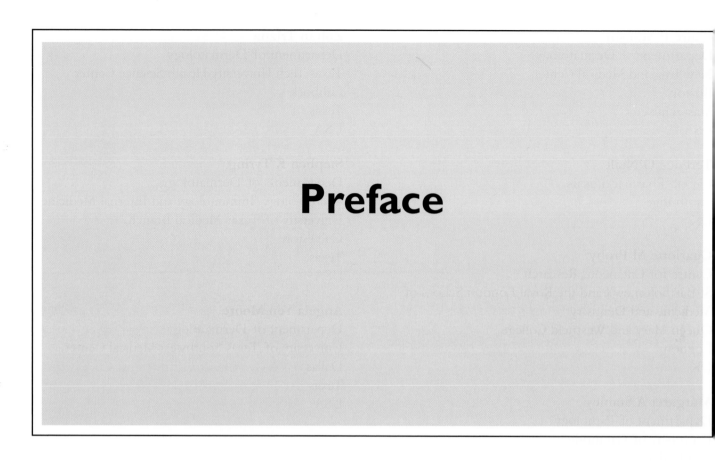

Preface

Warts of the skin and mucous membrane may be regarded as banal infections but the majority of the population is affected at some stage in their life, sometimes for prolonged periods. The causative infectious agents, the human papillomaviruses (HPVs), eluded laboratory culture and hence detailed study for many years, but the advent of molecular techniques has led to a rapid increase in the understanding of the biology of HPVs. Many of the advances in HPV research have stemmed from a focus on the propensity for certain types of HPV to contribute to malignant change. However, light has also been shed on the mechanisms leading to the benign epithelial proliferation induced by these viruses.

There is now the possibility of developing therapeutic approaches to HPV-induced or HPV-associated disease based on biological understanding of the nature of the infection and the body's response. The time is thus ripe for the practising clinician to have a firm grasp of the processes underlying warts and their behaviour and for the scientist to understand the current challenges of warts and HPV associated neoplasia.

The chapters of this book fall into three broad groups. First, the biology of the virus and the body's responses to the infection are presented. Knowing how the subcellular organism survives its passage through the environment and the skin and how it stimulates the changes we see as disease forms an essential basis for evolving management strategies. There are still many unknowns in the finely balanced nature of the virus-host cell interaction, but the current state of knowledge is presented in some detail. In the second section of the book, the clinical aspects of HPV disease of the skin and mucosae are described and the current methods of treatments explained. Finally, in the last three chapters, we look towards the future. The development of anti-viral approaches and of immune-stimulating vaccines to combat HPV disease are both promising, and the possible future of therapy is revealed. Basic research can develop in a huge number of directions and a taste of where advances are likely to be made in the next few years will be found in the last chapter.

In this book, our approach has been to marry up-to-the-minute science with clinical features and presently available treatments as well as potential future therapies. We have aimed to provide a text primarily for clinicians who treat patients with warts, but we hope that it will also serve as a detailed introduction for anyone with an interest in HPVs and their effects on epithelia, in particular for researchers entering or diversifying in the field. In order to achieve a balance between the art and the science of medicine, we have been very fortunate in having contributions to this book from a number of scientists eminent in their particular areas of HPV research as well as from clinicians with wide experience in dealing with the challenges of treating warts. The book can be used as an inclusive text defining where we are now in dealing with these infections and where we are going in the near future. It will also provide day to day reference for those practicing in fields where HPV infections cause disease and for researchers exploring the cellular and whole body interaction with these highly successful viruses.

Part I

Introduction

1

Introduction

Jane C. Sterling

1.1 INTRODUCTION AND HISTORY

In diseases caused by virus infections it has historically been difficult to establish the nature of the association and the proof of the causation. Although certain diseases were believed to be due to an infectious agent, the existence of many viruses was not proven until the technology of electron microscopy enabled visualization of the infectious particles. Human papillomaviruses (HPVs) are no exception to this rule and were first reported in 1949.[35] Prior to that, warts were recognized as a transmissible infection as a result of some bold experimentation of person to person inoculation.[8, 39]

Whereas research into the infectivity and other capabilities of viruses such as herpes simplex virus was able to progress during the middle part of the twentieth century, papillomavirus research was hampered by the fact that culture of the virus in a variety of potential host cells seemed impossible. Both animal and human wart tissue, when cultured *in vitro*, produced no on-going source of virions, and hence no system in which to observe the life cycle of the virus.[23, 27] However, in the late 1980s, the use of animal culture systems in which infected human epithelial cells could be grown in an immunosuppressed host permitted viral replication and reproduction.[14, 34] The growth conditions have now been defined whereby the virus can be propagated in cells cultured *in vitro*, thus allowing study of the virus within the environment of the natural host cell, the keratinocyte.[20] and, by this means, several genital HPV types have been successfully propagated (C. Meyers, 2000, personal communication).

It was always recognized, however, that warts affected several different body areas, could be of a variety of different shapes and sizes, and that not only humans were affected with papillomatous excrescences of skin and musosal surfaces. The advent of the molecular biology techniques and their widespread application in the 1970s were the main impetus to the evolution of our understanding of the biology of papillomavirus disease and have led to huge leaps forward in both basic research and clinical application.

In this book, we aim to bring together the current knowledge of the basic molecular and cellular aspects of the virus, of its interaction with host tissue and of the disease it causes. Clinicians involved in patient care will gain greater insight into the biology of the infection and the potential or otherwise for treatment, whilst basic researchers will appreciate the nature of HPV-induced disease and the areas in which treatment design might develop.

1.2 NATURE OF DISEASE CAUSED BY HPV

The ways in which the papillomaviruses can affect cells are detailed in Chapter 2. Papillomaviruses are able to produce disease in stratified squamous epithelia, showing species specificity as well as some degree of site specificity. Although much of our knowledge of these processes has come from the study of human disease, huge steps forward have been made from the study of animal papillomavirus infections, as well as with *in vitro* cell culture and molecular biology. It is tempting always to assume that what occurs in a non-human animal or in a cultured cell can be exactly transposed to humans, but this is not necessarily so. Other environmental factors (either internal or external) may affect the disease outcome. Animal papillomaviruses are widespread in nature (reviewed in reference 36). They appear to cause diseases of both skin and mucosa, but some may also infect fibroblasts, for example certain bovine papillomaviruses, in a way that does not seem to have a human equivalent.

Even within the group of viruses which infect humans, genomic sequencing has shown that the variation is large and nearly 100 different HPV types have now been identified, with several more suggested by sequencing of just a part of the genome. The variation and importance of these different genotypes are illustrated in the chapters of this book, with regard both to the diseases that are caused and also to the natural immunity to the virus and the prospects for therapy.

1.3. DISEASES CAUSED BY THE VIRUS

It was in cutaneous and later anogenital warts that HPV virions were first found, but it was not until DNA isolation and sequencing became readily available techniques that the virus was found not to be a single virus, but a group of closely related but molecularly distinct virus types. The distinction between these types was shown to correlate, at least in some cases, with the morphological appearance of the epithelial change and also with the evolution of the disease. In the early part of the 1970s, DNA analysis of virus in warts permitted the development of a different method of classifying the skin and mucosal lesions and the recognition of the variety of different sorts of warts and the body areas they infect. When HPV DNA was found in cervical cancer,[9] the possibility that the virus was acting as a carcinogen provided the impetus for a vast amount of research into the disease and other pre-malignant and malignant disorders of epithelia. Recently, HPVs have been linked with other proliferative conditions of the skin such as psoriasis.

1.3.1 Warts

A number of different types of human papillomaviruses cause warts when they gain access to keratinocytes and establish a productive infection. Following person-to-person transmission, the entry of the virus into the cell is essential before virus gene expression can influence the proliferation and maturation of the keratinocyte in a way which results in the growth of a benign tumor. The life cycle of the virus is completed by production of new sheddable virus and clearance of the infection by immunological attack. Warts can occur on any part of the skin or mucosa, but there is both a clinical and virological distinction between warts on keratinized epithelium, i.e., the skin, and those which occur on non-stratified mucosal surfaces. This distinction is not absolute and is more blurred in circumstances such as immunodeficiency.

1.3.2 Anogenital Cancer

The discovery of papillomavirus DNA in cervical cancer has been followed by numerous reports of the presence of viral DNA sequence, in other malignancies and premalignancies of the anogenital skin and mucosae,[17] and upper aero-digestive tract. The subgroup of HPVs which are found in association with such disease processes are termed 'high risk', and molecular and cellular analyses have demonstrated oncogenic properties of part of the viral genome (discussed more fully in Chapter 3). Invasive cancer of stratified squamous epithelium in these sites where skin abuts on mucosa frequently has a prolonged phase of intraepithelial dysplasia, which potentially could permit detection and treatment before frank malignancy.

1.3.3 Skin Cancer

The rare syndrome of epidermodysplasia verruciformis (EV) consists of a slightly depressed cell-mediated immunity plus the development of a variety of skin lesions, including flat warty lesions, erythematous scaly lesions, and also skin cancers, particularly in sun-exposed areas. HPV DNA was isolated from the skin lesions of these patients and several different types were identified[25] (reviewed in Chapter 9). In more recent years, types with a close genetic relationship to these original EV types have been detected in malignant and pre-malignant skin lesions in immunosuppressed individuals, again especially in ultraviolet-exposed sites.[3, 30] The role that the virus may play in the development of such lesions is currently debated and is discussed more fully in Chapter 10. The main reasons for uncertainty about the etiological relationship between the EV-related HPVs and skin cancer arise from both molecular and cellular studies of the E6 and E7 gene product function and also from the observation that these potentially 'high-risk' skin HPVs are found in the normal skin of both immunosuppressed and immunocompetent individuals without apparently causing disease.

1.3.4 Other skin disease associated with HPV

Several other skin conditions have been reported to harbour HPV DNA. Of greatest importance in recent years is the finding of EV-related HPV types in psoriasis, a T-cell-mediated skin condition in which the epidermis both hyperproliferates and matures abnormally in well-defined areas. Polymerase chain reaction (PCR) amplification of biopsies from affected skin and unaffected skin in psoriatic individuals has shown the presence of HPV 5, 20, 36 or 38 in over 80% of biopsies of psoriatic plaques, and in approximately 20% of skin biopsies from non-psoriatic individuals.[10, 38] Seropositivity to virus-like particles (VLPs) was found in 46% of individuals whose psoriasis had been treated with ultraviolet irradiation.[33] Although it has been hypothesized that the virus may be the antigenic stimulus for the immune response in psoriasis, the precise role the virus may be playing in the affected skin or in the psoriatic individual as a whole is not yet clear.

1.4 EXTENT OF THE PROBLEM OF HPV DISEASE

Human papillomavirus-related disease is a world-wide problem and no age group or race is spared. As a result, epidemiological studies of HPV-associated diseases have suggested that, at any one time, a significant proportion of the world's population may be infected with this virus. The severity of the abnormality produced by the infection is, however, very variable and depends on both viral and host factors as well as on environmental influences. Disease may be clinical, subclinical, and latent, and so epidemiological studies to define the extent and effect of infection with this virus must rely on detection methods other than clinical examination alone.

Detection of HPV infection is generally performed in two major ways: by the finding of viral nucleic acid in tissue and by detection of an immune response to a viral protein. Both of these methods are potentially applicable to large studies.

Firstly, the presence of the virus or the viral nucleic acid in the affected tissue suggests, but does not prove, an etiological relationship. DNA amplification by PCR permits detection of small amounts of viral DNA and is now the most frequently used method of ascertaining if the virus is present. Such a sensitive technique is prone to the problems of false positive results, due especially to contamination, but, with adequate control, can be a reliable diagnostic tool. Finding virus particles by electron microscopy, growing the virus in cell culture and transmission of the virus to animals are not possible routine methods for HPV detection. Detection of viral proteins can be used in certain circumstances and, although this is not a technique with a great degree of sensitivity, it would confirm that the virus is active within the host cell.

The second method for establishing whether or not an individual has had contact with the HPV is by means of serological responses to the virus or its proteins. Seroepidemiological studies have been performed for several different types. However, a seropositive response does not necessarily indicate that the virus is still present or that it has caused the current disease, but will suggest either a present or past infection. Human papillomavirus infection does not result in a viremia, which for many virus infections acts as the stimulus for development of an antibody response. However, local responses in the skin and mucosa are instead believed to be the starting point for an anti-HPV humoral response. The cell-mediated immune response is an important defense against active HPV infection, but methods to test the presence or strength of T-cell response to viral proteins are rather cumbersome and less easy to use in epidemiological studies.

1.4.1 Cutaneous warts

Warts of the skin are a common problem and affect a huge proportion of the population of the world, but usually for limited periods of time. Population studies suggest that cutaneous warts are most common in children and young adults, affecting between 3% and 20% of school-age children.[13, 15, 29] However, adults may also be affected and, in this older age group, the disease is often felt to be longer lived. Visible signs of infection in the form of warts may last just a few weeks or may persist for several years, sometimes despite treatment. The average duration of warts is of the order of 2 years.[29] Spontaneous clearance of skin warts in children occurs in 67% within 2 years.[19]

Cutaneous warts have a variety of different morphological forms, depending in part on the type of HPV, but also on the site affected and perhaps the response to trauma and treatment. In children with warts, the majority (70%) have common warts, a quarter have plantar warts, whilst plane and filiform warts are much rarer.[22]

1.4.2 Anogenital warts

Anogenital warts cause an increasingly large problem, particularly for young adults, who may become infected after commencing sexual activity. The incidence and prevalence may vary according to reporting as well as geography, but studies in several parts of the world have suggested a steady rise in the number of patients with genital warts over the last 30 years.[1, 31] In the UK, the incidence of the development of genital warts is highest in young adults aged 16 to 24, for whom the rate may be over 500 per 100 000, having reached a population rate of 300 per 100 000 in 1994.[31] Estimates of the number of people affected with warts are mainly dependent on self-referral and accurate diagnosis rather than on screening.

1.4.3 Intraepithelial neoplasia and squamous cell carcinoma

Anogenital intraepithelial neoplasia and cancer cause much more serious health problems and the incidence appears to vary geographically. Approximately 500 000 new cases of cervical cancer are diagnosed each year and, of these, about 80% are in developing countries where facilities for screening and early diagnosis and possibilities for treatment may be considerably less than in the developed nations.

HPV DNA has been found in the majority of invasive cervical cancers.[40] Studies of women in countries in South America, Europe, North Africa, and South-East Asia showed that an average of 91% of cancers were HPV positive.[21] (Muñoz, personal communication), although there was a slight variation of positivity rates from 75% in Columbia to 98% in Paraguay. Some feel that as many as 100% of cervical cancers harbor HPV genomes,[37] and that accurate and sensitive methods of detection will reveal almost no HPV-negative lesions. The majority (60–70%) of HPV-positive cervical cancers harbor HPV type 16, whilst HPV 18 is the second most common type in this disease (10–20%). The means by which a virus such as HPV could contribute to the process of carcinogenesis in this body area are discussed fully in Chapters 2 and 3.

Intraepithelial neoplasia of the cervix is frequently detectable visually as abnormal epithelium which whitens after application of diluted acetic acid and may be suggested by the finding of cytologically abnormal cells on a cervical smear test. However, diagnosis is not complete until a full-thickness sample of the epithelium is taken, to permit evaluation of the degree or grade of epithelial dysplasia. These pre-malignant stages of cervical disease are also frequently found to harbor HPV DNA. Several studies have not just evaluated the prevalence of HPV within normal and dysplastic cervix, but also have examined either retrospectively or prospectively the risk of the presence of certain HPV types and the future development of cancer. In high-grade cervical intraepithelial neoplasia, HPV is present in well over

50%, perhaps nearing 100% in some studies,[6] with HPV 16 being the predominant type.[16] From longer-term studies, it appears that the presence of high-risk HPVs in cervical intraepithelial neoplasia III gives an increased risk of the future development of cervical cancer.[24,26]

In addition to lesions of the uterine cervix, other sites, including the vagina, vulval, penis, and anal area as well as upper aero-digestive tract, may also be affected with pre-invasive intraepithelial neoplasia and cancer. In these situations, HPV may also be found, although reports to date have usually suggested a lower rate of HPV positivity than in equivalent lesions of the cervix (for review, see reference 17, and Chapters 7 and 8). However, more sensitive PCR detection may, in the future, give a story similar to that in the cervix.

1.4.4 Skin cancer

No large population studies of skin cancers and HPV DNA detection have yet been reported. There is some degree of correlation between circulating antibodies to EV types and skin cancer. Antibodies to HPV 8 VLPs were found in 46% of immunocompetent patients with skin cancers, in 21% of renal transplant patients who are at risk of skin cancers and in only 8% of the clinically normal population.[34] Although the ages of these three groups were not comparable, within the groups of individuals over the age of 50, the ratios of positive to negative remained similar.

1.4.5 HPV carriage without apparent disease

The sensitivity of the PCR has permitted many studies, which have found asymptomatic and subclinical carriage of HPV DNA in a variety of body sites. The cervix may certainly harbor both low-risk and high-risk types of genital HPVs and, although some may later develop into disease, in some the viral infection will clear. Women with clinically and cytologically normal cervices show a rate of HPV positivity averaging 13.7% in a world-wide study by Muñoz *et al.* (personal communication), with a range from 5.4% in Spain to 21.6% in Morocco. The carriage rate differs according to age, peaking in young adulthood (age 20–29), but even teenagers have a 5% carriage rate. However, the type of HPV found in clinically normal individuals is of consequence, with high-risk types greatly changing the future possibility of developing dysplastic cervical disease. Rozendaal and colleagues have demonstrated that the presence of a high-risk genital HPV in a cervix which shows no cytological abnormality leads to a hundred-fold increased risk of cervical cancer at some stage.[28]

HPV DNA can also be detected in normal skin and oral mucosa. It was in immunosuppressed transplant recipients that HPVs were found in plucked hairs and on the skin surface, but it was soon apparent that immunologically and clinically normal individuals could also carry the virus without apparent effect.[4] Low-risk genital HPVs can be found in plucked pubic hairs of up to 60% of individuals with genital warts, and also in a small number of people without apparent warts.[5]

The significance of the finding of viral DNA in situations in which disease is not apparent is not yet clear. The longer-term studies of cervical carriage have suggested that sub-clinical infection is of prognostic importance, but, in the skin and other anogenital sites, further prospective research will be necessary to establish whether the virus is active or having an effect on the cell which could lead to disease. Similarly, the possible role of the virus in diseases such as psoriasis, in which it is implicated to be associated, will need further investigation.

1.5 CONTROL AND MANAGEMENT OF HPV DISEASE

Compared to the treatment of bacterial infection, virus disease eradication from an infected individual is much more difficult, primarily due to the intracellular parasitic site of the virus. In addition, the HPV infects only the skin and mucous membranes and so maintains a relatively privileged position within the body, with the ability to evade many of the usual methods of immune attack. Control of an infectious virus disease may be achieved by preventing host-to-host transmission, eradication of the virus alone or within infected cells, blockage of the completion of the virus life cycle, or increasing the immune response either to prevent entry of the virus into the organism or to boost the methods of immune clearance of virus-infected cells.

1.5.1 Transmission

Person-to-person transmission of HPV occurs primarily via contact in which virus particles shed from an HPV-induced lesion pass to the epithelium of another individual. Interruption of such transfer could be achieved by physical means, such as the use of condoms for reducing the spread of genital warts or the use of 'verruca socks' for plantar warts. Alternatively, a vigorous mucosal or cutaneous immune response at the time of contact might prevent viral entry to cells or eliminate, at an early stage, virus-infected cells. This forms the basic tenet of prophylactic vaccination.

Acquisition of genital HPV infection is primarily by sexual contact, but there is growing evidence that other means of transmission may occur. Low-risk HPV types have been detected in fomites,[11] on underwear[2] and on the fingers of patients who have genital warts.[32] Vertical transmission of HPV occurs and may result in viral DNA being present in the oral cavity or the genital area. Analysis of HPV DNA present in scrapings from children of up to 6 months of age, avoiding the possibility of contamination of the infant with maternal cells, has shown a prevalence of HPV infection of 50% of children born to HPV 16-positive women, with evidence of identical genotypes of high-risk types in both child and mother.[12] Other studies have shown HPV DNA detection in children with a range of 0.25–52% (for review, see reference 18). Serological evaluation of antibodies to HPV 16 virus-like particles also suggests a degree of immunological competence to the high-risk virus type of up to 15% of children.[7]

1.5.2 Treatment

Traditionally, attempts to curtail HPV-induced disease have relied mainly on the concept that removal or destruction of virus-infected cells and tissue will remove the virus. However, the finding of viral DNA and RNA in many individuals and situations in which florid or even mild disease is detectable suggests that a purely surgical approach to therapy is unlikely to be uniformly successful. Other approaches to treatment, especially immunological, are under development and both current and future management strategies are described in several chapters of this book.

1.6 SCOPE AND AIMS OF THIS BOOK

We have aimed to present current research ideas alongside present-day approaches to patient management – essentially, a 'gene to clinic' approach. To do this, eminent scientists and clinicians have contributed to the various chapters, all adding their own perspectives on the world-wide problem of HPV disease, the ongoing lines of research into the virus and its interaction with its host, and also practical information to assist in patient care. The knowledge of HPV disease is expanding rapidly and in a few years we may have a very different approach to treatment. The final part is more speculative about the future, but may become a reality within the next decade or two. We hope that this book will serve both as a reference manual and also as an educational text for those involved in any field of HPV disease.

REFERENCES

1. Becker TM, Stone KM, Alexander ER. (1987) Genital human papillomavirus infection: a growing concern. *Obstet Gynecol Clin North Am* **14**: 389–96.
2. Bergeron C, Ferenczy A, Richart R. (1990) Underwear: contamination by human papillomavirus infection. *Epidemiol Rev* **10**: 122–63.
3. Berkhout RJ, Tieben LM, Smits HL, Bavinck JN, Vermeer BJ, ter Schegget J. (1995) Nested PCR approach for detection and typing of epidermodysplasia verruciformis-associated human papillomavirus types in cutaneous cancers from renal transplant recipients. *J Clin Microbiol* **33**: 690–5.
4. Boxman ILA, Berkhout RJM, Mulder LHC, *et al.* (1997) Detection of human papillomavirus DNA in plucked hairs from renal transplant recipients and healthy volunteers. *J Invest Dermatol* **108**: 712–15.
5. Boxman ILA, Hogewoning A, Mulder LHC, Bouwes Bavinck JN, ter Schegget J. (1999) Detection of human papillomavirus types 6 and 11 in pubic and perianal hair from patients with genital warts. *J Clin Microbiol* **37**: 2270–3.
6. Chua KL, Hjerpe A. (1997) Human papillomavirus analysis as a prognostic marker following conization of cervix uteri. *Gynaecol Oncol* **66**: 108–13.
7. Cubie H, Plumstead M, De Jesus O, Duncan LA, Stanley MA. (1998) Prevalence of antibodies to human papillomavirus type 16 in 11–13 year old schoolgirls. *J Med Virol* **56**: 210–16.
8. Cuiffo G. (1907) Innesto positivo confiltrado di verruca volgare. *G Ital Mal Vener* **48**: 12.
9. Dürst M, Gissmann L, Ikenberg H, zur Hausen H. (1983) A papillomavirus DNA from a cervical carcinoma and its prevalence in cancer samples from different geographic regions. *Proc Natl Acad Sci* **80**: 3812–15.
10. Favre M, Orth G, Majewski S, Baloul S, Pura A, Jablonska S. (1998) Psoriasis: a possible reservoir for human papillomavirus type 5, the virus associated with skin carcinomas of epidermodysplasia verruciformis. *J Invest Dermatol* **110**: 311–17.
11. Ferenczy A, Bergeron C, Richart RM. (1989) Human papillomavirus DNA in fomites on objects used for the management of patients with genital human papillomavirus infections. *Obstet Gynaecol* **74**: 950–4.
12. Kaye JN, Starkey WG, Kell B, *et al.* (1996) Human papillomavirus type-16 (HPV-16) in infants: use of DNA sequence analyses to establish the source of infection. *J Gen Virol* **77**: 1139–43.
13. Kilkenny M, Marks, R. (1996) The descriptive epidemiology of warts in the community. *Aust J Dermatol* **37**: 80–6.
14. Kreider JW, Howett MK, Leure-Dupree AE, Zaino RJ, Weber JA. (1987) Laboratory production *in vivo* of infectious human papillomavirus type 11. *J Virol* **61**: 590–3.
15. Larsson P-A, Lidén S. (1980) Prevalence of skin diseases among adolescents 12–16 years of age. *Acta Dermatovener* **60**: 415–23.
16. Lungu O, Sun XW, Felix J, Richart RM, Silverstein S, Wright TC. (1992) Relationship of human papillomavirus type to grade of cervical intraepithelial neoplasia. *JAMA* **267**: 2493–6.
17. Majewski S, Jablonska S. (1997) Human papillomavirus-associated tumors of the skin and mucosa. *J Am Acad Dermatol* **36**: 659–85.
18. Mant C, Cason J, Rice P, Best JM. (2000) Non-sexual transmission of cervical cancer-associated papillomaviruses: an update. *Pap Report* **11**: 1–5.
19. Massing AM, Epstein WL. (1963) Natural history of warts. *Arch Dermatol* **87**: 306–10.
20. Meyers C, Frattini MG, Hudson JB, Laimins LA. (1992) Biosynthesis of human papillomavirus from a continuous cell line upon epithelial differentiation. *Science* **257**: 971–3.
21. Muñoz N, Bosch FX. (1992) HPV and cervical neoplasia: review of case-control and cohort studies. In *The epidemiology of cervical cancer and human papillomavirus*, eds N Muñoz, FX Bosch, KV Shah, and A Meheus. Lyon, International Agency for Research and Cancer, 251–61.
22. Nagington J, Rook A, Highet A. (1986) Virus and related infections. In *Textbook of dermatology*, eds A Rook, DS Wilkinson, FJG Ebling, RH Champion, JL Burton. Oxford, Blackwell Scientific Publications 657–723.
23. Niimura M, Pass F, Wooley R, Souter CA. (1975) Primary tissue culture of human wart-derived epidermal cells. *J Natl Cancer Inst* **54**: 563–6.
24. Nobbenhuis MAE, Walboomers JMM, Helmerhorst TJM, *et al.* (1999) Relation of human papillomavirus status to cervical lesions and consequences for cervical screening: a prospective study. *Lancet* **354**: 20–5.
25. Orth G. (1987) Epidermodysplasia verruciformis. In *Papovaviridae*, Vol. 2, *The papillomaviruses*, eds NP Salzman and PM Howley. New York, Plenum Press, 199–243.

26. Remmink AJ, Walboomers JMM, Helmerhorst TJM, *et al.* (1995) The presence of persistent high risk HPV human papillomavirus genotypes in dysplastic cervical lesions is associated with progressive disease. Natural history up to 36 months. *Int J Cancer* **61**: 1–6.

27. Rose BR, Thompson CH, McDonald AM, Henderson BR, Cossart YE, Morris BJ. (1987) Cell biology of cultured anogenital warts. *Br J Dermatol* **116**: 311–22.

28. Rozendaal L, Westerga J, van der Linden JC, *et al.* (2000) PCR based high risk HPV testing is superior to neural network based screening for predicting incident CIN III in women with normal cytology and borderline changes. *J Clin Pathol* **53**: 606–11.

29. Rulison RH. (1942) Warts. A statistical study of nine hundred and twenty one cases. *Arch Dermatol Syphilol* **46**: 66–81.

30. Shamanin V, Glover M, Rausch C, *et al.* (1994) Specific types of human papillomavirus found in benign proliferations and carcinomas of the skin in immunosuppressed patients. *Cancer Res* **54**: 4610–13.

31. Simms I, Fairley CK. (1997) Epidemiology of genital warts in England and Wales: 1971–1994. *Genitourin Med* **73**: 365–7.

32. Sonnex C, Strauss S, Grey JJ. (1999) Detection of human papillomavirus DNA on the fingers of patients with genital warts. *Sex Transm Inf* **75**: 317–19.

33. Stark S, Petridis A, Ghim S, *et al.* (1998) Prevalence of antibodies against virus-like particles of epidermodysplasia verruciformis-associated HPV8 in patients at risk of skin cancer. *J Invest Dermatol* **111**: 696–701.

34. Sterling JC, Stanley MA, Gatward G, Minson AC. (1990) Production of human papillomavirus type 16 virions in a keratinocyte cell line. *J. Virol* **64**: 6305–7.

35. Strauss MJ, Shaw EW, Buntinh H, Melnick JL. (1949) 'Crystalline' virus-like particles from skin papillomas characterised by intranuclear inclusion bodies. *Proc Soc Exp Biol Med* **72**: 46–50.

36. Sundberg JP. (1987) Papillomavirus infection in animals. In *Papillomaviruses and human disease*, eds K Syrjänen, L Gissmann, LG Koss. Berlin, Springer Verlag 40–103.

37. Walboomers JMM, Jacobs MV, Manos MM, *et al.* (1999) Human papillomavirus is a necessary cause of invasive cervical cancer worldwide. *J Pathol* **189**: 12–19.

38. Weissenborn SJ, Höfpl R, Weber F, Smola H, Pfister HJ, Fuchs PG. (1999) High prevalence of a variety of epidermodysplasia verriciformis-associated human papillomaviruses in psoriatic skin of patients treated or not treated with PUVA. *J Invest Dermatol* **113**: 122–6.

39. Wile UJ, Kingery LB. (1919) The etiology of common warts. Preliminary report of an experimental study. *JAMA* **73**: 970–3.

40. Zur Hausen H. (1996) Papillomavirus infections – a major cause of human cancers. *Biochim Biophys Acta* **1288**: F55–79.

Part II

Molecular and cellular aspects

2

The biology of human papillomaviruses

John Doorbar and Jane C. Sterling

The human papillomaviruses (HPVs) are a group of closely related viruses which infect stratified squamous epithelia producing host cell proliferation. As well as exhibiting tissue specificity, they are also species specific, infecting only human tissue. Most also show a degree of site specificity, preferentially infecting or producing visible effects at certain body sites. The diseases they cause reflect not only altered epidermal growth but also the degree to which the host immune response is able to recognize and control the infection (discussed in Chapter 3).

2.1 VIRAL STRUCTURE AND DNA

Compared to other viruses which infect skin, such as herpes simplex virus and the poxviruses, HPV is small but it is a highly successful virus. The virus particle, or virion, consists of an icosahedral protein coat, or capsid, enclosing the viral genome, which is in the form of circular, double-stranded DNA (Figure 2.1). Electron microscopical analysis has shown the particle to be 55 nm in diameter and hence of similar size to polyoma virus and the vacuolating virus SV40.[123] The papillomavirus was therefore classified in a group with these other viruses, to constitute the papova (*pa*pillomavirus-*po*lyomavirus-*va*cuolating virus) family of viruses.

When the organization of the papillomavirus genome was discovered by sequencing, the arrangement of the genes was found to be quite different from that of other papova viruses. All the open reading frames (ORFs, i.e., the genes) are arranged on one strand. The DNA of approximately 8000 nucleotide base pairs encodes eight to ten genes, and

there is also a non-coding region (NCR) – also called the long control region (LCR) or upstream regulatory region (URR). Although there are variations in the size and sequence of the genes and the NCR between different papillomavirus types, they all have the same basic arrangement of the genome (Figure 2.2). Two proteins which make up the capsid are encoded by genes within the so-called late region and have been designated L1 (the major capsid protein) and L2 (the minor capsid protein). The early region (E region) encodes a series of proteins E1, E2, E4, E5, E6, and E7. In bovine papillomaviruses (BPVs), two other ORFs, E3 and E8, are also identified. The functions of the various genes were initially established from studies of BPV, but there are some important biological differences between the bovine and human papillomaviruses. Some BPVs (group A) can infect both keratinocytes and fibroblasts of the host and, as well as producing a warty surface growth, also induce a fibroblastic proliferation in the dermis. In contrast, group B BPVs and HPVs can only infect keratinocytes. In addition, one of the BPVs, BPV 4, infects the alimentary tract, where it can cause carcinoma.

The functions of the various genes are described in more detail below, in relation to the virus life cycle. The NCR between the end of the L1 gene and the start of the E6 gene is a stretch of approximately 480–950 nucleotides containing many regions which may bind cellular or viral factors. Short lengths of sequence with a recognized pattern of nucleotides (called motifs) can be identified as areas which are likely to bind certain known transcription factors, leading either to stimulation or depression of proteins produced downstream. The NCR therefore acts in the control of viral activity, connecting viral gene expression with the

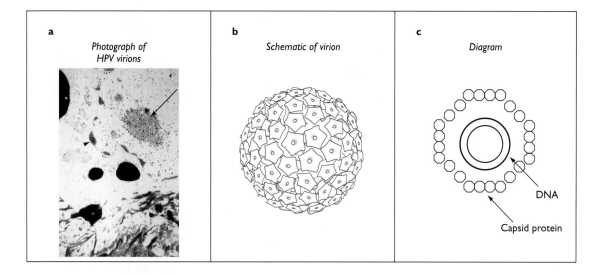

Figure 2.1

Structure of the human papillomavirus particle. (a) Immunoelectron microscopy of icosahedral papillomavirus particles (large arrow) within the nucleus of a cutaneous wart (arrowhead = nuclear membrane; small arrow = cell membrane). The capsid protein is identified by an antibody against the L1 protein and this antibody is localized by a second antibody labeled with gold particles. (b) The particle is icosahedral with 72 pentameric capsomers consisting predominantly of the L1 protein, with a smaller proportion of L2 embedded deeper within the protein shell. (c) Schematic representation of a cross-section through an intact virus particle. In the complete virion, the double-stranded, circular viral genome is contained within the protein coat.

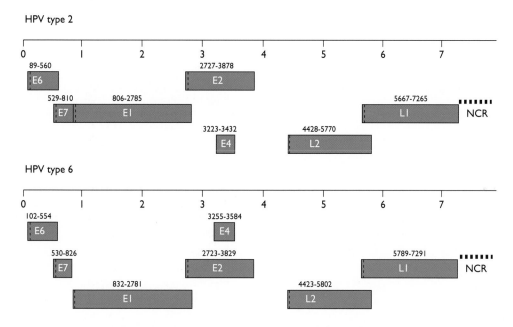

Figure 2.2

Papillomavirus genome arrangement of HPV 2 and HPV 6. All papillomaviruses, human and animal, have the same general arrangement of the genome. The genomes, which occur naturally as circular molecules, are shown here in linear form. The oblong boxes represent open reading frames (ORFs), distances of potential protein-coding sequence between one stop codon and the next. The terminology and gene functions are explained in the text. NCR = non-coding region; vertical dashed line within ORF = position of start codon.

modulating levels of cellular and also viral proteins. From detailed study of the NCRs of the genital HPVs, certain elements are known to be able to bind transcription factors and this binding has a functional effect. Computer analyses suggest that such motifs are also present in other HPV types and it may therefore be supposed that cutaneous HPVs will behave similarly. HPVs contain four or six potential binding sites for their own E2 protein and usually a site for E1 binding, providing the virus with feedback loops of transcriptional activity. In addition, over ten different known cellular transcription factors, including AP1, NF1, Oct-1, TEF-1, TEF-2, and YY1, are able to bind to this region.[89]

2.2 HPV TYPES

It was originally thought that all warts were caused by a single papilloma virus, and that the form of the lesion was influenced by body site or environmental factors. Only when molecular techniques such as hybridization and sequencing became established could different types of papillomavirus be distinguished. The initial slow identification of different types of HPV involved in the production of cutaneous warts has been followed by the discovery of numerous varieties of HPVs in a large number of different clinical situations.[36] (Table 2.1). HPVs can be broadly broken down into the types which preferentially infect muscosal surfaces and those which are most commonly found in skin. As well as the propensity to infect a particular form of epithelium, HPVs may also be subdivided by their association or lack of association with malignant disease of the stratified squamous integument.

Table 2.1

Human papillomavirus types reported and cloned

HPV type	Found in	Initial isolation from
1	Plantar and palmar warts	Plantar wart
2	Common skin warts	Hand wart
3	Plane warts, EV (benign lesions)	EV
4	Common warts, plantar warts	Plantar wart
5	EV (macular lesions, flat warts, SCC)	EV wart
6	Genital warts, laryngeal papillomas, CIN, Buschke–Löwenstein tumors	Genital wart
7	Butchers' warts, common Buschke–Löwenstein tumors	Butchers' wart
8	EV (macular lesions, plane warts, SCC)	EV
9	EV (macular lesions, plane warts)	EV
10	Plane warts, EV	EV
11	Genital warts, laryngeal papillomas, CIN, Buschke–Löwenstein tumors	Laryngeal papilloma
12	EV (benign lesions)	EV
13	Focal epithelial hyperplasia	Focal epithelial hyperplasia
14	EV (benign lesions, cutaneous SCC)	EV
15	EV (benign lesions)	EV
16	Genital intraepithelial neoplasia (CIN, VIN, AIN, PIN), genital SCC (cervical, vulval, anal, penile)	Cervical SCC
17	EV (benign lesions)	EV
18	CIN, cervical SCC	Cervical SCC
19	EV (benign lesions)	EV
20	EV (benign lesions)	EV
21	EV (benign lesions)	EV
22	EV (benign lesions)	EV
23	EV (benign lesions)	EV
24	EV (benign lesions)	EV
25	EV (benign lesions)	EV
26	Common and genital warts in immunosuppressed (rare)	Common wart, immunosuppressed
27	Common warts	Hand wart, immunosuppressed
28	Common warts, butchers' warts	Butchers' wart
29	Rare in cutaneous warts	Skin wart
30	Genital SCC, laryngeal SCC	Laryngeal SCC
31	Genital warts, CIN, cervical SCC	CIN
32	Focal epithelial hyperplasia, oral warts	Focal epithelial hyperplasia
33	CIN, cervical SCC	Cervical SCC
34	Anogenital warts, CIN	Cutaneous Bowen's disease
35	CIN, cervical SCC	Cervical adenocarcinoma
36	EV keratoses	Actinic keratosis
37		Keratoacanthoma
38		Malignant melanoma
39	CIN, cervical SCC	PIN
40	Genital warts, VIN	PIN
41	Cutaneous plane warts	Cutaneous SCC
42	CIN	Vulvar wart
43	Genital warts, CIN	Genital wart
44	Genital warts, CIN	Genital wart
45	CIN, cervical SCC	CIN
46	Reclassified as type 20b	
47	EV (benign lesions, cutaneous SCC)	EV (benign lesion)
48	Anogenital warts	SCC hand, immunosuppressed
49	Plane warts in immunosuppressed	Plane warts in immunosuppressed
50	EV	EV (benign lesions)
51	Anogenital warts, PIN, CIN, cervical SCC	Cervical SCC
52	CIN, cervical SCC	CIN
53	CIN, cervical SCC	Normal cervix
54	Anogenital warts, Buschke–Löwenstein tumors (rare)	Genital warts
55	Anogenital warts	VIN
56	CIN, cervical SCC	CIN
57	Mucosal warts and common warts in immunosuppressed	Inverted papilloma of the maxillary sinus
58	CIN, cervical SCC, PIN	Cervical SCC
59	Mucosal warts	VIN
60	Plantar epidermoid cyst	Plantar epidermoid cyst
61	VIN, CIN	VIN
62	VIN	VIN
63	Cutaneous warts (rare), multiple plantar punctate keratoses	Multiple plantar punctate keratoses
64	Anogenital warts, VIN	VIN
65	Pigmented plane warts, pigmented plantar and palmar warts	Pigmented wart
66	CIN, cervical SCC, PIN	Cervical SCC, normal cervix
67	CIN, cervical SCC	VIN
68	CIN, cervical SCC	Cervical carcinoma cell line ME180
69	CIN	Dysplastic tongue lesion
70	Anogenital warts	Cervical wart
72	CIN	Oral wart with atypia in HIV patient
73	Anogenital warts	Oral wart with atypia in HIV patient
74	Genital lesions in immunosuppressed	Vaginal lesions in immunosuppressed
75	Skin lesions in immunosuppressed	Dysplastic wart in immunosuppressed
76	Skin lesions in immunosuppressed	Skin SCC in immunosuppressed
77	Skin lesions in immunosuppressed	

AIN = anal intraepithelial neoplasia; CIN = cervical intraepithelial neoplasia; EV = epidermodysplasia verruciformis; HIV = human immunodeficiency virus; PIN = penile intraepithelial neoplasia; SCC = squamous cell carcinoma; VIN = vulval intraepithelial neoplasia.

Although the list of HPV types associated with the different clinical effects looks daunting, the majority of skin and mucosal diseases caused by the virus result from infection with just a small number of types. Table 2.2 offers a much simplified scheme for predicting which HPV is likely to cause a particular problem.

HPV types were originally distinguished one from another on the basis of hybridization in liquid medium.[24] If there was less than 50% homology under conditions of specified hybridization stringency, then HPV types were defined as different. It is important to point out that this comparison does not mean a precise concordance of sequence over 50% of the length. By 1991, the ease of polymerase chain reaction (PCR) permitted the ready sequencing of small areas of the genome following PCR, and the comparison between the E6, E7, and L1 parts of the genome was taken as the means of separation between types. A similarity of at least 90% in the nucleotide sequence in these three genes permitted HPVs to be classified as identical types. At the 1995 meeting of the International Papillomavirus Workshop, it was agreed that only the L1 portion need be amplified, sequenced, and compared and thus a greater than 10% dissimilarity in this region would allow a classification as a different type.

The phylogenetic relationships between HPV types on the basis of sequence variation within designated areas of the genome permit interpretation of how the different types and subtypes may have evolved. Using computer-assisted construction of phylogenetic trees of human and animal papillomaviruses, the genomic classification is shown to correlate with the clinical grouping of the virus types according to the particular type of epithelium infected (skin or mucosa) and the form of disease produced (benign or malignant).[15, 117] Comparison of the DNA sequence within the E1 and L1 regions of the genome allows the HPVs responsible for genital warts and neoplasia to be grouped together, the types responsible for lesions in epidermodysplasia verruciformis and immunosuppressed individuals to form another group, and the papillomaviruses which cause cutaneous warts in humans, cattle, or rabbits to be regarded as phylogenetically close (Figure 2.3). By this analysis, some HPV types which cause predominantly cutaneous warts, namely HPVs 2, 3, 7, and 10, are found to be more closely aligned with mucosal HPVs than with HPV 1 or HPV 4. HPV 2-induced lesions may, however, be found on both skin and mucosa, and HPV 7 warts are most frequent in individuals whose skin is frequently wet or macerated due to occupational circum-

stances. Thus, these HPVs with relationships with both cutaneous and mucosal types may represent examples of evolution from one disease niche to another. In addition, close scrutiny of the phylogeny of different variants of one HPV, type 16, isolated from different ethnic groups around the world, shows parallels with the prehistoric separation of human races and ancient migrations of populations.[62]

2.3 THE VIRUS LIFE CYCLE

HPVs have certain specific requirements to spread and grow. They are known to infect only human cells, exhibiting tight species specificity. In tissue culture, however, HPV virus-like particles (VLPs), which consist of the capsid proteins assembled in an icosahedral structure without viral DNA, can be taken up not only by human epithelial cells,[119] but also by other cells such as rat, rabbit, and monkey epithelial cells and mouse and hamster fibroblasts.[85] If such diverse possibilities for viral uptake exist *in vivo*, the lack of cross-species infection suggests that, in such situations, the virus is eliminated from the cell and cannot produce an active infection. Cellular tropism of the virus is therefore modulated not just by entry of the nucleic acid into the cell but also by control of viral gene expression and possibly by modification of translation of RNA. Thus, once inside a cell, a virus will only be able to propagate if the cell is permissive for the virus.

The virus also exhibits tissue specificity, producing disease almost entirely in stratified squamous epithelium such as skin and mucous membrane. Because such epithelia consist of a basal layer, in which cells have the capacity to divide, and more superficial layers, in which the cells have lost the ability to divide and are undergoing differentiation, it has long been assumed that the papillomavirus must initiate infection by entering the cells of the basal layer or possibly parabasal layer. If so, the virus would be present in a cell that has the capacity to divide and produce a proliferation of the epithelium. If the virus entered a non-dividing, differentiating cell, it might only exert a temporary effect on the cell, which was already programmed to die. In a study of very early times post-infection of cottontail rabbit papillomavirus (CRPV), it was observed that the keratinocytes within the bulge region of the hair follicle, the putative stem cells of the epidermis, are the first to be infected and to show evidence of viral gene transcription.[105]

2.3.1 Infection

The infectious nature of warts was first suggested over a century ago,[93] before confirmation and demonstration of their viral origin by Ciuffo in 1907.[23] Papillomavirus infection is thought to require a break in the epidermis, which allows the virus to infect the mitotically active basal cells. In the case of genital infections (such as those caused by HPV types 6 and 11), transmission appears to require direct contact, either as a result of sexual activity or from mother to child at delivery.[106] Cutaneous papillomavirus infection can be acquired either by personal contact or from the environment. The abrasive flooring present in swimming pools exacerbates the spread of plantar warts, while BPV1 can spread amongst cattle which scratch at the same fence post.[11, 19]

Table 2.2
Common human papillomavirus types

Lesions	Most common HPV types
Common hand warts	2, 4
Plantar warts	1, 2, 4
Flat cutaneous warts	3, 10
Genital warts	6, 11
CIN, cervical SCC	16, 18
Other anogenital neoplasias	16, 18

CIN = cervical intraepithelial neoplasia; SCC = squamous cell carcinoma.

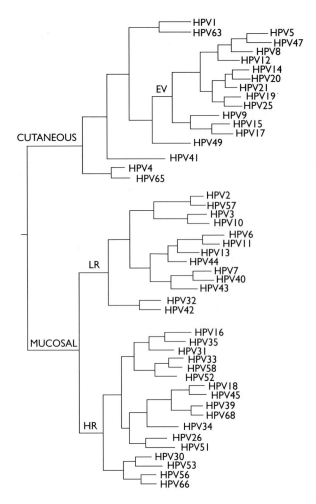

Figure 2.3
Phylogenetic relationships between papillomaviruses. Analysis of the DNA sequences of different HPV types reveals their phylogenetic similarities and differences. (*Reprinted from van Ranst et al., 1992*[117]).

Viruses gain entry to cells by interaction with a specific molecule on the surface of the cell which initiates the process of internalization. Virus receptors have only been identified for a few of the numerous viruses which infect humans, but knowledge of a receptor is an important aim in the development of specific antiviral therapy as the point of entry of a virus could theoretically be blocked. In the search for a cellular receptor for the human papillomavirus, initial *in vitro* work showed that there was an interaction at the cell surface between the virus and heparin. However, this was non-specific. More recent work has suggested that entry of the papillomavirus particle into the cell is mediated by binding to the α6 integrin, a molecule which is present on the surface of many cell types, including basal keratinocytes.[50, 84] Once within the cell, the viral DNA is uncoated and can be influenced by the enzymes of the host cell such that viral genes may be expressed. Following infection, the virus undergoes an incubation period of at least 2–3 weeks before tumor formation begins.[77, 91]

2.3.2 Latency

The HPV DNA may remain present but quiescent within cells either before or after active infection. HPV 16 has been detected using PCR in the cervical tissue of 5–40% women with no clinical or histological evidence of papillomavirus infection.[60, 115] In these individuals, the virus may have caused a subclinical or an un-noticed clinical infection before becoming latent or may have been acquired and held as a latent infection from the onset. The presence of such a high-risk HPV in the adult female genital tract gives an increased risk of development of dysplasia in the future. Men can also harbor HPV DNAs without any apparent clinical infection[61] and may serve as a reservoir of potential infection for sexual partners. Evidence is accumulating to support the concept that both low-risk and high-risk genital HPVs can be transmitted from mother to child by non-sexual routes, either at birth or in early infancy. Up to 40% of children have evidence of exposure to HPV infection as assessed by antibodies to HPV 16 proteins.[14, 72] HPV detection by PCR is of the order of 20% or more in oral samples taken from children,[70] further supporting the possibility of maternal-to-child transmission of the virus. It is not yet known how long perinatally acquired viral DNA may be retained in the epithelium, or what sort of risk, if any, there may be for the later development of lower genital tract dysplasia and cancer. Latent HPV infection also appears to occur in the skin. Hairs plucked from the eyebrows of a small proportion of normal individuals and a much higher proportion of immunosuppressed transplant recipients harbor HPVs which may act as a reservoir for overt infection in the future.[7]

2.3.3 Early events in the virus life cycle

Benign warts are thought to be clonal, arising from proliferation of a single basal cell (Figure 2.4).[53, 87] In the basal layer, the viral DNA is maintained as an episome which replicates in conjunction with cellular DNA at 20–50 copies per cell.[19] Transcripts arising from the early genes are detectable in these cells, and it is thought that proliferation is mediated by expression of viral early proteins.[59, 67] The viral transcripts produced in basal cells have not been mapped, but are likely to resemble the transcripts produced in HPV-immortalized keratinocytes grown in monolayer culture (figure 2.5).[44, 100] The HPV early genes are expressed from the early promoter (p1 in HPV 11, p97 in HPV 16) by differential splicing. At least four distinct RNAs are expressed from the E6 ORF, encoding variants of the E6 protein, each of which may have different roles in the virus life cycle.[95, 96] The E7 gene product has been implicated in the proliferation of infected keratinocytes, and binds to members of the AP1 family of transcription factors leading to activation of AP1-responsive promoters.[2] E7 can also associate with members of the retinoblastoma pocket protein family, including pRb, p107, and p130, and this is considered the mechanism by which E7 mediates its growth stimulatory effects (Figure 2.6).[16, 51] The Rb protein is a negative regulator of the cell cycle at the G1/S boundary, and in its hypophosphorylated state binds to the transcription factor E2F-1. During normal cell growth, Rb is phosphorylated by cyclin-dependent kinases (CDKs) in response to growth-promoting signals from outside the cell. The hyperphosphorylated form of pRb is unable to bind E2F-1, which is then able to transactivate genes involved in cell-cycle progression such as *c-myc* and *b-myb* (summarized in Figure 2.6). The binding of E7 to pRb mimics these events by displacing E2F-1 from pRb, so allowing progression through the cell cycle into S phase.[88] E7 also complexes with p107, p130, and other members of the E2F family.[122] Although Rb binding has been considered a major function for E7, it appears that the protein must have other roles in the virus life cycle,[13] and loss of the Rb binding motif in CRPV does not prevent the formation of benign warts in cottontail rabbits.[34] Complete loss of the E7 protein does, however, abolish wart formation, suggesting other important functions for E7 which are not related to its ability to bind pRb (discussed later).[8]

The second viral protein important in cellular proliferation is E6, which, in high-risk viruses, binds and inactivates p53 by ubiquitin-mediated degradation (Figure 2.6).[103] p53 is a tumor suppressor protein which is normally upregulated in response to DNA damage or virus infection.[80] It is a transactivator and can induce the expression of numerous cellular proteins, including p21waf1/cip1, a cyclin-dependent kinase inhibitor which mediates cell-cycle arrest (by preventing phosphorylation of members of the Rb family),[48] and bax, which is involved in the induction of apoptosis.[121] Although the E6 proteins of all genital HPVs probably have some p53-binding activity, only the high-risk types bind with high affinity and mediate p53 degradation.[30, 81] High-risk E6 proteins bind a cellular polypeptide, E6AP which is a ubiquitin ligase. This association is important for p53 interaction, and allows the cellular ubiquitin-conjugating enzymes specifically to target p53 for degradation (summarized in figure 2.6).[22, 64] Inhibition of pRb and p53 activities is a common characteristic of other viruses which induce cell proliferation, including adenoviruses,[120] polyomaviruses,[27] and certain herpesviruses.[58] It is clear that, like E7, E6 has other roles in the virus life cycle which remain to be established. Loss of E6 in CRPV results in an inability of the virus to produce benign tumors,[124] and E6 has been

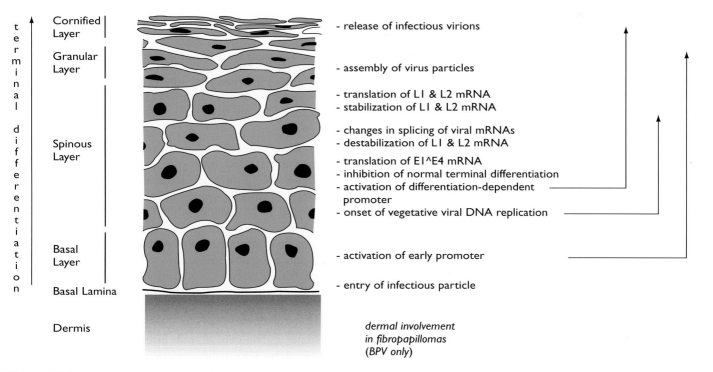

Figure 2.4
Life history of the papillomavirus within a differentiated epithelium. The life of the virus within epidermal keratinocytes begins with infection of a basal layer cell. As the keratinocyte differentiates, the viral gene expression changes and new particles are produced within the most superficial layers.

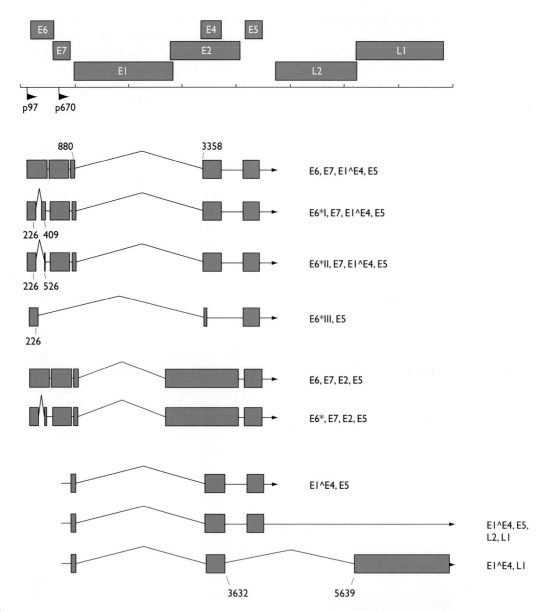

Figure 2.5

HPV 16 transcripts in keratinocytes grown in monolayer culture. Several different transcripts are produced in cells grown *in vitro*.[44,100] The use of different HPV 16 promoters and the variation in splicing patterns lead to a large series of RNAs which have the capability of coding for slightly different proteins. p97: HPV 16 promoter from which transcripts of early genes are derived; p742: HPV 16 differentiation-dependent promoter from which transcripts of late genes are produced; E6*I, E6*II, E6*III: transcripts encoding truncated E6 proteins; E1^E4: the E4 transcript is always fused at its 5′ end to a short portion of E1 RNA.

reported to activate cellular telomerase.[76, 111] High-risk E6 proteins can bind a range of cellular polypeptides, including E6BP – a calcium-binding protein[17] – and interferon response factor-3 – a transcription factor normally activated in response to virus infection.[101] There is evidence that these proteins may play an important role in the late stages of the virus life cycle. E7 expression in the upper layers of infected epidermis is thought to reactivate the host cells' DNA replication machinery to support viral replication,[18, 51] and E6 expression has been reported to interfere with terminal differentiation.[109, 112] Early gene expression is regulated to a large extent by the viral E2 protein, which binds a consensus motif present in multiple copies in the HPV URR.[83] Variants of this site have different affinities for E2, which can act as a transactivator or transrepressor depending on the proximity of the E2 binding sites to the HPV early promoter.[110] In HPV 16 infection, the full-length E2 protein is a repressor of E6 and E7 expression, and acts to control the level of

proliferation of the infected basal cells. E2 can also associate with E1, which on its own binds the viral origin of replication only poorly. E1 associates with the α subunit of DNA polymerase alpha, and is important for the initiation of viral DNA replication.[6, 25] The remaining early protein, E5, is a small, hydrophobic membrane protein which is thought to affect the rate of proliferation of the infected cell by inhibiting down-regulation of the epidermal growth factor (EGF) receptor,[113] and to affect cell–cell communication.[90] These effects may be mediated in part by the ability of E5 to associate stably with the 16 kDa subunit of the H⁺ vacuolar ATPase.[26] This prevents acidification of endosomes and inhibits receptor inactivation.[114] It has been suggested that E5 may be important for the proliferation of the underlying dermal cells in fibropapillomas such as those caused by BPV 1.[63, 78] The E5 protein of BPV 1, but not that of HPV 16, can activate the platelet-derived growth factor (PDGF) β receptor, which is abundant on dermal fibro-

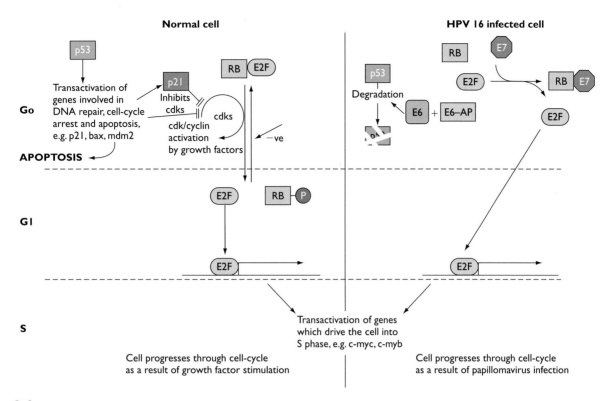

Figure 2.6
Effect of HPV E6 and E7 on cell-cycle control. HPV 16 E6 and E7 proteins are able to interact with cellular proteins (E6AP and pRB), which in turn have a modulating effect on the cell-cycle. Expression of E6 and E7 from high-risk HPV types causes degradation of p53 and inactivation of pRB, allowing progression through the cell-cycle. In the absence of papillomavirus infection, cell-cycle progression requires phosphorylation of pRB, which can occur in response to growth factor stimulation. RB= hypophosphorylated retinoblastoma gene product; RB-P= hyperphosphorylated retinoblastoma gene product.

blasts, and initiate their proliferation.[94] The E5 protein has, however, been detected in basal and differentiating keratinocytes, suggesting an additional role in epithelial cells.[5, 12]

2.3.4 Productive stages of the virus life cycle

The late stages of the virus life cycle occur within the infected keratinocyte as it migrates through the differentiating layers of the epidermis and include DNA amplification for the purpose of new particle formation (vegetative DNA replication) and the production of capsid proteins (see Figures 2.1 and 2.4),. These events are initiated as soon as the infected cell leaves the basal layer in veruccas caused by HPV 1[9, 43] but are usually retarded until higher layers in mucosal lesions such as those caused by HPV 6, 11, and 16.[10, 32] The E1 protein, which has DNA unwinding or helicase activity,[126] is thought to initiate replication of the viral episome. Activation of the papillomavirus differentiation-dependent promoter (p670 in HPV 16)[56] during migration of the infected keratinocyte toward the epithelial surface is thought to lead to an increase in the levels of E1 and E2, and to an increase in viral genome copy number from 20–50 copies per cell to around 10 000 copies per cell.[52,79] The viral early promoter, which controls E6 and E7 expression, is thought to be constitutively active during differentiation in order to maintain the cells in a 'pseudo' S phase state necessary for high-level replication of the viral episome.[39] Expression of the viral late genes, E4, L1, and L2, also depends on activation of a differentiation-dependent promoter, which

in most HPVs is contained within the E7 gene.[56,116] Differential splicing produces at least three late transcripts from this promoter,[20,21,65,66] and expression of the different proteins is controlled post-transcriptionally during differentiation (Figure 2.4). The first detectable late protein arises from the E4 gene, but is formed from a transcript which splices from the beginning of the E1 ORF into E4. The resulting E1^E4 fusion protein consists of approximately five amino acids from E1 at the C terminus, with the remainder of the polypeptide deriving from E4. E1^E4 protein is expressed in cells in which vegetative viral DNA replication has begun.[9,38] In HPV 1 warts, in particular, it is an abundant protein, accumulating to form up to 20–30% of total cell protein.[9,40] Its association with the intermediate filament cytoskeleton when expressed *in vitro*[42,97] has suggested a role in virus release by increasing the fragility of the infected cell.[41] The expression of E4 precedes that of capsid structural proteins,[43] and it has been suggested that E4's role may be to facilitate virus synthesis, perhaps by inhibiting cell death,[98,99] or by stimulating vegetative viral DNA replication.[9] In cutaneous warts, the abundant E4 proteins are concentrated in cytoplasmic inclusions which have a characteristic appearance dependent upon the infecting HPV type. Thus, HPV 4 and HPV 60 produce single large E4 inclusion granules, whereas HPV 1 produces numerous eosinophilic structures.[29,41,46] E4 inclusions have a fibrous appearance in warts caused by HPV 63.[47]

L1 and L2 are major and minor virion structural proteins, respectively, and their expression lags behind vegetative viral DNA replication and E4 synthesis to varying extents in different lesions.[38] Virus assembly begins in the granular layer of the epidermis (see Figure 2.4). The minor coat protein L2 is not essential for the formation of capsids *in vitro*[57] and is present at a L1:L2 molar ratio of around 30:1 following co-expression of both proteins *in vitro*, and following extraction from naturally occurring lesions caused by BPV 1,[75] suggesting a location for L2 at the 12 vertices of the virion. Only the N-terminus of L2 is exposed on the surface of the virion[82] and it has been suggested that L2 may have a role in DNA packaging or virus assembly, as capsid formation *in vitro* is enhanced up to 100-fold by the presence of L2.[57,75] Of the three spliced transcripts expressed from the differentiation-dependent promoter in the upper layers of the epidermis, those encoding L1 and L2 terminate at the late polyadenylation (poly A) site, and contain a negative regulatory element which prevents their efficient export into the cytoplasm until the infected cell reaches the granular layer.[54,73] Thus, although late transcripts are produced simultaneously during differentiation, only the abundant E1^E4.E5 message, which terminates at the early polyadenylation site, is expressed in the lower parabasal layers. Post-transcriptional control is further mediated by splice site selection[127] and poly A site usage[1] and is regulated by cellular factors involved in RNA processing.[37,127] All the viral late transcripts are polycistronic and contain E1^E4 as their first exon. The significance of this for the high-level production of infectious virions is unclear, but it suggests an important role for E1^E4 in virus synthesis. A promoter has been identified upstream of the L2 ORF which may be responsible for the expression of the minor capsid protein.[55] Virus particles produced in cells of the granular layer are ultimately shed from the surface of the lesion during desquamation.

2.4 EVENTS LEADING TO MALIGNANT PROGRESSION

Most papillomavirus infections are associated with purely benign tumors, which usually regress spontaneously after a period of months or years.[11,108] However, in some instances benign HPV infections may progress to neoplasia and cancer. The best-characterized association of HPVs with cancer is that of the high-risk mucosal HPV types such as HPV 16, 18, 31, 45, and 54 with cervical squamous cell carcinoma.[106]

Although these virus types can be detected in the general population, regression of the latent or subclinical infection commonly occurs[102] and only in a small number of cases are these lesions precursors of cervical cancer.[60] The time lag between primary infection and development of serious disease is several decades, suggesting a requirement for secondary mutagenic events in addition to virus infection.[128] In HPV-associated cervical cancers, the viral genome is often integrated into the host chromosome and, although integration leads to disruption of the viral genome, the E6 and E7 ORFs are preserved, and are transcriptionally active both in cervical cancer cell lines and in HPV-associated neoplasias (Figure 2.7).[45,107] Integration usually occurs in the E1/E2 region and has two consequences. The disruption of expression of the E2 transactivator leads to up-regulation of the HPV early promoter, and to increased production of the E6 and E7 proliferative proteins.[28] Integration in the E1/E2 region also prevents transcripts for E6 and E7 from terminating at the viral early polyadenylation site. These hybrid transcripts contain 3′ termini derived from cellular sequences and, as a consequence, lack viral 3′ destabilizing elements which regulate the levels of early proteins in normal infection (Figure 2.7).[71] The resulting overexpression of E7 leads to unscheduled progression through the cell cycle, whereas expression of E6 inhibits the apoptotic response by binding to *p53*. Mutations of *p53* are very common in human cancers,[118] but are not usually found in HPV-positive cervical malignancies,[31,104] suggesting that E6-mediated degradation of *p53* can substitute for its inactivation by mutation. Loss of *p53* function in HPV-transformed cells is a predisposing factor in malignant progression. *p53*-mediated growth arrest in response to DNA-damaging agents, which occurs in normal cells, is detrimentally affected in E6-expressing cells,[74] allowing the accumulation of secondary mutations which contribute to the development of cancer.

Of the other HPVs that infect humans, a subgroup is associated with malignancies in patients suffering from the rare inherited disease epidermodysplasia verruciformis (EV).[69] The lesions of the disease are associated with a range of HPV types, including HPV 3 and 10, which cause flat warts in the general population, as well as with a number of 'EV' types which are rare in normal individuals. These include HPV types 5, 8, 9, 12, 14, 15, 17, 19, 20, and 25, which can also be found in immunocompromised individuals such as renal allograft patients.[4] EV patients are thought

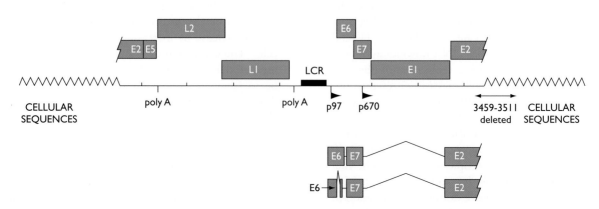

Figure 2.7
Integration of HPV 16. In malignant tissue which contains HPV 16, the viral DNA is usually integrated within the host cell DNA, breaking the E2 gene and consequently losing part of the HPV genome. The same viral promoters are used as in the episome, but the transcripts produced are truncated.

to be homozygous for a rare autosomal recessive gene which results in immunological deficiency and an inability to resolve HPV infection.[68,69] The disease begins in early childhood with the appearance of flat warts and reddish-brown macular plaques, the latter of which can develop into slow-growing carcinoma *in situ* or invasive cancer. Unlike cancers associated with HPV16, the genomes of the EV types do not generally integrate, but remain episomal.[92,125] Progression to cancer usually occurs at sun-exposed sites, and ultraviolet irradiation is considered a cofactor in the development of EV-associated malignancies. Indeed, a requirement for external cofactors is considered important in the development of many HPV-associated malignancies. For the progression of genital lesions to cervical cancer however, the use of oral contraceptives, smoking,[33] the presence of other sexually transmitted diseases[35] and specific HLA types[3,86] have been suggested, but a single risk factor has not been established.

REFERENCES

1. Andrews EM, DiMaio D. (1993) Hierarchy of polyadenylation site usage by bovine papillomavirus in transformed mouse cells. *J Virol* **67**: 7705–10.

2. Antinore MJ, Birrer MJ, Patel D, Nader L, McCance DJ. (1996) The human papillomavirus type 16 E7 gene product interacts with and trans-activates the AP1 family of transcription factors. *EMBO J* **15**: 1950–60.

3. Apple RJ, Erlich HA, Klitz W, Manos M, Becker TM, Wheeler CM. (1994) HLA DR-DQ associations with cervical carcinoma show papillomavirus type specificity. *Nat Genet* **6**: 157–62.

4. Benton C, Shahidullah H, Hunter JAA. (1992) Human papillomaviruses in the immunosuppressed. *Papillomavirus Rep* **3**: 23–6.

5. Biswas C, Kell B, Han X, *et al.* (1996) Human papillomavirus type 16 E5 expression in cervical neoplasia. *Br J Cancer* **74**: 26.

6. Bonneandrea C, Santucci S, Clertant P, Tillier F. (1995) Bovine papillomavirus E1 binds specifically DNA polymerase alpha but not replication protein A. *J Virol* **69**: 2341–50.

7. Boxman ILA, Berkhout RJM, Mulder LHC, *et al.* (1997) Detection of human papillomavirus DNA in plucked hairs from renal transplant recipients and healthy volunteers. *J Invest Dermatol* **108**: 712–15.

8. Brandsma JL, Yang Z, Barthold SW, Johnson EA. (1991) Use of a rapid, efficient inoculation method to induce papillomas by cottontail rabbit papillomavirus DNA shows that the E7 gene is required. *Proc Natl Acad Sci USA* **88**: 4816–20.

9. Breitburd F, Croissant O, Orth G. (1987) Expression of human papillomavirus type-1 E4 gene products in warts. In *Cancer Cells 5.* 115–22. Cold Spring Harbor, New York, Cold Spring Harbor Laboratory Press.

10. Brown DR, Chin MT, Strike DG (1988) Identification of human papillomavirus type 11 E4 gene products in human tissue implants from athymic mice. *Virology* **165**: 262–7.

11. Bunney MH. (1986). Viral warts: a new look at an old problem. *Br Med J* **293**: 1045–1047.

12. Burnett S, Jareborg N, and DiMaio D. (1992) Localization of bovine papillomavirus type 1 E5 protein to transformed keratinocytes and permissive differentiated cells in fibropapilloma tissue. *Proc Natl Acad Sci USA* **89**: 5665–9.

13. Caldeira, S, de Villiers EM, Tommasino M. (2000) Human papillomavirus E7 proteins stimulate proliferation independently of their ability to associate with retinoblastoma protein. *Oncogene* **19**: 821–6.

14. Cason J, Kambo PK, Shergill B, *et al.* (1994) Detection of class-specific antibodies to baculovirus derived human papillomavirus type 16 capsid proteins. In *Immunology of human papillomaviruses*, ed. MA Stanley. New York, Plenum Press, 155–60.

15. Chan S-Y, Bernard H-U, Ong C-K, *et al.* (1992) Phylogenetic analysis of 48 papillomavirus types and 28 subtypes and variants: a showcase for the molecular evolution of DNA viruses. *J Virol* **66**: 5714–25.

16. Chellappan S, Kraus VB, Kroger B, *et al.* (1992) Adenovirus E1A, simian virus 40 tumor antigen, and human papillomavirus E7 protein share the capacity to disrupt the interaction between transcription factor E2F and the retinoblastoma gene product. *Proc Natl Acad Sci USA* **89**: 4549–53.

17. Chen JJ, Reid CE, Band V, Androphy EJ. (1995) Interaction of papillomavirus E6 oncoproteins with a putative calcium binding protein. *Science* **269**: 529–31.

18. Cheng S, Schmidt-Grimminger D-C, Murant T, Broker T, Chow L. (1995) Differentiation-dependent up-regulation of the human papillomavirus E7 gene reactivates cellular DNA replication in suprabasal differentiated keratinocytes. *Genes Dev* **9**: 2335–49.

19. Chow LT, Broker TR. (1994) Papillomavirus DNA replication. *Intervirology* **37**: 150–8.

20. Chow LT, Nasseri M, Wolinsky SM, Broker TR. (1987) Human papillomavirus types 6 and 11 mRNAs from genital condylomata acuminata. *J Virol* **61**: 2581–8.

21. Chow LT, Reilly SS, Broker TR, Taichman LB. (1987) Identification and mapping of human papillomavirus type 1 RNA transcripts recovered from plantar warts and infected epithelial cell cultures. *J Virol* **61**: 1913–18.

22. Ciechanover A. (1994) The ubiquitin–proteasome proteolytic pathway. *Cell* **79**: 13–21.

23. Ciuffo G. (1907) Innesto positivo con filtrate di verruca vulgare. *G. Ital Mal Vener* **42**: 12–17.

24. Coggin JR, zur Hausen H. (1979) Workshop on papillomaviruses and cancer. *Cancer Res* **39**: 545–6.

25. Conger KL, Liu JS, Kuo SR, Chow LT, Wang TS. (1999) Human papillomavirus DNA replication. Interactions between the viral E1 protein and two subunits of human DNA polymerase alpha/primase. *J Biol Chem* **274**: 2696–705.

26. Conrad M, Bubb VJ, Schlegel R. (1993) The human papillomavirus type 6 and 16 E5 proteins are membrane-associated proteins which associate with the 16kd pore forming protein. *J Virol* **67**: 6170–8.

27. Conzen SD, Cole CN. (1994) The transforming proteins of simian virus 40. *Semin Virol* **5**: 349–56.

28. Cripe TP, Haugen TH, Turk JP, *et al.* (1987) Transcriptional regulation of the human papillomavirus 16 E6–E7 promoter by a keratinocyte dependent enhancer, and by viral E2 trans-activator and repressor gene products; implications for cervical carcinogenesis. *EMBO J* **6**: 3745–53.

29. Croissant O, Breitburd F, Orth G. (1985) Specificity of the cytopathic effect of cutaneous human papillomaviruses. *Clin Dermatol* **3**: 43–55.

30. Crook T, Tidy JA, Vousden KH. (1991) Degradation of p53 can be targeted by HPV E6 sequences distinct from those required for p53 binding and transactivation. *Cell* **67**: 547–56.

31. Crook T, Wrede D, Vousden KH. (1991) p53 point mutation in HPV negative human cervical carcinoma cell lines. *Oncogene* **6**: 873–5.

32. Crum CP, Barber S, Symbula M, Snyder K, Saleh AM, Roche JK. (1990) Coexpression of the human papillomavirus type 16 E4 and L1 open reading frames in early cervical neoplasia. *Virology* **178**: 238–46.

33. Daling JR, Sherman KJ, Hislop TG, *et al.* (1992). Cigarette-smoking and the risk of anogenital cancer. *Am J Epidemiol* **135**: 180–9.

34. Defeo-Jones D, Vuocolo GA, Haskell KM, *et al.* (1993) Papillomavirus E7 protein-binding to the retinoblastoma protein is not required for viral induction of warts. *J Virol* **67**: 716–25.

35. Desanjose S, Munoz N, Bosch FX, *et al.* (1994) Sexually transmitted agents and cervical neoplasia in Columbia and Spain. *Int J Cancer* **56**: 358–63.

36. de Villiers E-M. (1989) Heterogeneity of the human papillomavirus group. *J Virol* **63**: 4898–903.

37. Dietrich-Goetz W, Kennedy IM, Levins B, Stanley MA, Clements JB. (1997) A cellular 65-kDa protein recognizes the negative regulatory element of human papillomavirus late mRNA. *Proc Natl Acad Sci USA* **94**: 163–8.

38. Doorbar J. (1996) The E4 proteins and their role in the viral life cycle. *In Papillomavirus reviews: current research on papillomaviruses* ed. C Lacey. Leeds Medical Information, Leeds University Press, Leeds, 31–8.

39. Doorbar J. (1998) Late stages of the papillomavirus life cycle. *Papillomavirus Rep* **9**: 119–23.

40. Doorbar J, Campbell D, Grand RJA, Gallimore PH. (1986) Identification of the human papillomavirus-1a E4 gene products. *EMBO J* **5**: 355–62.

41. Doorbar J, Coneron I, Gallimore PH. (1989) Sequence divergence yet conserved physical characteristics among the E4 proteins of cutaneous human papillomaviruses. *Virology* **172**: 51–62.

42. Doorbar J, Ely S, Sterling J, McLean C., Crawford L. (1991) Specific interaction between HPV16 E1^E4 and cytokeratins results in collapse of the epithelial cell intermediate filament network. *Nature* **352**: 824–7.

43. Doorbar J, Foo C, Coleman N, *et al.* (1997) Characterisation of events during the late stages of HPV 16 infection in vivo using high affinity synthetic Fabs to E4. *Virology* **238**: 40–52.

44. Doorbar J, Parton A, Hartley K, *et al.* (1990) Detection of novel splicing patterns in a HPV 16-containing keratinocyte cell line. *Virology* **178**: 254–2.

45. Durst M, Glitz D, Schneider A, zur Hausen H. (1992) Human papillomavirus type 16 gene expression and DNA replication in cervical neoplasia: analysis by in situ hybridization. *Virology* **189**: 132–40.

46. Egawa K. (1994) New types of human papillomaviruses and intracytoplasmic inclusion bodies: a classification of inclusion warts according to clinical features, histology and associated HPV types. *Br J Dermatol* **130**: 158–66.

47. Egawa K, Delius H, Matsukura T, Kawashima M, de Villiers E-M. (1993) Two novel types of human papillomavirus, HPV63 and HPV65: comparison of their clinical and histological features and DNA sequences to other HPV types. *Virology* **194**: 51–62.

48. El-Deiry WS, Tokino T, Velculescu VE, *et al.* (1993) Waf1, a potential mediator of p53 tumour suppression. *Cell* **75**: 817–25.

49. Elston R, Napthine S, Doorbar J. (1998) The identification of a conserved binding motif within HPV16 E6 binding peptides, E6AP and E6BP. *J Gen Virol* **79**: 371–4.

50. Evander M, Frazer IH, Payne E, Mei Qi Y, Hengst K, McMillan NAJ. (1997) Identification of the alpha 6 integrin as a candidate receptor for papillomaviruses. *J Virol* **71**: 2449–56.

51. Flores ER, Allen-Hoffmann BL, Lee D, Lambert PF. (2000) The human papillomavirus type 16 E7 oncogene is required for the productive stage of the viral life cycle. *J Virol* **15**: 6622–31.

52. Frattini MG, Hurst SD, Lim HB, Swaminathan S, Laimins L. (1997) Abrogation of a mitotic checkpoint by E2 proteins from oncogenic human papillomaviruses correlates with increased turnover of the p53 tumour suppressor protein. *EMBO J* **16**: 318–31.

53. Friedman JM, Fialkow PJ. (1976) Viral tumorigenesis in man: cell markers in condylomata accuminata. *Int. J Cancer* **17**: 57–61.

54. Furth PA, Choe WT, Rex JH, Byrne JC, Baker CC. (1994) Sequences homologous to 5′ splice sites are required for the inhibitory activity of papillomavirus late 3′ untranslated regions. *Mol Cell Biol* **14**: 5278–89.

55. Geisen G, Khan T. (1996) Promoter activity of sequences located upstream of the human papillomavirus type 16 and type 18 late regions. *J Gen Virol* **77**: 2193–200.

56. Grassmann K, Rapp B, Maschek H, Petry KU, Iftner T. (1996) Identification of a differentiation-inducible promoter in the E7 open reading frame of human papillomavirus type 16 (HPV-16) in raft cultures of a new cell line containing high copy numbers of episomal HPV-16 DNA. *J Virol* **70**: 2339–49.

57. Hagensee ME, Yaegashi N, Galloway DA. (1993) Self-assembly of human papillomavirus type 1 capsids by expression of the L1 protein alone or by coexpression of the L1 and L2 capsid proteins. *J Virol* **67**: 315–22.

58. Henderson SA, Huen D, Rowe M. (1994) Epstein–Barr virus transforming proteins. *Semin Virol* **5**: 391–401.

59. Higgins GD, Uzelin DM, Phillips GE, McEvoy P, Marin R, Burrell CJ. (1992) Transcription patterns of human papillomavirus type 16 in genital intraepithelial neoplasia: evidence for promoter usage within the E7 open

reading frame during epithelial differentiation. *J Gen Virol* **73**: 2047–57.

60. Hildesheim A, Schiffman MH, Gravitt P. (1994) Persistence of type-specific human papillomavirus infection among cytologically normal women in Portland, Oregon. *J Infect Dis* **169**: 235–40.

61. Hippeläinen MI, Syränen S, Hippeläinen MJ, Saarikoski S, Syränen K. (1993) Diagnosis of genital human papillomavirus (HPV) lesions in the male. Correlation of peniscopy, histology and *in situ* hybridisation. *Genitourin Med* **69**: 346–51.

62. Ho L, Chan S-Y, Burk RD, *et al.* (1993) The genetic drift of human papillomavirus type 16 is a means of reconstructing prehistoric viral spread and the movement of ancient human populations. *J Virol* **67**: 6413–23.

63. Horwitz BH, Burkhardt AL, Schlegel R., DiMaio D. (1988) 44-amino acid E5 transforming protein of bovine papillomavirus requires a hydrophobic core and specific carboxyl terminal amino acids. *Mol Cell Biol* **8**: 4071–8.

64. Huibregtse JM, Scheffner M, Howley PM. (1991) A cellular protein mediates association of p53 with the E6 oncoprotein of human papillomavirus types 16 or 18. *EMBO J* **10**: 4129–35.

65. Hummel M, Hudson JB, Laimins LA. (1992) Differentiation-induced and constitutive transcription of human papillomavirus type 31b in cell lines containing viral episomes. *J Virol* **66**: 6070–80.

66. Hummel M, Lim HB, Laimins LA. (1995) Human papillomavirus type 31b late gene expression is regulated through protein kinase C-mediated changes in RNA processing. *J Virol* **69**: 3381–8.

67. Iftner T, Oft M, Bohm S, Wilczynski SP, Pfister H. (1992) Transcription of the E6 and E7 genes of HPV6 in anogenital condylomata is restricted to undifferentiated cell layers of the epithelium. *J Virol* **66**: 4639–46.

68. Jablonska S, Dabrowski J, Jakubowicz K. (1972) Epidermodysplasia verruciformis as a model in studies on the role of papovaviruses in oncogenesis. *Cancer Res* **32**: 583–9.

69. Jablonska S, Majewski S. (1994) Molecular pathogenesis of cancer of the cervix and its causation by specific human papillomavirus types. In *Human pathology papillomaviruses*, ed. H zur Hausen. Current topics in microbiology and immunology, Vol. 186. Berlin, Springer-Verlag, 157–75.

70. Jenison SA, Yu XP, Valentine JM, *et al.* (1990) Evidence of prevalent genital-type human papillomavirus infections in adults and children. *J Infect Dis* **162**: 60–9.

71. Jeon S, Lambert PF. (1995) Integration of HPV16 DNA into the human genome leads to increased stability of E6/E7 mRNAs: implications for cervical carcinogenesis. *Proc Natl Acad Sci USA* **92**: 1654–8.

72. Jochmus-Kudielka I, Schneider A, Braun R, *et al.* (1989) Antibodies against the human papillomavirus type 16 early proteins in human sera: correlation of anti-E7 reactivity with cervical cancer. *J Natl Cancer Inst* **81**: 1698–704.

73. Kennedy IA, Haddow JK, Clements JB. (1991) A negative regulatory element in the human papillomavirus type 16 genome acts at the level of late mRNA stability. *J Virol* **65**: 2093–7.

74. Kessis TD, Slebos RJ, Nelson WG. (1993) Human papillomavirus 16 E6 expression disrupts the p53-mediated cellular response to DNA damage. *Proc Natl Acad Sci USA* **90**: 3988–92.

75. Kirnbauer R, Taub J, Greenstone H, *et al.* (1993) Efficient self-assembly of human papillomavirus type 16 L1 and L1–L2 into virus like particles. *J Virol* **67**: 6929–36.

76. Klingelhutz AJ, Foster SA, McDougall JK. (1996) Telomerase activation by the E6 gene product of human papillomavirus type 16. *Nature* **380**: 79–82.

77. Kreider JW, Bartlett GL. (1981) The Shope papilloma–carcinoma complex of rabbits: a model system of neoplastic progression and spontaneous regression. *Adv Cancer Res* **35**: 81–110.

78. Kulke R, DiMaio D. (1991) Biological activities of E5 protein of the deer papillomavirus in mouse C127 cells: morphologic transformation, induction of cellular DNA synthesis and activation of the PDGF receptor. *J Virol* **65**: 4943–9.

79. Lambert PF. (1991) Papillomavirus DNA replication. *J Virol* **65**: 3417–20.

80. Lane DP. (1992) p53, guardian of the genome. *Nature* **358**: 15–16.

81. Lechner MS, Laimins LA. (1994) Inhibition of p53 DNA binding by human papillomavirus E6 proteins. *J Virol* **68**: 4262–73.

82. Liu WL, Gissman L, Sun XY, Kanjanahaluethai A, Doorbar J, Zhou J. (1997) The N-terminal portion of L2 protein is displayed on the surface of bovine papillomavirus type 1 virions. *Virology* **227**: 474–83.

83. McBride AA, Romanczuk H, Howley PM. (1991) The papillomavirus E2 regulatory proteins. *J Biol Chem* **266**: 18411–14.

84. McMillan NA, Payne E, Frazer IH, Evander M. (1999) Expression of the alpha6 integrin confers papillomavirus binding upon receptor-negative B-cells. *Virology* **261**: 271–9.

85. Müller M, Gissmann L, Cristiano RJ, *et al.* (1995) Papillomavirus capsid binding and uptake by cells from different tissues and species. *J Virol* **69**: 948–54.

86. Muñoz N, Bosch FX, deSanjose S, Shah KV. (1994) The role of HPV in the etiology of cervical cancer. *Mutat Res* **305**: 293–301.

87. Murray F, Hobbs J, Payne B. (1971) Possible clonal origin of common warts. *Nature* **232**: 51–2.

88. Nevins JR. (1992) E2F – a link between the Rb tumour suppressor protein and viral oncoproteins. *Science* **258**: 424–9.

89. O'Connor M, Chan S-Y, Bernard H-U. (1995) Review of the LCR. Transcription factor binding sites in the long control region of genital HPVs. *Human papillomavirus compendium* http://hpv-web.lanl.gov/COMPENDIUM_PDF/95PDF/3/oconnor.pdf

90. Oelze I, Kartenbeck J, Crusius K, Alonso A. (1995) human papillomavirus E5 protein affects cell–cell

communication in an epithelial cell line. *J Virol* **69**: 4489–93.

91. Oriel JD. (1971) Natural history of genital warts. *Brit J Vener Dis* **47**: 1–13.

92. Orth G. (1987) Epidermodysplasia verruciformis. The Papovaviridae. In *The papillomaviruses*, ed. NP Salzman, PM Howler. New York, Plenum Press, 199–243.

93. Payne J. (1891) On the contagious rise of common warts. *Br J Derm* **3**: 185.

94. Petti, L, DiMaio D. (1994) Specific interaction between the bovine papillomavirus E5 transforming protein and the B receptor for platelet derived growth factor receptor in stably transformed and acutely transfected cells. *J Virol* **68**: 3582–92.

95. Pim D, Banks L. (1999) HPV-18 E6*I protein modulates the E6-directed degradation of p53 by binding to full-length HPV-18 E6. *Oncogene* **18**: 7403–8.

96. Pim D, Massimi P, Banks L. (1998) Alternatively spliced HPV-18 E6* protein inhibits E6 mediated degradation of p53 and suppresses transformed cell growth. *Oncogene* **17**: 257–64.

97. Roberts S, Ashmole I, Johnson GD, Kreider JW, Gallimore PH. (1993) Cutaneous and mucosal human papillomavirus E4 proteins form intermediate filament-like structures in epithelial cells. *Virology* **197**: 176–87.

98. Rogel-Gaillard C, Breitburd F, Orth G. (1992) Human papillomavirus type 1 E4 proteins differing by their N-terminal ends have distinct cellular locations when transiently expressed in vitro. *J Virol* **66**: 816–23.

99. Rogel-Gaillard C, Pehau-Arnaudet G, Breitburd F, Orth G. (1993) Cytopathic effect in human papillomavirus type 1-induced inclusion warts: *in vitro* analysis of the contribution of two forms of the viral E4 protein. *J Invest Dermatol* **101**: 843–51.

100. Rohlfs M, Winkenbach S, Meyer S, Rupp T, Dürst M. (1991) Viral transcription in human keratinocyte cell lines immortalised by human papillomavirus type 16. *Virology* **183**: 331–42.

101. Ronco LV, Karpova AY, Vidal M, Howley PM. (1998) Human papillomavirus 16 E6 oncoprotein binds to interferon regulatory factor-3 and inhibits its transcriptional activity. *Genes Dev* **12**: 2061–72.

102. Rosenfeld WD, Rose E, Vermund SH, Schreiber K, Berk RD. (1992) Follow up evaluation of cervicovaginal human papillomavirus infection in adolescents. *J Pediatr* **121**: 301–11.

103. Scheffner M, Huibregtse JM, Howley PM. (1994) Identification of a human ubiquitin conjugating enzyme that mediates the E6AP-dependent ubiquitination of p53. *Proc Natl Acad Sci USA* **91**: 8797–801.

104. Scheffner M, Munger K, Byrne JC, Howley PM. (1991) The state of p53 and retinoblastoma genes in human cervical carcinoma cell lines. *Proc Natl Acad Sci USA* **88**: 5523–7.

105. Schmitt A, Rochat A, Zeltne R, *et al.* (1996) The primary target cells of the high-risk cottontail rabbit papillomavirus colocalise with the hair follicle stem cells. *J Virol* **70**: 1912–22.

106. Schneider A. (1994) Natural history of genital papillomavirus infections. *Intervirology* **37**: 201–14.

107. Schwarz E, Freese UK, Gissmann L, *et al.* (1985) Struc-

ture and transcription of human papillomavirus sequences in cervical carcinoma cells. *Nature* **314**: 111–14.

108. Shah KV, Howley PM. (1996) Papillomaviruses. In *Virology* Vol. 2, 3rd edn, ed. BN Fields, DM Knipe, PM Howley. Philadelphia, New York, Lippincott–Raven, 2077–109.

109. Sherman L, Schlegel R. (1996) Serum-induced and calcium-induced differentiation of human keratinocytes is inhibited by the E6 protein of human papillomaviruses. *J Virol* **70**: 3269–79.

110. Steger G, Ham J, Yaniv M. (1996) E2 proteins: modulators of papillomavirus transcription and replication. *Methods Enzymol* **274**: 173–85.

111. Stoppler H, Hartmann DP, Sherman L, Schlegel R. (1997) The human papillomavirus type 16 E6 and E7 oncoproteins dissociate cellular telomerase activity from the maintenance of telomere length. *J Biol Chem* **272**: 13332–7.

112. Stoppler MC, Ching K, Stoppler H, Clancey K, Schlegel R, Icenogle J. (1996) Natural variants of the human papillomavirus type 16 E6 protein differ in their abilities to alter keratinocyte differentiation and to induce p53 degradation. *J Virol* **70**: 6987–93.

113. Straight S, Hinckle PM, Jewers RJ, McCance DJ. (1993) The E5 oncoprotein of HPV16 transforms fibroblasts and effects the downregulation of the EGF receptor in keratinocytes. *J Virol* **69**: 4521–32.

114. Straight SW, Herman B, McCance DJ. (1995) The E5 oncoprotein of HPV16 inhibits the acidification of endosomes in human keratinocytes. *J Virol* **69**: 3185–92.

115. Syrjänen S, Saastamoinen J, Chang F, Ji H, Syrjänen K. (1990) Colposcopy, punch biopsy, *in situ* DNA hybridisation and polymerase chain reaction in searching for genital human papillomavirus (HPV) infections in women with normal PAP smears. *J Med Virol* **31**: 259–66.

116. Tomita Y, Shiga T, Simizu B. (1996) Characterization of a promoter in the E7 open reading frame of human papillomavirus type 11. *Virology* **225**: 267–73.

117. Van Ranst M, Kaplan JB, Burk RD. (1992) Phylogenetic classification of human papillomaviruses: correlation with clinical manifestations. *J Gen Virol* **73**: 2653–60.

118. Vogelstein B, Kinzler KW. (1992) p53 function and dysfunction. *Cell* **70**: 523–6.

119. Volpers C, Unckell F, Schirmacher P, *et al.* (1995) Binding and internalization of human papillomavirus type 33 virus-like particles by eukaryotic cells. *J Virol* **69**: 3258–63.

120. White E. (1994) Function of the adenovirus E1B oncogene in infected and transformed cells. *Semin Virol* **5**: 341–9.

121. White E. (1996) Life, death, and the pursuit of apoptosis. *Genes Dev* **10**: 1–15.

122. Whyte P. (1995) The retinoblastoma protein and its relatives. *Semin Cancer Biol* **6**: 83–90.

123. Williams MG, Howatson AF, Almeida JD. (1961) Morphological characterisation of the virus of the human common wart (verruca vulgaris). *Nature* **189**: 895–7.

124. Wu X, Xiao W, Brandsma JL. (1994) Papilloma forma-

tion by cottontail rabbit papillomavirus requires E1 and E2 regulatory genes in addition to E6 and E7 transforming genes. *J Virol* **68**: 6097–102.

125. Yabe Y, Tanimura Y, Sakai A, Hitsumoto T, Nohara N. (1989) Molecular characteristics and physical state of human papillomavirus DNA change with progressing malignancy: studies in a patient with epidermodysplasia verruciformis. *Int J Cancer* **43**: 1022–8.

126. Yang L, Mohr I, Fouts E, Lim DA, Nohaile M, Botchan M. (1993) The E1 protein of bovine papillomavirus 1 is an ATP-dependent DNA helicase. *Proc Natl Acad Sci USA* **90**: 5086–90.

127. Zheng Z-M, He P, Baker CC. (1996) Selection of the bovine papillomavirus type 1 nucleotide 3225 3′ splice site is regulated through an exonic splicing enhancer. *J Virol* **70**: 4691–9.

128. zur Hausen H, ed. (1994) Molecular pathogenesis of cancer of the cervix and its causation by specific human papillomavirus types. In *Human pathogenic papillomaviruses*, ed. H zur Hausen. Current topics in microbiology and immunology, Vol. 186. Heidelberg, Springer-Verlag, 131–56.

3

Molecular mechanisms of HPV-associated oncogenesis

Claire P. Mansur

3.1 INTRODUCTION

The papillomaviruses are small, double-stranded DNA viruses that infect a wide range of species. There are over 100 distinct genotypes of human papillomaviruses (HPVs), which have been identified based on differences in their nucleotide sequences.[35,182] Infection with most of these viruses causes benign epithelial proliferations called warts that have little serious impact on the host. However, infection with a specific subset of these viruses has been etiologically linked to the development of a growing number of epithelial cancers. HPVs have been associated with over 95% of all cervical cancers and over 50% of vulvar, vaginal, and penile cancers. The importance of this relationship is clear as cervical cancer is one of the most common causes of cancer death, but also of note is the growing association of HPVs with other epithelial cancers, including those of skin, larynx, and esophagus.[182] This cancer-associated subset of HPVs has been termed the 'high-risk' subset, and the types most commonly isolated from genital cancers are HPV 16 and 18. Those that have rarely been isolated from cancers are termed 'low-risk' viruses. In addition, specific HPV subtypes that have not been identified in immunocompetent hosts have been associated with the development of non-melanoma skin cancer in patients with epidermodysplasia verruciformis and also in some skin cancers in immunocompromised hosts. Now that methods for detecting a broad range of HPV subtypes have been developed, it has been reported that HPV DNA is detected in up to 30% of non-melanoma skin cancers even in immunocompetent hosts.[143] This is a surprising result but does not prove an etiologic role for HPV in these cancers. Investigation of whether the low-risk viruses may act as co-factors in the development of ultraviolet-induced cancers will be needed to clarify this issue. Because most HPV infections, even with the 'high-risk' genotypes, do not progress to cancer and because malignant transformation occurs only after a long latency, infection with HPV is believed to be necessary but not sufficient for the development of HPV-related cancers.

The viral genome is small, about 8000 base pairs, and encodes a small number of genes (Figure 3.1). The basic structure of the genome is the same for the different genotypes of papillomaviruses and consists of a regulatory region which controls gene transcription, an 'early gene' (E) region which encodes proteins that regulate viral function, and the 'late gene' (L) region which encodes the structural capsid proteins. The biological life cycle of the papillomaviruses differs from that of most other viral pathogens. These viruses are presumed to infect the basal or germ cells of the epithelium. Viral DNA transcription and replication are maintained at very low levels until the infected cells move to the higher strata of the epithelium. Only in the terminally differentiated epithelial cells, presumably in response to differentiation-specific signals, does viral transcription accelerate, DNA synthesis begin, and virions assemble. It is particularly important to note that it is within this terminally differentiating cellular environment that the virus must recruit the many cellular factors necessary for its reproduction. The virus presumably does this by stimulating non-dividing cells to divide so it can utilize the replicative machinery for its own replication. Thus, even in benign infections, the viruses have some ability to stimulate cellular growth and it is likely that the acquisition of transforming function in the 'high-risk' viruses may have come in part from a loss of regulation of this growth-promoting activity.

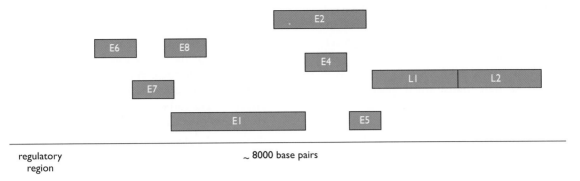

Figure 3.1
Schematic linear representation of the papillomavirus genome which is actuallly a closed circle of double-stranded DNA. The boxes indicate the protein coding regions. The regulatory region does not encode a viral protein, but is involved in the regulation of viral gene expression and the replication of viral DNA synthesis. While there are differences in protein function between the different viral genotypes, in general, E6, E7, and E5 are transforming genes, E1 and E2 co-ordinate replication and expression of the viral genome, and L1 and L2 are structural proteins which form the viral capsid. It is believed that E4 may actually be a late protein involved in the release of the virus from the cell's keratin framework. (Figure redrawn from reference 104.)

The detection of HPV DNA in human cancers did not prove that the viruses played an etiologic role in the development of cancer and evidence for this was a long time in coming. Part of the difficulty in proving a causal relationship has been due to the difficulty of developing laboratory models for the study of papillomaviruses. Because of the requirement for a differentiated environment for growth, it has not been possible to develop a simple means to culture HPVs *in vitro*.[92,150,152] Very limited production of HPV virions has been achieved *in vitro* using infected human cells in an organotypic culture system[43,109] However, introduction of cloned viral DNA into cells cultured in submerged monolayers has not led to synthesis of infectious viral particles. Papillomaviruses also show a strict species specificity. They do not undergo vegetative replication in cells of species other than their normal host *in vivo* and thus HPVs cannot readily be produced in an animal model. For years, epidemiological studies have debated the causal role of HPVs in human cancers, although carefully controlled studies have now clearly supported a role for HPVs in cancers (for review, see reference 134). Perhaps the most definitive proof of the etiologic role of HPVs in human cancers and some understanding of the molecular mechanisms by which these viruses exert transforming effects have come with the cloning of the viral genomes and molecular biologic studies of the functions of the high-risk and low-risk viral proteins.

This evidence for an etiologic association between papillomavirus infection and the development of cervical cancers has come from a number of lines of investigation. Isolation of new HPV types (HPV 6 and 11) from benign genital warts and of the HPV 16 and 18 subtypes from cervical cancers and the precursor lesions of cervical dysplasia and carcinoma *in situ* suggested the concept of 'low-risk' and 'high-risk' papillomavirus subtypes. Several established HPV-positive cervical carcinoma cell lines such as HeLa were found to continue to synthesize HPV proteins despite maintenance in culture for decades. Specifically, these cervical carcinoma cell lines selectively retain and express the early viral genes E6 and E7 which are now known to be the major transforming proteins of the high-risk HPVs (see below).[1,7,148] In addition, it was demonstrated that repression of HPV protein expression in cervical carcinoma cell lines led to decreased cell growth and loss of the transformed phenotype.[159,171,172] Using *in vitro* cellular transformation assays, with the introduction of HPV genomes or specific viral genes into cells grown in culture, various parameters of malignant transformation which are thought to mirror the *in vivo* transformation process have been measured (for review see reference 104). With numerous such assays, it was demonstrated that the 'high-risk' HPV genotypes could induce immortalization of primary cells[66,113] and malignant progression of immortalized cell lines.[169,174,178] These effects can be achieved with expression of only the E6 and E7 genes, thus identifying these as the major transforming proteins of the HPVs.[66,73,86] The E6 and E7 proteins from the low-risk HPVs show little or no activity in these transformation assays.[10,42,138,155]

Data such as these established a role for HPVs in epithelial cancers, but this work does not elucidate the mechanisms by which these viruses may exert their transforming effects. As mentioned above, the transformation assays identified the E6 and E7 genes as the major transforming oncogenes, with the probable additional contribution of E5. With identification of these HPV oncoproteins, it has been possible to investigate their interactions with the other cellular proteins and some potential molecular mechanisms by which they exert their transforming effects. The goal of this chapter is to examine our current understanding of the molecular mechanisms through which papillomavirus genes exert effects on cellular growth and transformation.

3.2 TRANSFORMATION ASSAYS

Much of our understanding of the effect of HPV oncoproteins on cellular functioning has come from cellular transformation assays. It is now understood that malignant transformation is a multistep process *in vivo,* with cellular dysplasia developing first, followed by carcinoma *in situ,* and finally development of invasive carcinoma. Using classical transformation assays, immortalization of cells corresponds to the early changes seen in carcinoma *in situ,* whereas measures of anchorage-independent growth and tumorigenicity in mice correspond to a more fully transformed phenotype. Immortalization of primary cervical epithelial cells, the natural target cells of HPVs, has been shown to require cooperation of both the E6 and E7 genes of high risk HPVs.[66,113] In culture, the morphological appearance of the immortalized cells closely mimics that which is seen in cervical intraepithelial neoplasia.[73,106] These cells are not tumorigenic, but when maintained for sustained periods in culture will evolve a fully transformed phenotype.[73,75] Thus, HPV-mediated extension of lifespan *in vitro* is thought to allow time for additional somatic alterations that must accumulate for a fully malignant phenotype to be manifest. All of these observations indicate that these transformation assays serve as an excellent model in which to understand the requirements of HPV-induced carcinogenesis. However, it is important to bear in mind that the cell culture systems upon which proliferation, immortalization, and transformation assays depend cannot reflect many aspects of the natural life cycle of the virus or the role of host immune surveillance in controlling infection and tumorigenic progression. Because we cannot produce mutant infectious papillomavirus *in vivo*, it is not yet possible to assess fully the contribution of the transforming genes to viral pathogenesis *in vivo*. Despite this, through cloning the viral oncogenes and genetic studies, it has been possible to identify a number of functions of these proteins. In general, as with other viral and cellular oncogenes, the HPV oncogenes have evolved mechanisms to disrupt the function of cellular tumor suppressors and growth regulators. Other functions appear to impact cell-cell adhesions and signaling and are important in later stages of tumor progression. The specific functions identified for these viral proteins are described below.

3.3 FUNCTIONS OF THE VIRUS-TRANSFORMING PROTEINS

3.3.1 The E7 Protein

The E7 oncoprotein is a zinc-binding, 98 amino acid phosphoprotein which is localized to both the cell cytoplasm[147] and the cell nucleus[62] (Figure 3.2). A critical finding that led to the elucidation of the biochemical properties of E7 was recognition of the amino acid similarities between the HPV

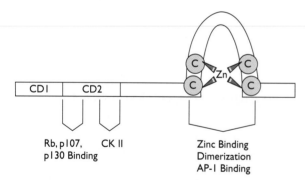

Figure 3.2
Schematic representation of the HPV E7 protein. CD 1 and CD 2 refer to the conserved domains of sequence homology with the adenovirus E1A protein. Retinoblastoma protein binds within a region of CD 1; the related proteins p107 and p130 bind to sequences which overlap but can be distinguished from the Rb-binding site. CK II represents a region which is phosphorylated by casein kinase II[8]. The carboxy-terminus contains a region which co-ordinates zinc binding, mediates E7 dimerization, and interacts with members of the AP-1 transcription factor family.

E7 proteins and other DNA tumor virus-transforming proteins.[125] The amino-terminal 37 amino acids bear marked sequence homology to conserved domains 1 and 2 (CD 1 and CD 2) of the adenovirus 5 E1A oncoprotein as well as to a homologous region of the SV 40 large T oncoprotein. Both of these domains contribute to E7's immortalizing effects.[124] The carboxy-terminal 60 amino acids contain two cysteine-x-x-cysteine repeats which have been shown to mediate zinc binding and dimerization of the E7 proteins.[107]

Like E1A and SV 40 large T, HPV 16 and 18 E7 proteins have been shown to bind to the family of cellular proteins which includes the retinoblastoma gene product (Rb) and the related p107 and p130 proteins[34,49,114] In the case of Rb, it was shown that E7 binding stimulates proteosome-mediated degradation of Rb.[15] The Rb binding domain of E7 has been localized to the region of homology with CD 2 of the adenovirus E1A protein[114] and, using synthetic peptides, amino acids 17 to 26 were sufficient for high-affinity binding.[83] The E7 proteins of the low-risk HPVs bind to Rb with much lower affinity than those of the high-risk HPVs.[67,131]

The Rb protein, p107, and p130 all function as cellular growth regulators. An important mechanism by which Rb and the related proteins act is through interaction with the family of E2F transcription factors (Figure 3.3). Rb is found in non-phosphorylated and phosphorylated forms that are specific for certain phases of the cell cycle.[18] The non-phosphorylated state is found in G1 and during growth arrest.[36] In its non-phosphorylated state, Rb acts to restrict cell proliferation, in part through binding to E2F.[144] It is believed that when E2F is complexed to Rb it is not able to activate promoters of genes, which encode positive signals for growth, such as c-myc and n-myc. During G2/S, Rb is phosphorylated, releases E2F, and thus releases its controls on cell growth.[18] The high-risk E7 proteins bind preferentially to the under-phosphorylated, activated form of Rb and induce release of E2F from the Rb complex,[78] freeing it to stimulate transcription of genes required for progression through the cell cycle. Similarly, the related proteins p107 and p130 complex with regulators of the cell cycle including other members of the E2F family, cyclin A, and cyclin E,[40,149] and participate in the regulation of both G1 and G2 cell cycle blocks. The high-risk E7 proteins bind to p107 and thus disrupt the regulation of cyclins A and E and to the cyclin dependent kinase, p33[CDK2] that are in complex with p107.[3,34,49,108,165] In addition, high-risk E7 has been shown to stimulate the constitutive expression of cyclins A and E when expressed in NIH 3T3 cells.[180] All of these interactions are mediated through the amino-terminus of E7 in the regions of CD1 and CD2, although the precise sequences required vary for the different complexes.[180] Mutational analyses have shown that the p107 binding site in E7 overlaps with, but can be distinguished from the Rb binding domain.[34] It has been reported that binding Rb correlates with E7's transforming activities.[8,23,124] although there is one report which suggests that, in the context of the full-length viral genome, E7 binding of Rb may not be strictly required for transformation.[81] The interactions with the Rb-related proteins might explain how an E7 mutant, which cannot bind Rb, might retain some transforming capability.

E7 has also been reported to activate transcription of the adenovirus E2 early promoter[123,125] and the B-myb promot-

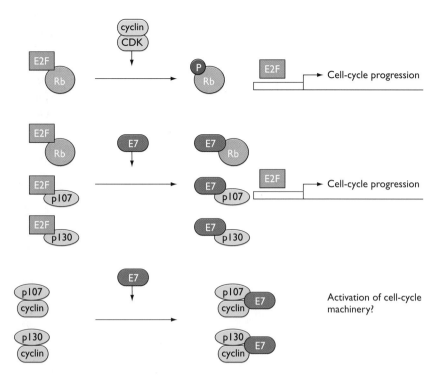

Figure 3.3
Interaction of HPV E7 with the retinoblastoma protein and related proteins p107 and p130. Activated Rb binds to E2F and inhibits gene expression required for progression through the G1 phase of the cell cycle. Similarly, p107 and p130 exert negative regulation of the cell cycle at other phases. With phosphorylation of Rb or the related proteins by CDks, or binding by HPV E7, E2F is released and can act to stimulate cell-cycle progression.

ers.[96] The cellular targets for transcriptional activation by E7 have not been identified, and transactivation may not be relevant to its transforming effects as it has been shown that co-transfection of the low-risk HPV E7 proteins with an adenovirus E2 promoter resulted in transactivation levels equal to those seen with the high-risk E7 proteins.[115,154] It may be that, during the course of viral infection, transactivation by the low-risk E7 proteins is not equal to that of the high-risk proteins, but this is artificially elevated by over-expression of the proteins in these assays. At this point, the relationship between E7's transactivation function and transformation remains to be fully elucidated.

Other studies have examined the functional role of the cysteine repeats in the carboxy-terminus which are necessary for binding of zinc and dimerization of E7 proteins.[27,107,183] While the amino-terminus of E7 is required for Rb binding, mutations of these cys-x-x-cys motifs eliminated keratinocyte immortalization[81] and led to partial or complete inhibition of transformation in rodent cells.[50,107,135,154] Proteins mutated in this region bound Rb efficiently but did not mediate release of E2F from complexes with Rb.[71,107,176] It has been proposed that release of E2F from Rb does not occur through binding by E7 alone, but also requires dimerization of the E7 protein mediated through the cysteine repeats. Because release of E2F from Rb is thought to be an important mechanism through which growth control is disrupted, these results may in part explain the requirement for the C-terminus in transformation assays.

Other work has demonstrated that the C-terminus may have additional, Rb-independent, transforming effects. The zinc-binding region of E7 was shown to complex with the AP-1 transcription factors c-jun, jun-B, jun-D, and c-fos, and activate transcription of AP-1-driven genes. When a

transcription-defective c-jun mutant was bound to E7, it was found to abrogate E7-induced immortalization of cells.[2] It has further been reported that the C-terminus of E7 is required for interaction with inhibitors of cyclin-dependent kinases, p21[82] and p27.[181] These C-terminal interactions offer further mechanisms by which E7 could deregulate control of cell-cycle progression.

In functional assays, it has been shown that E7 expression can overcome cellular G1 arrest induced by several mechanisms including growth factor withdrawal,[111] loss of cell adhesion,[139] DNA damage,[37] and differentiation signals.[130] It is clear that there are multiple mechanisms through which E7 functions to disrupt normal cellular growth.

3.3.2 The E6 Protein

The E6 proteins have about 150 amino acids with four cysteine-x-x-cysteine motifs that have been shown to mediate zinc binding[9,64,136] and are believed to form two large zinc binding fingers (Figure 3.4). The high-risk E6 proteins, in cooperation with high-risk E7, are able to immortalize

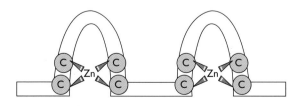

Figure 3.4
Schematic representation of the putative zinc finger structure of the E6 protein. Extensive mutation analyses of the E6 protein suggest that domains for p53 binding and degradation are not represented by a linear peptide.

human keratinocytes[66,73,86] and alone are sufficient for immortalization of primary human mammary epithelial cells.[5,6]

Unlike E7, the high-risk E6 proteins have not been found to have significant sequence homology with other transforming proteins, but they have been found to be functionally similar to the adenovirus 5 E1B and SV 40 large T oncoproteins in that they also interact with a cellular tumor suppressor, p53.[175] Binding of p53 by E6 leads to the selective degradation of the p53 protein via the ubiquitin proteolysis pathway.[133] The low-risk E6 proteins do not induce degradation of p53.[32,133] The ubiquitin pathway is a mechanism by which the cell can regulate the levels of short-lived cellular proteins. Specific cellular enzymes interact with proteins that are to be degraded and ligate chains of a small molecule called ubiquitin. Thus tagged, the targeted proteins are degraded by the 26S proteosome (for review, see reference 68). This interaction between the high-risk E6 proteins and p53 is mediated via a cellular protein called E6-AP (for E6 associated protein),[74] and together E6 and E6-AP function as a ubiquitin ligase, binding and ligating ubiquitin to p53.[132] It has been reported that p53 is normally targeted and degraded through the ubiquitin pathway independent of E6,[25] and further that p53 levels rise in a mutant cell line which is defective for ubiquitin degradation.[24] Thus, it appears that E6 stimulates accelerated turnover of p53 or perhaps stimulates degradation of p53 in the face of signals that would normally induce stabilization and activation of p53. Studies using antisense E6-AP suggest that E6-AP is not normally involved in the turnover of p53.[12] Using *in vivo* assays, it has been shown that HPV 16 E6 induces a shortened half-life of p53 in human keratinocytes,[72] and that decreased p53 levels are invariably seen in human mammary epithelial cells immortalized with HPV 16 E6,[33] supporting the idea that p53 degradation is important to the transforming effect of E6.

The significance of E6-mediated degradation of *p53* is becoming clearer as more is understood of the function of the tumor suppressor p53 (for review, see reference 61). The wild-type *p53* (*wt p53*) gene encodes a nuclear phosphoprotein that acts as a tumor suppressor and cellular growth regulator. Mutation of p53 is the most common mutation detected in human cancers,[70] and cellular transfection studies have shown that *wt p53* is able to suppress cell growth and oncogene-mediated cellular transformation.[4,21,51,55] Whereas p53 is not essential for basal cellular growth and development,[44] it does play a critical role in the response of cells to stress, mediating a G1/S cell-cycle arrest and/or apoptosis (programmed cell death) following damage to DNA.[26,84,85,93,103] When DNA is damaged, p53 levels rise and induce G1 cell-cycle arrest, presumably allowing time for the DNA to be repaired. Conversely, cells with mutant *p53* continue to divide, thus perpetuating DNA mutations. Loss of the G1 checkpoint leads to genomic instability, as demonstrated by the increase in gene amplification seen in p53-defective cells.[102,179] In other cases, presumably with more extensive DNA damage, p53 signals apoptosis or programmed cell death.

An important mechanism by which p53 mediates at least some of these effects is through transcriptional regulation. Wild-type, but not mutant, p53 exerts strong transcriptional activation of promoters containing p53-binding sites[53,58,87,128]

and represses the transcription of several growth-regulated genes which lack a p53 response element.[157] An important transactivational target of p53 in the mediation of the G1 checkpoint is p21/WAF1, a protein that has been termed a universal inhibitor of cyclin dependent kinases (CDKs). CDKs play a critical role in mediating progression through the cell-cycle.[65,177] Among other functions, CDKs stimulate the phosphorylation of Rb, which, as outlined above, leads to the release of E2F from complexes with Rb and stimulates progression through the cell-cycle (Figure 3.5). This linking of the p53 and Rb pathways may in part explain why both E6 and E7 are required for immortalization of primary cells. Another mechanism by which p53 participates in the response to DNA damage is through binding to proteins such as RPA, TFIIH and CSB, which have functions in both DNA replication and repair.[46,48,173] Although the pathways are not completely worked out, it is thought that p53 may inhibit the DNA replication functions of these proteins but localize them to sites of DNA damage and perhaps participate directly in facilitating the DNA repair process.

With elucidation of the transcriptional function of p53, it has been possible to explore the impact of interactions between HPV E6 proteins and p53. p53-mediated activation of p53-responsive reporters is markedly inhibited by co-expression of HPV 16 E6, but no inhibition is seen with low-risk HPV 6 E6.[110] With promoters at which p53 has a repressive effect, co-transfection of E6 releases the repression of growth-stimulating genes.[98] While it is likely that E6's inhibition of p53-mediated transcriptional regulation is related to the stimulation of degradation of p53, it has also been shown that E6 can directly inhibit sequence-specific DNA binding by p53 *in vitro*.[97,163] In other studies it has been demonstrated that high-risk E6 proteins block p53-mediated G1 growth arrest following DNA damage, inhibit p53-induced apoptosis, and induce genomic instability.[88,102,164] The p53-dependent growth arrest and apoptotic pathways are also an important means by which cells show sensitivity to chemotherapeutic agents and ionizing radiation. The interaction of E6 with p53 appears to be a means through which cells acquire drug resistance, as it has been shown that, by stimulating the degradation of p53, the high-risk E6 proteins release cells from actinomycin D-induced growth arrest.[56] Similarly, HPV 16 E6-expressing fibroblasts show a loss of p21/Waf1 induction and a loss of radiosensitivity in response to ionizing radiation.[168]

While it is clear that E6-mediated degradation of p53 is important for growth promotion and the induction of genetic instability, there are a number of other functions which have been identified for the E6 protein which are likely to be relevant to both the viral life cycle and viral transformation. Mutational analyses of HPV 16 E6 have found that there are E6 mutants which retain p53 binding and degradation capability but which have lost the ability to stimulate the growth of embryonic fibroblasts and transform primary cells in cooperation with E7.[79,116] As has been found with E7, one potential additional function for E6 is the regulation of transcription as it has been shown to have both activating and repressive effects at a number of viral and cellular promoters.[39,52,141] However, cellular targets for transcriptional regulation by E6 have not been identified.

A number of other proteins that are degraded by E6 have been identified. HPV E6 proteins have been shown to bind

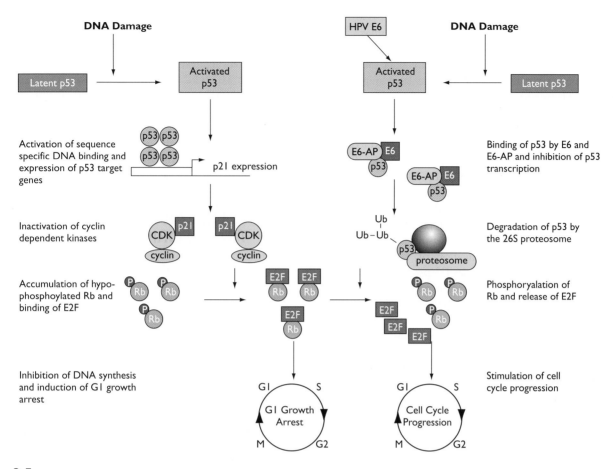

Figure 3.5
Activation of p53 by DNA damage leads to p53-dependent gene expression, increased expression of growth-inhibiting genes, and cell-cycle arrest. With interaction with the high-risk HPV E6 proteins, p53 is degraded and G1 growth arrest is lost.

and degrade DLG protein.[90,99] DLG is the human homolog of the *Drosophila* discs large protein. This protein functions to recruit cytoskeletal proteins to regions of cell–cell contact and also mediates contact between cytoskeletal proteins and signaling molecules. By disrupting cell adhesion and signaling, targeted degradation of this protein might be important in the later stages of tumor progression. Another protein targeted for ubiquitin-mediated degradation by E6 is E6 TP1 (E6-targeted protein 1), a protein which is thought to function as a negative regulator of mitotic signaling.[59] E6 has also been shown to mediate the degradation of Mcm7.[94] In complex with other proteins, Mcm7 functions to regulate chromosomal replication and ensure that the DNA is replicated only once with each cell division. Finally, E6 also induces the degradation of c-Myc and Bak proteins, both of which can function to induce cellular apoptosis.[63,161,162] These results help explain how E6 proteins can function to block cellular apoptosis by both p53-dependent and independent means.[118]

Other proteins are bound by E6 but not targeted for degradation. One of these is the ERC-55 homolog E6BP (E6-binding protein).[20] This calcium-binding protein is associated with vitamin D receptor[77] and may play a role in cellular differentiation. Because E6 can inhibit cellular differentiation in keratinocytes, this effect may be mediated through E6BP binding. E6 also binds to paxillin without inducing degradation.[166,167] Paxillin is another protein involved in signal transduction between the plasma membrane and cell contacts.

Finally, E6 proteins have been shown to up-regulate telomerase during the immortalization of cells.[54,89,91,153] Telomeres are short DNA repeats at the ends of chromosomes that help position and protect chromosomes during DNA replication and cell division. Telomerase is an enzyme that adds telomeric sequences to DNA and is normally active only in germ cells. With normal aging and senescence of cells, telomere ends gradually shorten. Up-regulation of telomerase has been detected in immortalized cells and tumor cells, suggesting telomerase activation may allow cells to proliferate beyond their normal lifespan. Consistent with the immortalizing activities of E6, it was found that E6 can up-regulate telomerase activity in human keratinocytes and that this activity may be more critical to immortalization than p53 degradation. At this time, the precise role of telomerase activation in cellular transformation is not clear and so one cannot conclude which of E6's activities are most critical to cellular transformation. However, it is clear that this is a multi-functional protein with many activities that can impact normal cellular growth.

3.3.3 The E5 Protein

Using transformation assays, it has been shown that the bovine papillomavirus (BPV) E5 protein is the major transforming protein for BPVs,[41,137] but the HPV E5 is relatively weakly transforming,[100,101,127,170] and the role of HPV E5 in malignant conversion *in vivo* is uncertain. While cervical intraepithelial neoplasias have been reported to express relatively high levels of E5,[151], the HPV E5 gene is often deleted or its gene not expressed in cervical carcinomas.[140] It would thus appear that the biological impact of HPV E5 in malignant progression would be at an early stage of viral infection and may be dispensable for the later stages of malignant transformation.

The E5 protein is a very small, hydrophobic protein that is localized to the Golgi apparatus and the plasma membrane.[19] The BPV E5 protein has been shown to bind to and activate the receptors for epidermal growth factor (EGF-R) and platelet-derived growth factor (PDGF-R). However, reports vary on whether HPV 16 E5 can complex with these receptors.[28,30,60,76,121,122] More recent evidence suggests that the HPV 16 E5 does enhance the activity of these and other receptors and may do so through decreasing their degradation rate by delaying the acidification of cellular endosomes.[127,156] Both BPV and HPV 16 E5 proteins have also been shown to complex with a membrane-bound proton-ATPase which is part of the gap junction complex[29] and participates in cell–cell communication. Over-expression of E5 has been reported to induce the dephosphorylation of a gap junctional protein, connexin 43, and consequently induce impairment of gap-junction-mediated dye coupling.[117] These effects suggest the E5 protein functions to increase unscheduled cell cycling and disrupt normal cellular communication.

3.3.4 The E2 Protein

Although the HPV E2 proteins are not transforming proteins, some understanding of their function is relevant to the oncogenic potential of these viruses as the E2 proteins act as regulators of viral gene transcription and, importantly, this gene is frequently deleted in cervical cancer cells.[140] The E2 open reading frame encodes two or three proteins which can exert both transcriptional activating and repressing effects[11,14,31,123,160] and are thought to be important in regulating the expression of the other viral proteins. Expression of E2 has been shown to down-regulate the level of expression of E6 and E7 in cells which contain HPV 18 DNA.[38] Thus, the loss of E2 expression in cervical cancers has led to the speculation that this may be important in the induction of transformation. In benign HPV infections, the viral genome exists as a circular episome, separate from the host DNA, but in cervical cancers the HPV frequently becomes integrated into the host DNA and this integration frequently leads to disruption of the E2 gene.[140] It has been shown that disruption of the E2 gene leads to increased expression of the E6 and E7 proteins[80,140] and increases the immortalization capacity of HPV 16.[129] Evidence indicates that viral DNA integration and disruption of the E2 gene are neither necessary nor sufficient for malignant transformation, as a number of cervical cancers with episomal viral DNA have been identified,[105] and, conversely, cells with integrated viral DNA and active viral gene expression do not always display a malignant phenotype.[13] Nonetheless, it is likely that the loss of E2's regulatory function serves to enhance the transforming capability of these viruses. There is also evidence that E2 may directly contribute to growth dysregulation. Over-expression of HPV 31 E2 in keratinocytes can induce a marked decrease in the half-life of the p53 protein and S phase arrest of cells with ongoing DNA synthesis.[57]

Whether the decrease in p53 half-life by E2 is due to a mechanism similar to that induced by the high-risk E6 proteins or another means is unknown at present. However, these interesting data suggest that the targeting of p53 may be a means through which E2 can stimulate cellular DNA replication to facilitate viral replication. Presumably, if this targeting of p53 is accelerated or unregulated, as seen with the E6 proteins, the loss of G1 growth arrest leads to an increased likelihood of accumulating genetic alterations which might lead to full malignant transformation.

3.4 CELLULAR RESPONSES TO HPV-TRANSFORMING EFFECTS

The interactions of the high-risk E6 and E7 transforming proteins with cellular tumor suppressors clearly induce many downstream abnormalities in the growth regulation of the cell that are critical to their transforming effects. Having examined these thus far identified molecular functions of the transforming proteins of the high-risk HPVs, it is important to put this information back into the context of what we understand about cellular transformation *in vivo*. Infection with the high-risk HPV viruses does not immediately or necessarily lead to cancer, despite their activity in acute transformation assays *in vitro*. Warts and cervical papillomas that are infected with high-risk HPVs such as types 16 or 18 progress toward a malignant phenotype only after a long latent period, estimated to be from 5 to 20 years. This implies the existence of important cellular, immune, and/or viral modulators of their transforming activities. Using somatic cell hybridization studies, it has been shown that, when cells which have been immortalized by E6 and E7 are hybridized with primary cells, despite the fact that these cells continue to express E6 and E7, they frequently undergo senescence.[22] When fully transformed cervical cells are grafted onto nude mice they show no change in the expression of E6 and E7 genes, but when immortalized, but not fully transformed, cells are grafted onto mice, expression of E6 and E7 genes is down-regulated.[47] These results support the evidence that infection with the high-risk HPVs is not sufficient for the development of cancer and that the cell has mechanisms by which it can interfere with the function of the viral oncogenes (i.e., by inducing cellular senescence in the presence of viral oncogene expression) as well as act to down-regulate their expression. In order for malignant progression to occur, these cellular growth suppressive functions must be inactivated and thus other mutational events would be expected to occur. It is clear that the viral oncogenes do induce genetic instability, most profoundly through the interaction between high-risk E6 proteins and p53, but the exact mutations that occur to allow malignant progression have not been identified.

In order to search for other likely mechanisms by which inhibition of cell growth is overcome, investigators have searched for genetic alterations which may be found in HPV-transformed cells and potential co-factors which may contribute to malignant progression. When cervical cancer cells have been subjected to cytogenetic analysis, a number of chromosomal abnormalities at a number of different sites have been found,[12,145,146] although no one mutation was consistently identified. However, one commonly detected candidate mutation that may have an impact on the regulation of viral gene transcription is a deletion of the short arm of chromosome 11. This region is thought to be important in the regulation of protein phosphatase 2A and deletions here are associated with both up-regulation of a regulatory subunit of protein phosphatase 2A and enhanced HPV gene transcription in cells.[146] The precise signaling pathway by which this protein might impact upon viral gene transcription has not been identified, although there is other work that indicates that paracrine growth factors may regulate viral gene expression. It has been reported that tumor necrosis factor-α (TNFα), interleukin-1, and transforming growth factor-β (TGFβ) can all induce the down-regulation of viral early gene expression.[16,95] In other reports it has been shown that HPV transformed cells have evolved resistance to the growth suppressive effects of TGFβ,[126] thus suggesting that, with malignant progression, additional mutational events allow escape from this paracrine regulation. Glucocorticoids are co-factors that may act in a positive way to stimulate HPV-transforming capability. The high-risk HPVs have glucocorticoid-responsive elements within the regulatory region of their genome and the addition of glucocorticoids to transformation assays is reported to enhance the immortalizing effects of HPV 16.[119] In another report, it was shown that HPV 16-mediated transformation was inhibited by the exposure of cells to a glucocorticoid antagonist.[120] Whereas none of these reports elucidates the precise signaling pathways through which the cell interacts with and responds to the HPV proteins, they do make it clear that these interactions are complex and that, while the high-risk viruses encode potent transforming proteins, there are a number of cellular mechanisms that act to safeguard the genome and prevent malignant transformation.

The study of HPVs and human cancer has taught us a great deal about both the interaction of the virus with the cell and the mechanisms of cellular growth regulation in general. It is hoped that, with greater understanding of the interactions of viral proteins with cellular proteins, chemotherapeutic drugs might be devised which would interfere with the function of these viral oncoproteins. Through the use of 'virus-like particles' constructed from the structural late papillomavirus proteins, other researchers are making the possibility of a vaccine against these viruses an excellent likelihood.[17,45,69,142,158] The development of such therapies for these very common human cancers would be of obvious importance.

REFERENCES

1. Androphy EJ, Hubbert NL, Schiller JT, Lowy DR. (1987) Identification of the HPV-16 E6 protein from transformed mouse cells and human cervical carcinoma cell lines. *EMBO J* **6**: 989–92.
2. Antinore MJ, Birrer MJ, Patel D, Nader L, McCance DJ. (1996) The human papillomavirus type 16 E7 gene product interacts with and trans-activates the AP1 family of transcription factors. *EMBO J* **15**: 1950–60.
3. Arroyo M, Bagchi S, and Raychaudhuri P. (1993) Association of the human papillomavirus type 16 E7 protein with the S-phase-specific E2F-cyclin A complex. *Mol Cell Biol* **13**: 6537–46.
4. Baker SJ, Markowitz S, Fearon ER, Willson JKV, Vogelstein B. (1990) Suppression of human colorectal carcinoma cell growth by wild-type p53. *Science* **249**: 912–15.
5. Band V, DeCaprio J, Delmolino L, Kulesa V, Sager R. (1991) Loss of p53 protein in human papillomavirus type 16 E6-immortalized human mammary epithelial cells. *J Virol* **65**: 6671–6.
6. Band V, Zajchowski D, Kulesa V, Sager R. (1990) Human papilloma virus DNAs immortalize normal human mammary epithelial cells and reduce their growth factor requirements. *Proc Natl Acad Sci* **87**: 463–7.
7. Banks L, Spence P, Androphy E, Hubbert N, Matlashewski G, Murray A, Crawford L. (1987) Identification of human papillomavirus type 18 E6 polypeptide in cells derived from human cervical carcinomas. *J Gen Virol* **68**: 1351–9.
8. Barbosa MS, Edmonds C, Fisher C, Schiller JT, Lowy DR, Vousden KH. (1990) The region of the HPV E7 oncoprotein homologous to adenovirus E1a and Sv40 large T antigen contains separate domains for Rb binding and casein kinase II phosphorylation. *EMBO J* **9**: 153–60.
9. Barbosa MS, Lowy DR, Schiller JT. (1989) Papillomavirus polypeptides E6 and E7 are zinc-binding proteins. *J Virol* **63**:1404–7.
10. Barbosa MS, Vass WC, Lowy DR, Schiller JT. (1991) In vitro biological activities of the E6 and E7 genes vary among human papillomaviruses of different oncogenic potential. *J Virol* **65**: 292–8.
11. Barsoum J, Prakash SS, Han P, Androphy EJ. (1992) Mechanism of action of the papillomavirus-E2 repressor – repression in the absence of DNA binding. *J Virol* **66**: 3941–5.
12. Beer-Romero P, Glass S, Rolfe M. (1997) Antisense targeting of E6AP elevates p53 in HPV-infected cells but not in normal cells. *Oncogene* **14**: 595-602.
13. Bosch F, Schwarz E, Boukamp P, Fusenig NE, Bartsch D, zur Hausen H. (1990) Suppression in vivo of human papillomavirus type 18 E6–E7 gene expression in non-tumorigenic HeLa × fibroblast hybrid cells. *J Virol* **64**: 4743–54.
14. Bouvard V, Storey A, Pim D, Banks L. (1994) Characterization of the human papillomavirus E2 protein: Evidence of trans-activation and trans-repression in cervical keratinocytes. *EMBO J* **13**: 5451–9.
15. Boyer SN, Wazer DE, Band V. (1996) E7 protein of human papilloma virus-16 induces degradation of retinoblastoma protein through the ubiquitin–proteosome pathway. *Cancer Res* **56**: 4620–4.
16. Braun L, Durst M, Mikumo R, Crowley A, Robinson M. (1992) Regulation of growth and gene expression in human papillomavirus-transformed keratinocytes by transforming growth factor-beta: implications for the control of papillomavirus infection. *Mol Carcinogen* **6**: 100-11.

17. Breitburd F, Kirnbauer R, Hubbert NL, *et al.* (1995) Immunization with viruslike particles from cottontail rabbit papillomavirus (CRPV) can protect against experimental CRPV infection. *J Virol* **69**: 3959-63.

18. Buchkovich K, Duffy LA, Harlow E. (1989) The retinoblastoma protein is phosphorylated during specific phases of the cell cycle. *Cell* **58**: 1097–105.

19. Burkhardt A, Willingham M, Gay C, Jeang, R. Schlegel. 1989. The E5 oncoprotein of bovine papillomavirus is oriented asymmetrically in Golgi and plasma membranes. *Virology* **170**: 334–9.

20. Chen JJ, Reid CE, Band V, Androphy EJ. (1995) Interaction of papillomavirus E6 oncoproteins with a putative calcium-binding protein. *Science* **269**: 529–31.

21. Chen P-L, Chen Y, Bookstein R, Leu W-H. (1990) Genetic mechanisms of tumor suppression by the human p53 gene. *Science* **250**: 1576–9.

22. Chen TM, Pecoraro G, Defendi V. (1993) Genetic analysis of in vitro progression of human papillomavirus-transfected human cervical cells. *Cancer Res* **53**: 1167–71.

23. Chesters PM, Vousden KH, Edmonds C, McCance DJ. (1990) Analysis of human papillomavirus type 16 open reading frame E7 immortalizing function in rat embryo fibroblast cells. *J Gen Virol* **71**: 449–53

24. Chowdary DR, Dermody JJ, Jha KK, Ozer HL. (1994) Accumulation of p53 in a mutant cell line defective in the ubiquitin pathway. *Mol Cell Bio* **14**: 1997–2003.

25. Ciechanover A, DiGiuseppe JA, Bercovich B, *et al.* (1991) Degradation of nuclear oncoproteins by the ubiquitin system. *Proc Natl Acad Sci* U *USA* **8**: 139–43.

26. Clarke AR, Purdie CA, Harrison DJ, *et al.* (1993) Thymocyte apoptosis induced by p53-dependent and independent pathways. *Nature* **362**: 849–52.

27. Clemens KE, Brent R, Gyuris J, Münger K. (1995) Dimerization of the human papillomavirus E7 oncoprotein in vivo. *Virology* **214**: 289–93.

28. Cohen BD, Goldstein DJ, Rutledge L, *et al.* (1993) Transformation-specific interaction of the bovine papillomavirus E5 oncoprotein with the platelet-derived growth factor receptor transmembrane domain and epidermal growth factor receptor cytoplasmic domain. *J Virol* **67**: 5303–11.

29. Conrad M, Bubb VJ, Schlegel R. (1993) The human papillomavirus type 6 and 16 E5 proteins are membrane-associated proteins which associate with the 16-kilodalton pore-forming protein. *J Virol* **67**: 6170–8.

30. Conrad M, Goldsteins D, Andresson T, Schlegel R. (1994) The E5 protein of HPV-6, but not HPV-16, associates efficiently with cellular growth factor receptors. *Virology* **200**: 796–800.

31. Cripe TP, Haugen TH, Turk JP, *et al.* (1987) Transcriptional regulation of the human papillomavirus-16 E6–E7 promoter by a keratinocyte-dependent enhancer, and by viral E2 trans-activator and repressor gene products: implications for cervical carcinogenesis. *EMBO J* **6**: 3745–53.

32. Crook T, Tidy JA, Vousden KH. (1991) Degradation of p53 can be targeted by HPV E6 sequences distinct from those required for p53 binding and trans-activation. *Cell* **67**: 547–56.

33. Dalal S, Gao Q, Androphy EJ, Band V. (1996) Mutational analysis of HPF-16 E6 demonstrates that p53 degradation is necessary for immortalization of human mammary epithelial cells. *J Virol* **70**: 683–8.

34. Davies R, Hicks R, Crook T, Morris J, Vousden K. (1993) Human papillomavirus type 16 E7 associates with a histone H1 kinase and with p107 through sequences necessary for transformation. *J Virol* **67**: 2521–8.

35. de Villiers EM, Lavergne D, McLaren K, Benton EC. (1997) Prevailing papillomavirus types in non-melanoma carcinomas of the skin in renal allograft recipients. *Int J Cancer* **73**: 356–61.

36. DeCaprio JA, Ludlow JW, Figge *et al.* (1988) SV40 large tumor antigen forms a specific complex with the product of the retinoblastoma susceptibility gene. *Cell* **54**: 275–83.

37. Demers G W, Foster SA, Halbert CL, Galloway DA. (1994) Growth arrest by induction of p53 in DNA damaged keratinocytes is bypassed by human papillomavirus 16 E7. *Proc Natl Acad Sci USA* **91**: 4382–6.

38. Desaintes C, Demeret C, Goyat S, Yaniv M, Thierry F. (1997) Expression of the papillomavirus E2 protein in HeLa cells leads to apoptosis. *EMBO J* **16**: 504–14.

39. Desaintes C, Hallez S, VanAlphen P, Burny A. (1992) Transcriptional activation of several promoters by the E6 protein of human papillomavirus type 16. *J Virol* **66**: 325–33.

40. Devoto SH, Mudryj M, Pines J, Hunter T, Nevins JR. (1992) A cyclin A–protein kinase complex possesses sequence-specific DNA binding activity: p33cdk2 is a component of the E2F–cyclin A complex. *Cell* **68**: 167–76.

41. DiMaio D, Guralski D, Schiller JT. (1986) Translation of open reading frame E5 of bovine papillomavirus is required for its transforming activity. *Proc Natl Acad Sci* **83**: 1797–801.

42. DiPaolo JA, Popescu NC, Woodworth CD, Zimonjic DB. (1996) Papillomaviruses and potential copathogens. *Toxicol Lett* **88**: 1–7.

43. Dollard SC, Wilson JL, Demeter LM, *et al.* (1992) Production of human papillomavirus and modulation of the infectious program in epithelial raft cultures. *Genes Devel* **6**: 1131–42.

44. Donehower LA, Harvey M, Slagle BL, *et al.* (1992) Mice deficient for p53 are developmentally normal but susceptible to spontaneous tumors. *Nature* **356**: 215–21.

45. Donnelly JJ, Martinez D, Jansen KU, Ellis RW, Montgomery DL, Liu MA. 1996. Protection against papillomavirus with a polynucleotide vaccine. *J Infect Dis* **173**: 314–20.

46. Drapkin R, Reardon JT, Ansari A, *et al.* (1994) The dual role of TFIIH in DNA excision repair and in transcription by RNA polymerase II. *Nature* **368**: 769–72.

47. Durst M, Bosch FX, Glitz D, Schneider A, zur Hausen H. (1991) Inverse relationship between human papillomavirus (HPV) type 16 early gene expression and cell differentiation in nude mouse epithelial cysts and tumors induced by HPV-positive human cell lines. *J Virol* **65**: 796–804.

48. Dutta A, Ruppert JM, Aster JC, Winchester E. (1993) Inhibition of DNA replication factor RPA by p53. *Nature* **365**: 79–82.

49. Dyson N, Guida P, Munger K, Harlow E. (1992) Homologous sequences in adenovirus E1a and human papillomavirus E7 proteins mediate interaction with the same set of cellular proteins. *J Virol* **66**: 6893–902.

50. Edmonds C, Vousden KH. (1989) A point mutational analysis of human papillomavirus type 16 E7 protein. *J Virol* **63**: 2650–6.

51. Eliyahu D, Michalovitz D, Eliyahu S, Pinhasi-Kimhi O, Oren M. (1989) Wild-type p53 can inhibit oncogene-mediated focus formation. *Proc Natl Acad Sci USA* **86**: 8763–7.

52. Etscheid BG, Foster SA, Galloway DA. (1994) The E6 protein of human papillomavirus type 16 functions as a transcriptional repressor in a mechanism independent of the tumor suppressor protein, p53. *Virology* **205**: 583–5.

53. Farmer G, Bargonetti J, Zhu H, Friedman P, Prywes R, Prives C. (1992) Wild-type p53 activates transcription in vitro. *Nature* **358**: 83–6.

54. Filatov L, GolubovskayaV, Hurt JC, Byrd LL, Phillips JM, Kaufmann WK. (1998) Chromosomal instability is correlated with telomere erosion and inactivation of G2 checkpoint function in human fibroblasts expressing human papillomavirus type 16 E6 oncoprotein. *Oncogene* **16**: 1825–38.

55. Finlay CA, Hinds PW, Levine AJ. (1989) The p53 proto-oncogene can act as a suppressor of transformation. *Cell* **57**: 1083–93.

56. Foster SA, Demers GW, Etscheid BG, Galloway DA. (1994) The ability of human papillomavirus E6 proteins to target p53 for degradation in vivo correlates with their ability to abrogate actinomycin D-induced growth arrest. *J Virol* **68**: 5698–705.

57. Frattini MG, Hurst SD, Lim HB, Swaminathan S, Laimins LA. (1997) Abrogation of a mitotic checkpoint by E2 proteins from oncogenic human papillomaviruses correlates with increased turnover of the p53 tumor suppressor protein. *EMBO J* **16**: 318–31.

58. Funk WD, Kern SE, Zambetti GP, *et al.* (1992) Wild-type p53 mediates positive regulation of gene expression through a specific DNA sequence element. *Genes Dev* **6**: 1143–52.

59. Gao QS, Srinivasan S, Boyer SN, Wazer DE, Band V. (1999) The E6 oncoproteins of high-risk papillomaviruses bind to a novel putative GAP protein, E6TP1, and target it for degradation. *Mol Cell Biol* **19**: 733–44.

60. Goldstein DJ, Andresson T, Sparkowski JJ, Schlegel R. (1992) The BPV-1 E5 protein, the 16 kDa membrane pore-forming protein and PDGF receptor exist in a complex that is dependent on hydrophobic transmembrane interactions. *EMBO J* **11**: 4851–9.

61. Gottlieb TM, Oren M. (1996) p53 in growth control and neoplasia. Biochim. Biophys. Acta 1287:77–102.

62. Greenfield I, Nickerson J, Penman S, Stanley M. (1991) Human papillomavirus 16E7 protein is associated with the nuclear matrix. *Proc Natl Acad Sci* **88**: 11217–21.

63. Gross-Mesilaty S, Reinstein E, Bercovich B, *et al.* (1998) Basal and human papillomavirus E6 oncoprotein-induced degradation of Myc proteins by the ubiquitin pathway. *Proc Natl Acad Sci USA* **95**: 8058–63.

64. Grossman SR, Laimins LA. (1989) E6 protein of human papillomavirus type 18 binds zinc. *Oncogene* **4**: 1089–93.

65. Harper JW, Adami GR, Wei N, Keyomarsi K, Elledge SJ. (1993) The p21 Cdk-interacting protein Cip1 is a potent inhibitor of G1 cyclin-dependent kinases. *Cell* **75**: 805–16.

66. Hawley-Nelson P, Vousden KH, Hubbert NL, Lowy DR, Schiller JT. (1989) HPV16 E6 and E7 proteins cooperate to immortalize human foreskin keratinocytes. *EMBO J* **8**: 3905–10.

67. Heck DV, Yee CL, Howley PM, Munger K. (1992) Efficiency of binding the retinoblastoma protein correlates with the transforming capacity of the E7 oncoproteins of the human papillomaviruses. *Proc Natl Acad Sci USA* **89**: 4442–6.

68. Hershko A, Ciechanover A. (1992) The ubiquitin system for protein degradation. *Annu Rev Biochem* **61**: 761–807.

69. Hines JF, Ghim SJ, Schlegel R, Jenson AB. (1995) Prospects for a vaccine against human papillomavirus. *Obstet Gynecol* **86**: 860–6.

70. Hollstein M, Rice K, Greenblatt MS, *et al.* (1994) Database of p53 gene somatic mutations in human tumors and cell lines. *Nucl Acids Res* **22**: 3551–5.

71. Huang PS, Patrick DR, Edwards G, *et al.* (1993) Protein domains governing interactions between E2F, the retinoblastoma gene product, and human papillomavirus type 16 E7 protein. *Mol Cell Biol* **13**: 953–60.

72. Hubbert NL, Sedman SA, Schiller JT. (1992) Human papillomavirus type 16 increases the degradation rate of p53 in human keratinocytes. *J Virol* **66**: 6237–41.

73. Hudson JB, Bedell MA, McCance DJ, Laiminis LA. (1990) Immortalization and altered differentiation of human keratinocytes in vitro by the E6 and E7 open reading frames of human papillomavirus type 18. *J Virol* **64**: 519–26.

74. Huibregtse JM, Scheffner M, Howley PM. (1991) A cellular protein mediates association of p53 with the E6 oncoprotein of human papillomavirus types 16 or 18. *EMBO J* **10**: 4129–35.

75. Hurlin PJ, Kaur P, Smith PP, Perez RN, Blanton RA, McDougall JK. (1991) Progression of human papillomavirus type 18-immortalized human keratinocytes to a malignant phenotype. *Proc Natl Acad Sci USA* **88**: 570–4.

76. Hwang ES, Nottoli T, Dimaio D. (1995) The HPV16 E5 protein: expression, detection, and stable complex formation with transmembrane proteins in COS cells. *Virology* **211**: 227–33.

77. Imai T, Matsuda K, Shimojima T, *et al.* (1997) ERC-55, a binding protein for the papilloma virus E6 oncoprotein, specifically interacts with vitamin D receptor among nuclear receptors. *Biochem Biophys Res Commun* **233**: 765–9.

78. Imai Y, Matsushima Y, Takashi S, Terada M. (1991) Purification and characterization of human papillomavirus type 16E7 protein with preferential binding capacity to the underphosphorylated form of retinoblastoma gene product. *J Virol* **65**: 4966–72.

79. Ishiwatari H, Hayasaka N, Inoue H, Yutsudo M, Hakura A. (1994) Degradation of p53 only is not sufficient for the growth stimulatory effect of human

papillomavirus 16 E6 oncoprotein in human embryonic fibroblasts. *J Med Virol* 44:243–9.

80. Jeon S, Lambert PF. (1995) Integration of human papillomavirus type 16 DNA into the human genome leads to increased stability of E6 and E7 mRNAs: implications for cervical carcinogenesis. *Proc Natl Acad Sci USA* **92**: 1654–8.

81. Jewers RJ, Hildebrandt P, Ludlow JW, Kell B, McCance DJ. (1992) Regions of human papillomavirus type 16 E7 oncoprotein required for immortalization of human keratinocytes. *J Virol* **66**: 1329–35.

82. Jones DL, Alani RM, Münger K. (1997) The human papillomavirus E7 oncoprotein can uncouple cellular differentiation and proliferation in human keratinocytes by abrogating p21Cip1-mediated inhibition of cdk2. *Genes Dev* **11**: 2101–11.

83. Jones R, Wegrzyn R, Patrick D, *et al*. 1990. Identification of HPV-16 E7 peptides that are potent antagonists of E7 binding to the retinoblastoma suppressor protein. *J Biol Chem* **265**: 12782–5.

84. Kastan MB, Onyekwere O, Sidransky D, Vogelstein B, Craig RW. (1991) Participation of p53 protein in the cellular response to DNA damage. *Cancer Res* **51**: 6304–11.

85. Kastan MB, Zhan Q, El-Deiry WS, *et al*. (1992) A mammalian cell cycle checkpoint pathway utilizing p53 and GADD45 is defective in ataxia-telangectasia. *Cell* **71**: 587–97.

86. Kaur P, McDougall JK, Cone R. (1989) Immortalization of primary human epithelial cells by cloned cervical carcinoma DNA containing human papillomavirus type 16 E6/E7 open reading frames. *J Gen Virol* **70**: 1261–6.

87. Kern SE, Kinzler KW, Bruskin A, *et al*. (1991) Identification of p53 as a sequence-specific DNA-binding protein. *Science* **252**: 1708–11.

88. Kessis TD, Slebos RJ, Nelson WG, *et al*. (1993) Human papillomavirus 16 E6 expression disrupts the p53-mediated cellular response to DNA damage. *Proc Natl Acad Sci USA* **90**: 3988–92.

89. Kiyono T, Foster SA, Koop JI, McDougall JK, Galloway DA, Klingelhutz AJ. (1998) Both Rb/p16INK4a inactivation and telomerase activity are required to immortalize human epithelial cells [see comments]. *Nature* **396**: 84–8.

90. Kiyono T, Hiraiwa A, Fujita M, Hayashi Y, Akiyama T, Ishibashi M. (1997) Binding of high-risk human papillomavirus E6 oncoproteins to the human homologue of the *Drosophila* discs large tumor suppressor protein. *Proc Natl Acad Sci USA* **94**: 11612–6.

91. Klingelhutz AJ, Foster SA, McDougall JK. (1996) Telomerase activation by the E6 gene product of human papillomavirus type 16. *Nature* **380**: 79–82.

92. Kreider JW, Howett MK, Leure-Dupree AE, Zaino RJ, Weber JA. (1987) Laboratory production in vivo of infectious human papillomavirus type 11. *J Virol* **61**: 590–3.

93. Kuerbitz SJ, Plunkett BS, Walsh WV, Kastan MB. (1992) Wild-type p53 is a cell cycle checkpoint determinant following irradiation. *Proc Natl Acad Sci USA* **89**:7491–5.

94. Kuhne C, Banks L. (1998) E3-ubiquitin ligase/E6-AP links multicopy maintenance protein 7 to the ubiquitination pathway by a novel motif, the L2G box. *J Biol Chem* **273**: 34302–9.

95. Kyo S, Inoue M, Hayasaka N, *et al*. (1994) Regulation of early gene expression of human papillomavirus type 16 by inflammatory cytokines. *Virology* **200**: 130–9.

96. Lam E W-F, Morris JDH, Davies R , Crook T, Watson RJ, Vousden KH. (1994) HPV16 E7 oncoprotein deregulates B-myb expression: correlation with targeting of p107/E2F complexes. *EMBO J* **13**: 871–8.

97. Lechner MS, Laimins LA. (1994) Inhibition of p53 DNA binding by human papillomavirus E6 proteins. *J Virol* **68**: 4262–73.

98. Lechner MS, Mack DH, Finicle AB, Crook T, Vousden KH, Laimins LA. (1992) Human papillomavirus E6 proteins bind p53 in vivo and abrogate p53-mediated repression of transcription. *EMBO J* **11**: 3045–52.

99. Lee SS, Weiss RS, Javier RT. (1997) Binding of human virus oncoproteins to hDlg/SAP97, a mammalian homolog of the *Drosophila* discs large tumor suppressor protein. *Proc Natl Acad Sci USA* **94**: 6670–5.

100. Leechanachai P, Banks L, Moreau F, Matlashewski G. (1992) The E5 gene from human papillomavirus type 16 is an oncogene which enhances growth factor-mediated signal transduction to the nucleus. *Oncogene* **7**: 19–25.

101. Leptak C, Ramon y Cajal S, Kulke R, *et al*. (1991) Tumorgenic transformation of murine keratinocytes by the E5 genes of bovine papillomavirus type 1 and human papillomavirus type 16. *J Virol* **65**: 7078–83.

102. Livingstone LR, White A, Sprouse J, Livanos E, Jacks T, Tlsty TD. (1992) Altered cell cycle arrest and gene amplification potential accompany loss of wild-type p53. *Cell* **70**: 923–35.

103. Lowe SW, Schmitt EM, Smith SW, Osborne BA, Jacks T. (1993) p53 is required for radiation-induced apoptosis in mouse thymocytes. *Nature* **362**: 218–19.

104. Mansur CP, Androphy EJ. (1993) Cellular transformation by papillomavirus oncoproteins. Biochim. *Biophys Acta Cancer Rev* **1155**: 323–45.

105. Matsukura T, Koi S, Sugase M. (1989) Both episomal and integrated forms of human papillomavirus type 16 are involved in invasive cervical cancers. *Virology* **172**: 63–72.

106. McCance DJ, Kopan R, Fuchs E, Laimins LA. (1988) Human papillomavirus type 16 alters human epithelial cell differentiation in vitro. *Proc Natl Acad Sci USA* **85**: 7169–73.

107. McIntyre M, Frattini M, Grossman S, Laimins L. (1993) Human papillomavirus type 18 E7 protein requires intact cys-x-x-cys motifs for zinc binding, dimerization, and transformation but not for Rb binding. *J Virol* **67**: 3142–50.

108. McIntyre MC, Ruesch MN, Laimins LA. (1996) Human papillomavirus E7 oncoproteins bind a single form of cyclin E in a complex with cdk2 and p107. *Virology* **215**: 73–82.

109. Meyers C, Frattini MG, Hudson JB, Laimins L. (1992) Biosynthesis of human papillomavirus from a continuous cell line upon epithelial differentiation. *Science* **257**: 971–3.

110. Mietz J, Unger T, Huibregtse J, Howley P. (1992) The transcriptional transactivation function of wild-type p53 is inhibited by SV40 large T-antigen and by HPV-16 E6 oncoprotein. *EMBO J* **11**: 5013–20.

111. Morozov A, Shiyanov P, Barr E, Leiden JM, Raychaudhuri P. (1997) Accumulation of human papillomavirus type 16 E7 protein bypasses G1 arrest induced by serum deprivation and by the cell cycle inhibitor p21. *J Virol* **71**: 3451–7.

112. Mullokandov MR, Glass KNG., Atkin NB, Burk RD, Johnson AB, Klinger HP. (1996) Genomic alterations in cervical carcinoma: losses of chromosome heterozygosity and human papilloma virus tumor status. *Cancer Res* **56**: 197–205.

113. Munger K, Phelps WC, Bubb V, Howley PM, SR, (1989) The E6 and E7 genes of the human papillomavirus type 16 together are necessary and sufficient for transformation of primary human keratinocytes. *J Virol* **63**: 4417–21.

114. Munger K, Werness BA, Dyson N, Phelps WC, Harlow E, Howley PM. (1989) Complex formation of human papillomavirus E7 proteins with the retinoblastoma tumor suppressor gene product. *EMBO J* **8**: 4099–105.

115. Munger K, Yee CL, Phelps WC, Pietenpol JA, Moses HL, Howley PM. (1991) Biochemical and biological differences between E7 oncoproteins of the high- and low-risk human papillomavirus types are determined by amino-terminal sequences. *J Virol* **65**: 3943–8.

116. Nakagawa S, Watanabe S, Yoshikawa H, Taketani Y, Yoshiike K, Kanda T. (1995) Mutational analysis of human papillomavirus type 16 E6 protein: transforming function for human cells and degradation of p53 in vitro. *Virology* **212**: 535–42.

117. Oelze I, Kartenbeck J, Crusius K, Alonso A. (1995) Human papillomavirus type 16 E5 protein affects cell-cell communication in an epithelial cell line. *J Virol* **69**: 4489–94.

118. Pan HC, Griep AE. (1995) Temporally distinct patterns of p53-dependent and p53-independent apoptosis during mouse lens development. *Genes Dev* **9**: 2157–69.

119. Pater MM, Hughes GA, Hyslop DE, Nakshatri H, Pater A. (1988) Glucocorticoid-dependent oncogenic transformation by type 16 but not type 11 human papilloma virus DNA. *Nature* **335**: 832–5.

120. Pater MM, Pater A. (1991) RU486 inhibits glucocorticoid hormone-dependent oncogenesis by human papillomavirus type 16 DNA. *Virology* **183**: 799–802.

121. Petti L, Dimaio D. (1992) Stable association between the bovine papillomavirus-E5 transforming protein and activated platelet-derived growth factor receptor in transformed mouse cells. *Proc Natl Acad Sci USA* **89**: 6736–40.

122. Petti L, Nilson LA, DiMaio D. (1991) Activation of the platelet-derived growth factor receptor by the bovine papillomavirus E5 transforming protein. *EMBO J* **10**: 845–55.

123. Phelps WC, Howley PM. (1987) Transcriptional transactivation by the human papillomavirus type 16 E2 gene product. *J Virol* **61**: 1630–8.

124. Phelps WC, Munger K, Yee CL, Barnes JA, Howley PM. (1992) Structure-function analysis of the human papillomavirus type 16 E7 oncoprotein. *J Virol* **66**: 2418–27.

125. Phelps WC, Yee CL, Munger K, Howley PM. (1988) The human papillomavirus type 16 E7 gene encodes transactivation and transformation functions similar to those of adenovirus E1A. *Cell* **53**: 539–47.

126. Pietenpol JA, Stein RW, Moran E, *et al.* (1990). TGF-beta 1 inhibition of c-myc transcription and growth in keratinocytes is abrogated by viral transforming proteins with pRB binding domains. *Cell* **61**: 777–85.

127. Pim D, Collins M, Banks L. (1992) Human papillomavirus type 16 E5 gene stimulates the transforming activity of the epidermal growth factor receptor. *Oncogene* **7**: 27–32.

128. Raycroft L, Wu H, Lozano G. (1990) Transcriptional activation by wild-type but not transforming mutants of the p53 anti-oncogene. *Science* 249:1049–51.

129. Romanczuk H, Howley PM. (1992) Disruption of either the E1 or the E2 regulating gene of human papillomavirus type 16 increases viral immortalization capacity. *Proc Natl Acad Sci USA* **89**: 3159–63.

130. Ruesch MN, Laimins LA. (1998) Human papillomavirus oncoproteins alter differentiation-dependent cell cycle exit on suspension in semisolid medium. *Virology* **250**: 19–29.

131. Sang BC, Barbosa MS. (1992) Single amino acid substitutions in low-risk human papillomavirus (HPV) type-6 E7 protein enhance features characteristic of the high-risk HPV E7 oncoproteins. *Proc Natl Acad Sci USA* **89**: 8063–67.

132. Scheffner M, Huibregtse JM, Vierstra JD, Howley PM. (1993) The HPV-16 E6 and E6-AP complex functions as a ubiquitin-protein ligase in the ubiquitination of p53. *Cell* **75**: 495–505.

133. Scheffner M, Werness BA, Huibregtse JM, Levine AM, Howley PM. (1990) The E6 oncoprotein encoded by human papillomavirus types 16 and 18 promotes the degradation of p53. *Cell* **63**: 1129–36.

134. Schiffman MH, Brinton LA. (1995) The epidemiology of cervical carcinogenesis. *Cancer* **76**: 1888–901.

135. Schiller J, Vousden K, Hawley-Nelson P, *et al.* (1990) Analysis of papillomavirus E6 and E7 gene products. In *UCLA Symposium Papillomaviruses*, ed. D. Lowy. New York, Wiley-Liss; Los Angeles, UCLA, 271–83.

136. Schiller JT, Vass WC, Lowy D. (1984) Identification of a second transforming region in bovine papillomavirus DNA. *Proc Natl Acad Sci USA* **81**: 7880–4.

137. Schiller JT, Vass WC, Vousden KH, Lowy DR. (1986) E5 open reading frame of bovine papillomavirus type 1 encodes a transforming gene. *J Virol* **57**: 1–6.

138. Schlegel R, Phelps WC, Zhang YL, Barbosa M. (1988) Quantitative keratinocyte assay detects two biological activities of human papillomavirus DNA and identifies viral types associated with cervical carcinoma. *EMBO J* **7**: 3181–7.

139. Schulze A, Mannhardt B, Zerfass TK, Zwerschke W, Jansen DP. (1998) Anchorage-independent transcription of the cyclin A gene induced by the E7 oncoprotein of human papillomavirus type 16. *J Virol* **72**: 2323–34.

140. Schwarz E, Freese UK, Gissmann L, Mayer W, *et al.* 1985. Structure and transcription of human papillomavirus sequences in cervical carcinoma cells. *Nature* **314**: 111–4.

141. Sedman SA, Barbosa MS, Vass WC, Hubbert NL, Haas JA, Lowy DR, Schiller JT. (1991) The full-length E6 protein of human papillomavirus type 16 has transforming and trans-activating activities and cooperates with E7 to immortalize keratinocytes in culture. *J Virol* **65**: 4860–66.

142. Selvakumar R, Borenstein LA, Lin YL, Ahmed R, Wettstein FO. (1995) Immunization with nonstructural proteins E1 and E2 of cottontail rabbit papillomavirus stimulates regression of virus-induced papillomas. *J Virol* **69**: 602–5.

143. Shamanin V, zur Hausen H, Lavergne D, *et al.* (1996) Human papillomavirus infections in nonmelanoma skin cancers from renal transplant recipients and non-immunosuppressed patients. *J Natl Cancer Inst* **88**: 802–11.

144. Shirodkar S, Ewen M, DeCaprio JA, Morgan J, Livingston DM, Chittenden T. (1992) The transcription factor E2F interacts with the retinoblastoma prodict and a p107–cyclin A complex in a cell cycle-regulated manner. *Cell* **68**: 157–66.

145. Smith PP, Bryant EM, Kaur P, McDougall JK. (1989) Cytogenetic analysis of eight human papillomavirus immortalized human keratinocyte cell lines. *Int J Cancer.* **44**: 1124–31.

146. Smits PH, Smits HL, Minnaar RP, *et al.* (1992) The 55 kDa regulatory subunit of protein phosphatase 2A plays a role in the activation of the HPV 16 long control region in human cells with a deletion in the short arm of chromosome 11. *EMBO J* **11**: 4601–6.

147. Smotkin D, Wettstein FO. (1987) The major human papillomavirus protein in cervical cancers is a cytoplasmic phosphoprotein. *J Virol* **61**: 1686–9.

148. Smotkin D, Wettstein FO. (1986) Transcription of human papillomavirus type 16 early genes in a cervical cancer and a cancer-derived cell line and identification of the E7 protein. *Proc Natl Acad Sci USA* **83**: 4680–4.

149. Starostik P, Chow KN, Dean DC. (1996) Transcriptional repression and growth suppression by the p107 pocket protein. *Mol Cell Biol* **16**: 3606–14.

150. Sterling J, Stanley M, Gatward G, Minson T. (1990) Production of human papillomavirus type 16 virions in a keratinocyte cell line. *J Virol* **64**: 6305–7.

151. Stoler MH, Rhodes CR, Whitbeck A, Wolinsky SM, Chow LT, Broker TR. (1992) Human papillomavirus type 16 and 18 gene expression in cervical neoplasias. *Hum Pathol* **23**: 117–28.

152. Stoler MH, Whitbeck A, Wolinsky SM, *et al.* (1990) Infectious cycle of human papillomavirus type 11 in human foreskin xenografts in nude mice. *J Virol* **64**: 3310–18.

153. Stoppler H, Hartmann DP, Sherman L, Schlegel R. (1997) The human papillomavirus type 16 E6 and E7 oncoproteins dissociate cellular telomerase activity from the maintenance of telomere length. *J Biol Chem* **272**: 13332–7.

154. Storey A, Almond N, Osborn K, Crawford L. (1990) Mutations of the human papillomavirus type 16 E7 gene that affect transformation, transactivation and phosphorylation by the E7 protein. *J Gen Virol* **71**: 965–70.

155. Storey A, Pim D, Murray A, Osborn K, Banks L, Crawford L. (1988) Comparison of the in vitro transforming activities of human papillomavirus types *EMBO J* **7**: 1815–20.

156. Straight SW, Herman B, McCance DJ. (1995) The E5 oncoprotein of human papillomavirus type 16 inhibits the acidification of endosomes in human keratinocytes. *J Virol* **69**: 3185–92.

157. Subler MA, Martin DW, Deb S. (1992) Inhibition of viral and cellular promoters by human wild-type p53. *J Virol* **66**: 4757–62.

158. Suzich JA, Ghim SJ, Palmer HF, *et al.* (1995) Systemic immunization with papillomavirus L1 protein completely prevents the development of viral mucosal papillomas. *Proc Natl Acad Sci USA* **92**: 11553–7.

159. Tan T, Ting R. (1995) *In vitro* and *in vivo* inhibition of human papillomavirus type 16 E6 and E7 genes. *Cancer Res* **55**: 4599–605.

160. Thierry F, Yaniv M. (1987) The BPV-1 trans-acting protein can be either an activator or a repressor of the HPV 18 regulatory region. *EMBO J* **6**: 3391–7.

161. Thomas M, Banks L. (1999) Human papillomavirus (HPV) E6 interactions with Bak are conserved amongst E6 proteins from high and low risk HPV types. *J Gen Virol* **80**: 1513–17.

162. Thomas M, Banks L. (1998) Inhibition of Bak-induced apoptosis by HPV-18 E6. *Oncogene* **17**: 2943–54.

163. Thomas M, Massimi P, Jenkins J, Banks L. (1995) HPV-18 E6 mediated inhibition of p53 DNA binding activity is independent of E6 induced degradation. *Oncogene* **10**: 261–8.

164. Thomas M, Matlashewski G, Pim D, Banks L. (1996) Induction of apoptosis by p53 is independent of its oligomeric state and can be abolished by HPV-18 E6 through ubiquitin mediated degradation. *Oncogene* **13**: 265–73.

165. Tommasino M, Adamczewski JP, Carlotti F, *et al.* (1993) HPV 16 E7 protein associates with the protein kinase p33-cdk2 and cyclin A. *Oncogene* **8**: 195–202.

166. Tong X, Salgia R, Li JL, Griffin JD, Howley PM. (1997) The bovine papillomavirus E6 protein binds to the LD motif repeats of paxillin and blocks its interaction with vinculin and the focal adhesion kinase. *J Biol Chem* **272**: 33373–6.

167. Tong XA, Howley PM. (1997). The bovine papillomavirus E6 oncoprotein interacts with paxillin and disrupts the actin cytoskeleton. *Proc Natl Acad Sci USA* **94**: 4412–17.

168. Tsang NM, Nagasawa H, Li C, Little JB. (1995) Abrogation of p53 function by transfection of HPV16 E6 gene enhances the resistance of human diploid fibroblasts to ionizing radiation. *Oncogene* **10**: 2403–8.

169. Tsunokawa Y, Takebe N, Kasamatsu T, Terada M, Sugimura T. (1986) Transforming activity of human papillomavirus type 16 DNA sequences in a cervical cancer. *Proc Natl Acad Sci USA* **83**: 2200–3.

170. Valle GF, Banks L. (1995) The human papillomavirus (HPV)-6 and HPV-16 E5 proteins co-operate with HPV-16 E7 in the transformation of primary rodent cells. *J Gen Virol* **76**: 1239–45.

171. von Knebel Doeberitz, M, Rittmuller C, Aengeneyndt F, Jansen-Durr P, Spitkovsky D. (1994)

Reversible repression of papillomavirus oncogene expression in cervical carcinoma cells: consequences for the phenotype and E6-p53 and E7-pRB interactions. *J Virol* **68**: 2811–21.

172. von Knebel Doeberitz M, Rittmuller C, zur Hausen H, and Durst M. (1992) Inhibition of tumorigenicity of cervical cancer cells in nude mice by HPV E6-E7 antisense RNA. *Int J Cancer* **51**: 831–4.

173. Wang XW, Yeh H, Schaeffer L, *et al*. (1995) p53 modulation of TFIIH-associated nucleotide excision repair activity. *Nat Genet* **10**:188–95.

174. Watts SL, Phelps WC, Ostrow RS, Zachow KR, Faras JA. (1984) Cellular transformation by human papillomavirus DNA in vitro. *Science* **225**: 634–6.

175. Werness BA, Levine AJ, Howley PM. (1990) Association of human papillomavirus types 16 and 18 E6 proteins with p53. *Science* **248**:76–9.

176. Wu EW, Clemens KE, Heck DV, Munger K. (1993) The human papillomavirus E7 oncoprotein and the cellular transcription factor E2F bind to separate sites on the retinoblastoma tumor suppressor protein. *J Virol* **67**: 2402–7.

177. Xiong Y, Hannon GJ, Zhang H, Casso D, Kobayashi R, Beach D. (1993) p21 is a universal inhibitor of cyclin kinases. *Nature* **366**: 701–4.

178. Yasumoto S, Burkhardt AL, Dongier J, DiPaolo J. (1986) Human papillomavirus type 16 DNA-induced malignant transformation of NIH 3T3 cells. *J Virol* **57**: 572–7.

179. Yin Y, Tainsky MA, Bischoff FZ, Strong LC, Wahl GM. (1992) Wild-type p53 restores cell cycle control and inhibits gene amplification in cells with mutant p53 alleles. *Cell* **70**: 937–48.

180. Zerfass K, Schulze A, Spitkovsky D, Friedman V, Henglein B, Jansen-Durr P. (1995) Sequential activation of cyclin E and cyclin A gene expression by human papillomavirus type 16 E7 through sequences necessary for transformation. *J Virol* **69**: 6389–99.

181. Zerfass-Thome, K., W. Zwerschke, B. Mannhardt, R. Tindle, J. W. Botz, and D. P. Jansen. 1996. Inactivation of the cdk inhibitor p27KIP1 by the human papillomavirus type 16 E7 oncoprotein. *Oncogene* **13**: 2323–30.

182. zur Hausen H. (1996) Papillomavirus infections – a major cause of human cancers. *Biochim Biophys Acta* **1288**: F55–F78.

183. Zwerschke W, Joswig S, Jansen-Durr P. (1996) Identification of domains required for transcriptional activation and protein dimerization in the human papillomavirus type-16 E7 protein. *Oncogene* **12**: 213–20.

4

Immune responses to human papillomaviruses

Margaret A. Stanley

4.1 INTRODUCTION

Human papillomaviruses (HPVs) are exclusively intraepithelial pathogens with a replication cycle which is both time dependent and differentiation dependent. The viral replication cycle is one in which viral infection is targeted to basal keratinocytes, but high-level expression of viral proteins and viral assembly occur only in differentiating keratinocytes in the stratum spinosum and granulosum of squamous epithelium. These cells are destined for death and desquamation and are distant from sites of immune activity. Crucially, the viruses are not cytolytic and no inflammation accompanies infection and viral replication, a phenomenon which may retard the initiation of, or even prevent, an effective immune response. Productive infections are chronic and the lesions may persist for months or even years. The central questions, therefore, are:

- Does natural infection with HPV evoke an effective host defence response?
- What is the nature of this response?
- When and how does it occur?
- What is the role of humoral and cell-mediated responses in the natural history of HPV-induced disease?
- With respect to the oncogenic HPVs, how does this influence oncogenesis?

4.2 IMMUNE RESPONSES TO VIRAL PROTEINS

Before discussing the host defence to HPVs, it might be useful to outline briefly the current knowledge of how the immune system, particularly T lymphocytes, recognizes antigen and the consequences of this for responses to viral proteins. B lymphocytes, which produce antibody, recognize antigenic determinants on macromolecules and can therefore interact with proteins in the native conformation. However, these interactions, with certain well-known exceptions, are not sufficient to activate the B-cell differentiation program and generate mature antibody-secreting plasma cells. Antigen-primed B-cells require further help from a subset of T lymphocytes which themselves have been activated by antigen presented by professional antigen-presenting cells (APCs).

T-cells cannot recognize macromolecules, but require antigen to be processed into short peptides, some of which are then presented in association with major histocompatibility complex (MHC) molecules as a membrane-bound receptor complex on the cell surface. The selection of which of the processed peptides is presented on the cell surface depends upon the MHC molecule itself to a large extent and, because these molecules are polymorphic, in an outbred population, different peptides from any individual protein will be presented by different individuals. Polymorphic MHC molecules fall into two groups, class I (HLA-A, B, C) and class II (HLA-DR, DP, DQ). MHC class I is expressed to varying extents on all somatic cells except red cells, but class II is expressed constitutively only on professional APCs, which are, in the main, dendritic cells.

Antigen presented in the context of class II is exogenous antigen taken up by APC from the extracellular environment by pinocytosis and/or phagocytosis (Figure 4.1). Inside the cell, antigen is processed within the endosomal compartment into small peptide fragments, 10–20 amino acids in

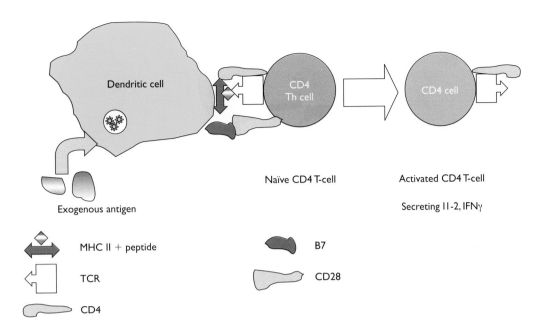

Figure 4.1
Antigen presentation to CD4 T-cells. The dendritic cell processes exogenous antigen and presents it to the CD4 cell in the context of MHC class II. Activation of the T-cell occurs via the T-cell receptor and with co-stimulatory signals via the B7–CD28 interaction.

length; these then associate with class II molecules and are presented on the cell surface as a MHC–peptide complex. This complex represents the epitope for a specific T-cell receptor (TCR) and only T-cells with this specific TCR will recognize and bind to the complex. The subset of T-cells recognizing antigen expressed in the context of class II MHC express the cell surface marker CD4, a molecule which binds to all class II glycoproteins. The interaction between the CD4 T-cell and the APCs is complex: it requires several other adhesion events which must occur in a regulated fashion, but, in particular, activation requires a second signal (in addition to antigen) mediated via the interaction of CD80 on the APC and CD28 on the T-cell. Failure to receive this second signal can cause clonal inactivation, which confers a state of clonal anergy or unresponsiveness on the T-cell, precluding any subsequent response to antigen. Activation of the T-cell results in clonal proliferation and the secretion of a repertoire of small polypeptides or cytokines which 'help' and regulate the activities of other cells. The pattern of cytokine secretion defines two subsets of CD4-T cells

1. T-helper 2 (Th2) lymphocytes, which secrete interleukin-4 (IL-4), IL-5, IL-10. Th2 cells help B-cells to differentiate and produce antibody, generating humoral immunity.
2. Th1 lymphocytes which secrete interferon-γ (IFN-γ). Th1 cells activate macrophages and help natural killer (NK) cells and cytotoxic T lymphocytes (CTLs), generating cell-mediated immunity.

This helper T-cell response is central to the initiation and activation of the immune response to a specific pathogen, and the microenvironment in which the cellular interactions occur, together with the interaction of the pathogen and the APC, are crucial in determining the subsequent pattern of the response.

Antigen presented in the context of class I MHC is endogenous antigen derived usually, but not always, from the intracellular synthesis of pathogen proteins (Figure 4.2). Within the APC, proteins are broken down into small peptides, about eight to nine amino acids in length, which associate with class I glycoproteins and are presented on the cell surface as a specific MHC class I–peptide complex. This complex represents the epitope for a specific TCR and cells bearing this TCR recognize this epitope and bind to it. The subset of T-cells recognizing antigen expressed in the context of class I express the CD8 surface marker, which binds to all class I glycoproteins. CD8 cells after antigen activation and help (usually in the form of cytokines) from CD4 cells are predominantly cytotoxic effector cells which seek out and kill any cell expressing the specific MHC–peptide epitope against which they were activated. Recent studies[1,73] have clarified some aspects of CD4 help for CD8 cells (Figure 4.3) in the situation in which pathogen proteins are **not** synthesized within the APC. In this scenario, antigen from virally infected necrotic or apoptotic cells is taken up by APCs, processed, and presented to CD4 cells, which then signal back to the APC via CD40L/CD40 interaction. This activates the APC, which can then directly present to and activate naïve CD8 cells to differentiate into CTL effectors. Because HPV infects and replicates only within keratinocytes, it is likely that this scenario applies in HPV infections.

4.3 HUMORAL IMMUNITY

The role of the humoral immune response in the natural history of HPV infection is becoming clearer. Disorders of humoral immunity do not result in an increased susceptibility to HPV-induced lesions,[57] suggesting that antibody has little to do with the maintenance of infection. However, data from animal models such as the rabbit and ox show that antibodies directed against the major capsid protein L1 are protective.[13] Serological studies of HPV infection and the relevance of antibody in the natural history of HPV-induced

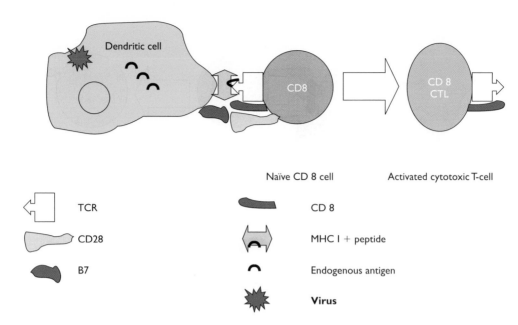

Figure 4.2
Antigen presentation to CD8 T-cells. CD8-positive T-cells are activated by endogenously produced viral antigens presented in the context of MHC class I molecules. Activated CD8 cells are predominantly cytotoxic in effector action.

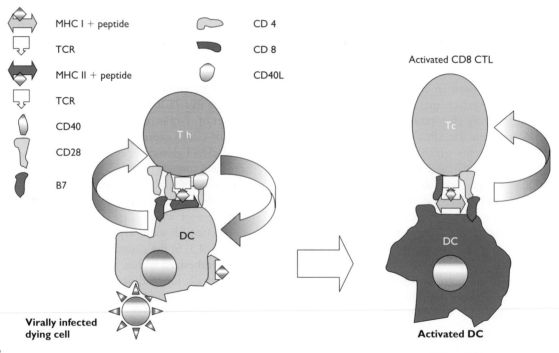

Figure 4.3
T-cell help from T-killer cells. Viral antigens from dying cells can be taken up by dendritic cells and processed for presentation to T-helper cells in the context of MHC class II. The Th cell can activate the dendritic cell and stimulate the presentation to and activation of cytotoxic CD8 cells.

disease have been hampered, until recently, by the lack of appropriate antigen targets for serological assays. *In vitro* systems permissive for viral replication generate little virus and few lesions contain enough virus to be a practical source of antigen. The exceptions to this are plantar warts from which HPV 1 virions can be harvested in amounts adequate for serological assay.[85] These studies showed that antibody responses to capsid proteins occurred in infected individuals and that these were both to conformational and linear epitopes. However, the dominant immune response was to native conformational determinants on the intact particle, demonstrating that antigen targets for serological assays must include correctly folded native protein. This objective

has been met by the recent development of expression systems in which either co-expression of the capsid proteins L1 and L2[97] or expression of L1 alone,[53] via vaccinia, baculovirus or yeast expression vectors, results in the *in vitro* assembly of empty capsids or virus-like particles (VLPs). Expression of the L1 protein alone is sufficient for the assembly of a particle,[53] which appears to be identical to the native virion. These VLPs are highly immunogenic, and when injected into rabbits, induce high titers of antibody which is type specific[18] and neutralizing.[19] Furthermore, the responses measured in enzyme-linked immunosorbent assay (ELISA) using VLPs as the target antigen indicate that these are type specific with little or no cross-reactivity with other types. Thus, assays using HPV 6 and 11 VLPs could distinguish between infections with these closely related viruses,[46] even though these viral types share neutralizing epitopes.[56]

A small number of studies have been reported in which VLPs have been used as the antigen in ELISA in patients with genital warts or a history of these lesions. In the largest of these,[14] a total of 901 sera derived from a population-based, case-control study and two longitudinal cohort studies of genital HPV infection were screened using HPV 6 VLPs in the ELISA. In this study, individuals with genital warts had significantly higher titers than those without lesions; seropositivity was associated with warts diagnosed in the first episode and an increased proportion of those with recurrent disease were seropositive compared to controls with no history of lesions. Serum IgG and IgA levels correlate well with disease, but IgM levels are not informative.[31] Widely varying seroprevalences have been reported ranging from 23%,[31] 50%,[14, 46] to 100%.[43,95] Men and women differ, it appears, in their serum response to HPV 6/11. Little or no relationship between seropositivity and disease in men was found in two studies.[14,43] Sex-specific differences in seropositivity were not found in a more recent study,[31] but women had higher antibody titers than men, an observation confirmed in a large, population-based, control study which found that, while males were more frequently seropositive, their responses were not as vigorous and did not correlate significantly with previous sexual activity (Carter JJ, personal communication).

Several studies have examined seropositivity to the capsid proteins of the high-risk genital viruses, particularly HPV 16, in women known to be HPV 16 DNA positive. The data indicate that about 50–60% of women currently infected with HPV 16 have serum antibodies to HPV 16 VLPs. Cervical IgA antibodies to HPV 16 VLPs have been detected and the pattern of the mucosal humoral response with respect to disease progression correlates well with serum antibody.[91] As was found for HPV 6/11, viral persistence is associated with seropositivity, because 83% of women positive for HPV 16 DNA on more than one occasion were seropositive, compared with 22% found to be DNA positive only once.[94] Prospective studies[95] indicate that 70–90% of women acquiring HPV 16 DNA seroconvert, with a mean time of 8 months elapsing between the acquisition of HPV DNA and seroconversion (Carter JJ, personal communication).

Seropositivity to capsid proteins is associated with increasing severity of cervical intraepithelial disease,[9,78,94] but decreases in patients with frank carcinoma.[71] Interestingly, in a cohort study of women with cervical intraepithelial neoplasia (CIN), systemic IgG responses to VLPs were more frequently detected in those with persistent infection, whereas systemic, but not mucosal, IgA responses correlated with virus clearance.[9] Seropositivity to HPV 16 VLPs is associated with an increased risk for the development of cervical carcinoma,[55] supporting the notion that viral persistence is a key factor in disease progression. However, when compared with HPV DNA detection, seropositivity is significantly less sensitive as a predictor of progression.[20]

Overall, the evidence from these studies is that specific antibody responses to the L1 capsid protein, as measured in a VLP ELISA, are common during and after infection with the genital HPVs and this assay has proved to be valuable in

sero-epidemiological and natural history studies. However, the relatively low sensitivity of this assay and the variability of the interval between infection and seroconversion suggest that serum antibody responses are not useful for diagnosis of infection in the individual patient.

Antibody reactivity to proteins other than the structural proteins L1 and L2 has been reported in individuals with both benign and malignant HPV-associated disease, but in the majority of these studies the target antigen was either bacterially expressed fusion protein or synthetic peptide and the significance of much of these data remains uncertain (for review, see reference 83). However, there is good evidence for antibody reactivity to the early proteins E6 and E7 in patients with cervical carcinoma. This was first shown in studies using fusion proteins as the target antigen in Western blotting assays,[51] in which 20% of sera from patients with HPV 16 containing cervical carcinoma had antibodies to HPV 16 E7, compared to 1.4–3.8% in controls. Other investigators also found E7 seroreactivity in patients as compared to controls using either peptides[60] or protein.[29] Studies in which full-length *in vitro* translated protein[66] or baculovirus-expressed protein[82] was used in radio-immunoprecipitation assay (RIPA) support these observations. However, the relationship between seroreactivity to E7 and cervical cancer was not supported in another study[40] in which no significant differences were found between E7 antibody status in cervical cancer patients when compared to other malignancies. Nonetheless, overall, the data show that seroreactivity to E7 is associated with HPV-containing cervical cancer but not with HPV-negative cancer.

Seroreactivity to the immunodominant region of the HPV 16 E7 was examined using a peptide-based ELISA[28] in a cohort study of women all initially presenting with mild to moderate dyskaryosis. During follow-up, the cohort could be divided into those who cleared virus, those with fluctuating infection, and those with persistent infection. The highest proportion of seropositive responders (29%) and those with the highest titers were found amongst patients who cleared the infection. Patients with persistent infection were more consistently seronegative. Analysis of the IgG subclass in this study revealed that IgG_2 was dominant in CIN patients who cleared, whereas IgG_1 and IgG_2 were equally produced in patients with frank invasive cancer, suggesting that clearance in the seropositive subset was associated with a cell-mediated or Th1-type response, and progression involved a shift to an antibody-associated or Th2-type response.

Responses to the E2 protein of the high-risk viruses have been reported in several studies (for review, see reference 83), although the significance of these studies, many of which were peptide based, is difficult to assess. Recently, however, using a baculovirus-derived protein in a RIPA, a relationship between serum IgA anti-E2 antibodies and stage and progression of cervical neoplasia was shown,[74] with a decrease in IgA anti-E2 correlating with progression.

An intriguing relationship between the humoral response to HPV and skin cancer risk in renal transplant patients has been shown.[5] In this study, the prevalence of antibodies to the E7 and L1 proteins of HPV 8 was examined using gel-purified bacterial fusion proteins in a Western blot assay. Allograft recipients who had anti-L1 IgM antibodies but no anti-L1 IgG antibodies had skin cancer in 50% of cases, whereas recipients with IgG anti-L1 antibodies had skin cancer in only 18% of cases. These data suggest that the failure to class switch (and, by implication, deficiency in T-cell help) increases cancer risk in renal transplant recipients.

4.4 CELL-MEDIATED IMMUNITY TO HPV

The role of the cellular immune response in the pathogenesis of HPV is shown by the incidence and progress of HPV infections in immunosuppressed individuals which suggest strongly that the immune system is central.[57] Generalized warts have been reported in individuals with inherited immune deficiencies, specifically those in whom the T-cell arm of the response is in deficit.[54] Cutaneous and genital warts are two of the most frequent viral complications in patients suppressed as a consequence of renal transplantation and these lesions are refractory to most therapeutic strategies.[6] Similar findings are reported for individuals immunosuppressed as a consequence of HIV infection.[12] Overall, the evidence from allograft recipients, inherited immunodeficiencies, and HIV-infected individuals suggests that it is the absolute deficit in CD4 cells which is important in HPV-induced disease and associated neoplastic progression, implying a central role for CD4-mediated mechanisms in the control of HPV infection.

4.4.1 Histological studies

The involution and regression of genital warts are accompanied histologically by a pronounced mononuclear cell infiltrate dominated by CD4 T-cells and macrophages, an appearance characteristic of a type 1V or delayed-type hypersensitivity (DTH) response. The response to genital warts represents the host response to HPV-induced lesions which are not complicated by the genetic instability of true neoplasia.[84] Immunohistological studies show that non-regressing genital or cutaneous warts are characterized by a lack of immunocytes, the few intraepithelial lymphocytes are mainly CD8 T-cells, and mononuclear cells are present predominantly in the stroma.[21] Spontaneously regressing genital warts are characterized by a mononuclear cell infiltrate in both the stroma and epithelium. This infiltrate is dominated by CD4 T-cells although a large number of CD8 T-cells are present. The infiltrating lymphocytes express activation markers such as CD25 and have an 'antigen experienced' phenotype expressing CD45RO.[21] The wart keratinocytes express HLA-DR and ICAM-1, and endothelial cells in the stromal capillaries immediately underneath the infected epithelium express the adhesion molecules E-selectin and VCAM and the chemokine RANTES. Analysis of cytokine mRNA expression in these lesions supports the morphological evidence for a Th1-biased response, with increased expression of the pro-inflammatory cytokines IFNγ, IL-2, and TNFα, and the induction of expression of the p40 chain of IL-12. Immunohistological studies show that bioactive IL-12 is expressed in regressing lesions and that, in addition to the expression by macrophages and dendritic cells in the lesion, the infected keratinocytes also express this molecule (Scarpini CG *et al*, personal communication).

Interestingly, no statistical differences in Langerhans cell number in regressors as opposed to non-regressors were found in this study, although the morphology of Langerhans cells in the non-regressing warts was characterized by a loss of dendritic arborizations, a phenomenon reported also for HPV-associated cervical lesions.[65] However, in a recent careful study,[36] an increased density of Langerhans cells was measured in laryngeal epithelium infected with HPV 6/11 compared to adjacent normal epithelium. Cross-sectional studies, however, can only provide a snapshot in what is a dynamic process. In a recent study examining the mechanism of action of imiquimod, a topical preparation with immunomodulatory properties, a decrease in CD1a mRNA was observed during wart regression post-treatment.[3a] This was reflected morphologically by a decrease in CD1a-positive intraepithelial dendritic cells as warts regressed (Stanley M, unpublished observations).

The situation in HPV-infected cervical epithelium differs from that observed in genital warts. Low-grade cervical lesions – cervical intraepithelial lesions (CIN 1) and low-grade squamous intraepithelial lesions (LGSILs) – are, overall, immunologically quiescent, with decreased numbers of morphologically altered Langerhans' cells.[45] High-grade cervical lesions (CIN 2/3, HGSIL) also exhibit a decrease in Langerhans cell number intraepithelially.[90] Several studies have documented T-cell numbers in both LGSIL and HGSIL, but with differing results. A significant reduction in intraepithelial T-cell numbers, particularly the CD4 subset, was found in all grades of CIN by Tay and colleagues,[88] but, in other studies, an increase in the intraepithelial CD8 subset was documented, with equal numbers of CD4 and CD8 T-cells in the stroma.[90] These discrepancies are not surprising if the biology of HPV-associated cervical disease is considered. HGSILs are aneuploid, genetically unstable lesions exhibiting heterogeneity in the expression of immunologically relevant molecules such as adhesion molecules and cytokines which must affect recruitment of lymphocyte subsets to the epithelium. In addition, all studies reported have been cross-sectional and the stage in the natural history of the disease cannot be known.

Surveillance and defence against viral infection and tumours are mediated via a range of effector mechanisms. An important group of effectors have the morphology of large granular lymphocytes (LGLs); these include the NK subset. LGLs with the NK phenotype CD56+, CD16+, CD3−, CD2variable, CD57variable are rarely found within either normal cervical epithelium or CIN, but are found in the stroma, particularly in the endocervix. A separate subset of LGLs with the phenotype CD56+, CD16−, CD3+, CD2+ is found within the ectocervical epithelium and this subset dominates the intraepithelial population in high-grade CIN,[62] a phenomenon related to neoplasia rather than HPV infection.

4.4.2 Helper T-cell responses

Immunohistological studies indicate that HPV-associated lesions induce an immune response which has the features of a DTH response, but the target antigens in this response are not known. The evidence from both experimental models and human studies indicates that viral proteins are immune targets. In a murine model, which mimics the natural route of infection, keratinocytes expressing HPV 16 E6 or E7 genes are grafted onto the flanks of syngeneic immunocompetent recipients reforming a differentiated epithelium. Subsequent challenge of the engrafted animals by intradermal inoculation in the ear with E7 or E6 protein expressed via recombinant vaccinia virus vectors results in a DTH response which is CD4 dependent.[15,63] In this murine model, the ability to prime the immune system and elicit a DTH response is critically dependent upon antigen dose and there is a threshold graft inoculum of keratinocytes expressing E7 below which a DTH response cannot be elicited upon subsequent challenge.[16] This immune non-responsiveness is associated with a Th1–Th2 switch in cytokine expression in the CD8 T-cell fraction in the draining lymph node 5 days post-grafting suggestive of a suppresser effect.[55a]

The analysis of T-cell responses to HPV proteins in humans has been hampered by the heterogeneity of the circulating T-cell population. In an early study,[86] proliferative responses to peptides from the E6 and L1 proteins of HPV 16 were tested in peripheral blood mononuclear cells (PBMC) from healthy donors. Peptide-specific clones and T-cell lines were used to define the HLA restriction of these responses. A similar protocol was used,[2] to identify three Th epitopes in HPV 16 E7 recognized in association with at least two different HLA haplotypes. Specific T-cell responses to HPV 16 E7 and L1 have been identified in patients with CIN of various grades in cross-sectional studies. Shepherd and colleagues[81] found that all patients with current HPV 16 infection exhibited lymphoproliferative responses to one or more HPV 16 L1 peptides including 92% of the HGSIL group. The majority of peptide-specific T-cells were CD4 lymphocytes. In a study examining proliferative responses to HPV 16 E7 peptides, 47% of healthy controls responded to N′ and C′ terminal peptides. However, only 33% of women with SIL of all grades showed a response to E7, and the response to the N′ and C′ terminal peptides was significantly reduced in this group.[58] The HGSIL group in this study contained a higher proportion of responders than the LGSIL group, but patients with frank invasive carcinoma showed diminished responses to both E7 and L1. T-cell proliferative responses to HPV 16 E7 were determined in a cohort study of women all initially presenting with mild to moderate dyskaryosis.[27] During follow-up, the cohort could be divided into those who cleared virus, those with fluctuating infection, and those with persistent infection. Interestingly, the strongest T-cell responses were observed in women with persisting HPV infection and progressing cervical lesions (99% reactive) compared to those with clearing or fluctuating infection (41% reactive).

Few studies have determined the antigen specificity of lymphocytes infiltrating HPV-infected lesions. However, in a recent study,[49] wart-infiltrating lymphocytes (WILs) isolated from HPV-6-infected anogenital warts were characterized for their response to HPV 6 E7 and L1 proteins in a lymphoproliferation assay. HPV 6 E7-specific or L1-specific WILs could be isolated from more than 75% of the patients studied ($n=24$). Interestingly, despite the huge variation between patients in surface markers of the WILs (CD4, CD8, TCRαβ or TCRγδ) the HPV 6 E7 and L1 peptides recognized by WILs differed from those recognized by

peripheral T-cells. No CTL activity against L1 or E7 could be demonstrated in this study and, because the warts were surgically excised, whether these lesions would have persisted or regressed is not known.

In the context of these data, it is of interest that in cottontail rabbit papillomavirus (CRPV) infection in the rabbit, which provides a good model for papilloma/carcinoma progression, the induction of T-cell proliferative responses to the E2 protein was the best predictor of lesion regression,[79] and immunization with E1 or E2 protein before viral challenge resulted in enhanced regression of lesions.[80] In the ox, immunization with E2 has no effect on the regression of BPV-induced lesions, but immunization with E7 enhances regression.[61] These data suggest that, although HPV early proteins may not induce strong immune responses during the natural infection, deliberate immunization with them could be an effective vaccination strategy. This thesis receives some support from a recent Phase I/II trial in which patients with anogenital warts were immunized with a HPV 6 E7/L2 fusion protein in alum adjuvant. Patients were conventionally treated in addition to vaccination in most cases. The vaccine preparation was immunogenic[89] and no recurrences were reported in those vaccinated patients whose warts had regressed and who were available for follow-up (HSG Thompson personal communication).

4.4.3 Cell-mediated cytotoxicity

Cell-mediated cytotoxicity, a phenomenon mediated by a range of effector cells, including CTLs, NK cells, and lymphocyte-activated killer cells (LAKs), is the most important effector mechanism for the control and clearance of viral infections. Classically, CTLs are CD8 T-cells which 'see' endogenously processed protein antigen presented on the infected cell surface as small peptides (8–10 amino acids in length) complexed with MHC class I glycoproteins. The role of these CD8 CTLs in HPV infection is a topic of intense contemporary interest and, until recently, a paradox existed between the data generated from experimental murine models and studies on infections in humans. Murine experiments showed that the E6 and E7 proteins of HPV 16 contained CTL epitopes and conventional immunization procedures generated CTLs which recognized these epitopes.[37,76] Furthermore, HPV 16 E6 and E7, when expressed in murine tumor cells, acted as tumor rejection antigens, eliciting a CTL response.[17,35] Mice transgenic for HLA-A2 immunized with recombinant HPV proteins generated HLA-A2 restricted HPV-specific CTLs.[7] Potential HLA-A-restricted CTL epitopes for HPV 16 E6 and E7 were identified for several HLA-A alleles,[52] and putative CTL epitopes for HLA-A2.1 in HPV 11 E7 were identified using motif predictions. The authenticity of one of these nonapeptides was confirmed.[87] However, despite these data from experimental studies, there was no convincing evidence for CTLs which recognized HPV antigens in the context of HLA-A2 or any other allele.

This scenario has now changed with evidence that HPV-specific CTLs can be detected in patients with previous[68] or on-going HPV infection.[33, 34,72] Nakagawa and colleagues[68] report data on a small group of patients, including nine with previously documented HPV 16 infection and 11 with newly diagnosed HPV 16 positive CIN. In this study, PBMCs were restimulated with soluble, bacterially synthesized HPV 16 E6 or E7 fusion proteins in the presence of recombinant interleukin-2 (rIL-2) for 7 days; the target cells were recombinant vaccinia E6-infected or E7-infected autologous B-cells. CTL responses to both antigens were detected in both groups of patients, but those who had cleared infection were more frequent responders (63%) than those with current CIN (14%), implying that an effective CTL response is important for the clearance of HPV infection. Both CD4 and CD8 cytotoxic effectors have been shown to be involved in these responses.[69] CTL responses have been described in 6/10 CIN3 patients in an assay in which PBMC restimulated with adenovirus recombinants expressing an HPV16 and 18 E6/E7 fusion protein lysed autologous targets infected with a recombinant vaccinia virus expressing the same fusion protein.[70] No CTL responses were identified in control subjects. However, the HPV status of controls and patients was not defined in this study. Recent studies show that high-affinity HPV E7-specific CTLs are rare in patients with carcinoma or HGSIL, but can be detected with increased sensitivity using the technology involving fluorescently labeled HLA peptide complexes (tetramers).[96] HPV-specific CD4 and CD8 lymphocytes can be induced by E7 pulsed dendritic cells in patients with HPV-positive cervical carcinoma,[67,77] suggesting that immunotherapy of HPV-induced malignancies could be possible.

Increased numbers of T-cells are seen locally in squamous cell carcinoma of the cervix,[38] with a dominance of CD8 cells. However, bulk cultures of these tumor-infiltrating lymphocytes showed non-MHC-restricted cytotoxicity in the majority of cases,[38] and T-cell clones derived from two cases showed low cytotoxicity to autologous tumor cells.[39] Recently, however,[34] HPV 16 and 18 E6/E7-specific CTLs were detected in PBMC, draining lymph nodes, and tumor of cervical cancer patients. Limiting dilution analysis was used to determine the frequency of the HPV-specific CTLs and these were present in significantly higher numbers in the tumors and lymph nodes than in peripheral blood. These data strongly suggest that HPV-specific CTLs are generated in HPV infections and are important in the natural history. However, a cautionary note is sounded by the studies of Jochmus and colleagues.[50] These workers established CTL lines by *in vitro* stimulation of T-cells with autologous dendritic cells loaded with HLA-A*0201-restricted HPV 16 E6 and E7 peptides. A small number of low-affinity peptide-specific CTL lines were generated which specifically lysed HLA-A*0201 B-cells loaded with the relevant peptides. Cytotoxicity was also observed against two HLA-A*0201 HPV 16 E7-positive keratinocytes lines, (Caski and HPK1A) but none of the CTLs recognized both of the keratinocyte lines and none recognized a cell line transfected with E7, suggesting that the responses were not E7 specific, but rather against cellular antigens expressed on the immortalized keratinocytes.

Further caveats about the effectiveness of HPV-specific CTLs in patients with neoplastic lesions are raised by studies on mice transgenic for HPV 16 E6 and E7 in which expression of the transgene is restricted to keratinized epithelia.[64] Epithelial cells from these mice can present at least one E7-encoded CTL epitope, but CTLs from these mice were neither primed nor made tolerant to this epitope.

Immunization of mice with the peptide protected them against subcutaneous challenge with tumor cells expressing a transfected E7 gene, but the skin remained unaffected and was not a target for the E7-specific CTLs. Herd *et al*[47] also report that transgenic mice expressing E7 constitutively remain immunologically naive to E7 epitopes presented by immunization. It does seem clear from these and other data[33] that autologous keratinocyte cell lines expressing the relevant HPV antigens are the appropriate targets in CTL assays and will need to be included if unequivocal evidence for HPV-specific CTLs is to be obtained.

Cytotoxic effector mechanisms also include NK cells, a subset of lymphocytes which kill virally infected or tumor cells lacking surface expression of MHC class I molecules, the so-called 'altered self' hypothesis.[30] There is evidence for defective NK cell function in HPV-16-associated disease. PBMCs from patients with active HPV 16 neoplastic disease display a reduced NK cell activity against HPV-16-infected keratinocytes, although their response to K562 cells is not affected[59] and *in vitro* expression of the E7 protein of HPV 16/18 precludes the lysis of HPV-transformed cells by interferon-stimulated NK cells.[75] Target recognition by NK cells does not involve classical antigen receptors because these cells do not express T-cell or B-cell antigen receptors, nor do they rearrange their immunoglobulin or T-cell receptor genes. This apparent lack of antigen-specific receptors and MHC recognition originally led to the view that NK-mediated killing was broad and non-MHC restricted. Recent studies, however, have shown that NK cells express clonally distributed receptors specific for MHC class I type molecules, and functionally these receptors can be inhibitory or stimulatory. Inhibitory receptors block NK-mediated cytotoxicity upon binding to HLA ligands. Stimulatory receptors also bind HLA class I motifs but trigger NK-cell mediated cytotoxicity. NK-mediated cytolysis of a virally infected or tumor cell depends upon the balance between the negative and positive signals received by the NK cell.[30] It is evident that MHC class I expression is critical for both CTL and NK effector mechanisms, and specific down-regulation, or loss, of class I alleles would be a way of evading cytotoxic effector mechanisms and is, indeed, a well-recognized mechanism whereby viruses evade host defenses.

4.5 MHC EXPRESSION

4.5.1 MHC class I expression

There is no published evidence for MHC class I modulation in anogenital condylomata, although down-regulation of class I expression has been reported in recurrent respiratory papillomatosis.[8] However, there is evidence from *in vitro* studies that HPV 16 E7 gene expression can down-regulate class I expression when HPV 16 sequences are integrated into the host genome, but this effect is lost if the virus is present as the episome.[4] Studies on CIN lesions have produced conflicting results. No evidence for modulation of class I expression was found in an immunohistological study using frozen sections of CIN lesions and the monoclonal antibody (Mab) W6/36 which recognizes monomorphic determinants of heterodimeric class I determinants.[41] However, studies of paraffin wax-embedded material using a polyclonal antibody RaHC specific for HLA A, B and C heavy chains and HC10 convincingly showed disturbed class I heavy chain expression in all grades of CIN and cervical carcinoma.[25] A recent report examining HLA B expression in a cohort of women with mild or moderate dyskaryosis at entry suggests that allele-specific down-regulation may be a comparatively early event in the CIN spectrum and is associated with clinical progression.[10,11]

Down-regulation of MHC class I expression in cervical squamous cell carcinomas has been well documented.[41] These changes have been shown in a proportion of tumors to be post-transcriptionally regulated,[26] and in HPV 16-positive or HPV 18-positive lesions this post-transcriptional deregulation is related to down-regulation of transporters associated with antigen processing (TAP) protein.[24] It is unlikely that all class I down-regulation is due to this single mechanism. β_2-microglobulin expression in cervix cancer is often accompanied by HLA heavy chain loss and the regulation of any one of several MHC gene products may be disturbed in invasive cancer. Whatever the mechanism of down-regulation is, functionally these changes may be crucial in neoplastic progression. Allele-specific down-regulation or the absence of class I would interfere with both NK cell and CTL recognition of targets, whether of viral or cellular origin, disabling the major cytotoxic effector mechanisms.

4.5.2 MHC Class II expression

The keratinocytes of the squamous epithelium of the genital tract do not express MHC class II antigens, but can be induced to do so by pro-inflammatory cytokines such as IFNγ and TNFα.[23] When anogenital warts regress spontaneously, the keratinocytes express HLA-DR and ICAM-1, and this is thought to be related to the release of pro-inflammatory cytokines by infiltrating lymphocytes and macrophages.[21] A variable expression of class II antigens is seen in LGSIL ranging from no[93] to patchy focal expression.[23] Class II expression is seen in HGSIL and is visualized as predominantly extensive, diffuse staining.[23,25] At least 80% of cervical cancers express class II antigens on the malignant keratinocytes.[25,41] It is likely that the expression of class II on neoplastic keratinocytes is induced rather than constitutive. Increased numbers of T-cells are observed in the stroma underneath HLA-DR-positive CIN[23] and there is an increase in tumor-infiltrating lymphocytes in DR-positive regions of carcinomas.[48] A significant proportion of HGSIL express ICAM-I as well as HLA-DR, although the expression of these molecules is not co-ordinate.[84] Evidence from *in vitro* studies suggests that expression of ICAM-I in immortal HPV-16-expressing keratinocytes is constitutive rather than induced[22] and is more likely to be a consequence of neoplastic transformation than a virally induced phenomenon.

4.6 HLA POLYMORPHISM AND HPV INFECTION

The recognition of foreign or 'dangerous' as opposed to self molecules depends upon the recognition by the T-cell receptor of subtle changes in the architecture of the MHC–peptide complex presented on the cell surface. There is an increasing realization of the importance of the dynamic interaction between the host MHC and the permissivity for presentation of pathogen-derived peptides in determining resistance or susceptibility to infectious agents. For any one protein, different alleles of the MHC will present different peptides to the immune system. Thus, the HLA haplotype of the individual can clearly influence the natural history of HPV infection in that individual and could be a major determinant of whether infection is cleared or persists, which, in the case of the oncogenic viruses, could influence the risk of neoplastic progression. If this thesis is correct, then it could be reflected in different HLA frequencies in patients with persistent or chronic HPV infections (including carcinoma) compared to the appropriate control populations.

Data from the rabbit strongly support this supposition because the regression or progression of papillomas induced by CRPV is strongly linked to the MHC DR or DQ phenotypes, respectively, of the animals.[44] Recurrent respiratory papillomatosis represents an extreme form of persistent HPV infection and an over-representation of HLA-DQ3 and DQ-11 alleles has been reported in these patients.[8] A number of studies have examined associations between HLA haplotype and cervical carcinoma, with differing results. Using serological typing, an association between HLA-DQw3 and increased risk for cervical cancer was shown.[92] However, this was not confirmed in a subsequent study.[42] The possibility that the association might be between HPV type and HLA class II loci was examined[3] in a case-control study which included biopsies from 98 Hispanic patients with cervical cancer and cervical scrapes from 220 Hispanic women with normal Pap smears, all from the same geographic area. In this study, certain HLA class II haplotypes, including DB1*150 - DQB1*0602, were significantly associated with HPV-16-containing cancer, whereas DR13 haplotypes were negatively associated.

Although class II haplotype associations with HPV-16-associated cervical carcinoma have been described, it is MHC class I alleles which are down-regulated in cervical carcinoma biopsies, indicating that these locus products may be important for the presentation of target host or viral peptides. This is supported by a recent study[32] in which the E6 gene in HPV 16 isolates derived from HLA-B7 cervical cancer patients was sequenced. A consistent mutation in the N terminus of E6 was identified in a site corresponding to a putative HLA-B7-restricted CTL epitope. This mutation, although not preventing binding to the TCR, would alter the affinity of the TCR/MHC interaction and could compromise the CTL response. The 'mutant' virus is a true HPV 16 variant with a wide geographic distribution and its over-representation in HLA-B7 patients may reflect immune evasion.

4.7 SUMMARY

HPV infection in the genital tract is common in young, sexually active individuals, the majority of whom clear the infection without overt clinical disease. Those who develop warts, also, in most cases, mount an effective cell-mediated immune response and the lesions regress. Anogenital warts and LGSILs are not associated with inflammation or histological evidence of immune activity. Regression of anogenital warts is accompanied histologically by a response characteristic of a type IV hypersensitivity; animal models support this and provide evidence that the response is regulated by CD4 T-cell-dependent mechanisms. The central importance of the CD4 T-cell population in the control of HPV infection is shown by the increased prevalence of HPV infections in individuals immunosuppressed as a consequence of either organ transplantation or HIV infection. Although it seems clear that the CD4 T-cell subset is critical for the induction and regulation of the host response to HPV, the nature of the effector response remains obscure. There is increasing evidence that both NK cells and antigen-specific CTLs are important effectors, but these responses are poorly understood.

Humoral responses to the capsid proteins accompany the induction of successful cell-mediated immunity and these responses are certainly protective against subsequent viral challenge in natural infections in animals, suggesting that prophylactic immunization against the capsid protein will be effective in controlling HPV-induced genital disease. If the cell-mediated response fails to induce lesion regression and viral clearance, then a persistent viral infection results which is, in part, due to operational immune tolerance. This seems to be reflected by the detection *in vitro*, in persistently infected individuals, of enhanced cellular and humoral responses to early viral proteins but the failure to clear these *in vivo*. The importance of the MHC in susceptibility to or protection from papillomavirus infection and associated neoplastic disease is supported by data from animal models and clinical studies, but this area remains a crucial one for further investigation.

The increasing understanding of the mechanisms by which the host responds effectively to HPV infection and of the reasons for the failure of these defense mechanisms in a minority of circumstances has led to the development of prophylactic and therapeutic immunologically based strategies targeted to both high-risk and low-risk viruses. There is now reason for optimism that control of these infections and the cancers associated with them will be achieved within the foreseeable future.

REFERENCES

1. Albert ML, Sauter B, Bhardwaj N. (1998) Dendritic cells acquire antigen from apoptotic cells and induce class I-restricted CTLs. *Nature* **392**: 86–9.
2. Altmann A, Jochmus-Kudielka I, Frank R, *et al.* (1992) Definition of immunogenic determinants of the human papillomavirus type 16 nucleoprotein E7. *Eur J Cancer* **28**: 326–33.
3. Apple RJ, Erlich HA, Klitz W, *et al.* (1994) HLA DR DQ associations with cervical carcinoma show papillomavirus type specificity. *Nat Genet* **6**: 157–62.
3a. Aranyi I, Tyring SK, Stanley MA, *et al.* (1999) Enhancement of the innate and cellular immune response in patients with genital warts treated with topical imiquimod cream 5%. *Antiviral Res* **43**: 55–63.
4. Bartholomew JS, Glenville S, Sarkar S, *et al.* (1997) Integration of high-risk human papillomavirus DNA is linked to the down-regulation of class I human leukocyte antigens by steroid hormones in cervical tumor cells. *Cancer Res* **57**: 937–42.
5. Bavinck JN, Gissmann L, Claas FH, *et al.* (1993) Relation between skin cancer, humoral responses to human papillomaviruses, and HLA class II molecules in renal transplant recipients. *J Immunol* **151**: 1579–86.
6. Benton C, Shahidullah H, Hunter JAA. (1992) Human papillomaviruses in the immunosuppressed. *Papillomavirus Rep* **3**: 23–6.
7. Beverley PC, Sadovnikova E, Zhu X, *et al.* (1994) Strategies for studying mouse and human immune responses to human papillomavirus type 16. *Ciba Found Symp* **187**: 78–86.
8. Bonagura VR, Siegal FP, Abramson AL, *et al.* (1994) Enriched HLA DQ3 phenotype and decreased class I major histocompatibility complex antigen expression in recurrent respiratory papillomatosis. *Clin Diagn Lab Immunol* **1**: 357–60.
9. Bontkes HJ, de Gruijl TD, Walboomers JMM, *et al.* (1999) Immune responses against human papillomavirus (HPV) type 16 virus-like particles in a cohort study of women with cervical intra-epithelial neoplasia. II Systemic but not local IgA responses correlate with clearance of HPV 16. *J Gen Virol* **80**: 409–14.
10. Bontkes HJ, van Duin M, de Gruijl TD, *et al.* (1998) HPV 16 infection and progression of cervical intra-epithelial neoplasia: analysis of HLA polymorphism and HPV 16 E6 sequence variants. *Int J Cancer* **79**: 166–71.
11. Bontkes HJ, Walboomers JM, Meijer CJ, Helmerhorst TJ, Stern PL. (1998) Specific HLA class I down-regulation is an early event in cervical dysplasia associated with clinical progression. *Lancet* **351**: 187–8.
12. Braun L. (1994) Role of human immunodeficiency virus infection in the pathogenesis of human papillomavirus associated cervical neoplasia. *Am J Pathol* **144**: 209–14.
13. Campo MS. (1994) Towards vaccines for papillomavirus. In *Human papillomaviruses and cervical cancer*, eds PL Stern, MA Stanley. Oxford, Oxford University Press, 177–91.
14. Carter JJ, Wipf GC, Hagensee ME, *et al.* (1995) Use of human papillomavirus type 6 capsids to detect antibodies in people with genital warts. *J Infect Dis* **172**: 11–18.
15. Chambers MA, Stacey SN, Arrand JR, *et al.* (1994) Delayed type hypersensitivity response to human papillomavirus type 16 E6 protein in a mouse model. *J Gen Virol* **75**: 165–9.
16. Chambers MA, Wei Z, Coleman N, *et al.* (1994) 'Natural' presentation of human papillomavirus type 16 E7 protein to immunocompetent mice results in antigen specific sensitization or sustained unresponsiveness. *Eur J Immunol* **24**: 738–45.
17. Chen LP, Thomas EK, Hu SL, *et al.* (1991) Human papillomavirus type 16 nucleoprotein E7 is a tumor rejection antigen. *Proc Natl Acad Sci U S A* **88**: 110–14.
18. Christensen ND, Höpfl R, DiAngelo SL, *et al.* (1994) Assembled baculovirus expressed human papillomavirus type 11 L1 capsid protein virus like particles are recognized by neutralizing monoclonal antibodies and induce high titres of neutralizing antibodies. *J Gen Virol* **75**: 2271–6.

19. Christensen ND, Kirnbauer R, Schiller JT, *et al.* (1994) Human papillomavirus types 6 and 11 have antigenically distinct strongly immunogenic conformationally dependent neutralizing epitopes. *Virology* **205**: 329–35.

20. Chua KL, Hjerpe A. (1997) Human papillomavirus analysis as a prognostic marker following conization of the cervix uteri. *Gynecol Oncol* **66**: 108–13.

21. Coleman N, Birley HD, Renton AM, *et al.* (1994) Immunological events in regressing genital warts. *Am J Clin Pathol* **102**: 768–74.

22. Coleman N, Greenfield IM, Hare J, *et al.* (1993) Characterization and functional analysis of the expression of intercellular adhesion molecule 1 in human papillomavirus related disease of cervical keratinocytes. *Am J Pathol* **143**: 355–67.

23. Coleman N, Stanley MA. (1994) Analysis of HLA DR expression on keratinocytes in cervical neoplasia. *Int J Cancer* **56**: 314–9.

24. Cromme FV, Airey J, Heemels M-T, *et al.* (1994) Loss of transporter protein encoded by the TAP-1 gene, is highly correlated with loss of HLA expression in cervical carcinomas. *J Exp Med* **179**: 335–40.

25. Cromme FV, Meijer CJ, Snijders PJ, *et al.* (1993) Analysis of MHC class I and II expression in relation to presence of HPV genotypes in premalignant and malignant cervical lesions. *Br J Cancer* **67**: 1372–80.

26. Cromme FV, Snijders PJ, Van Den Brule AJ *et al.* (1993) MHC class I expression in HPV 16 positive cervical carcinomas is post transcriptionally controlled and independent from c myc overexpression. *Oncogene* **8**: 2969–75.

27. de Gruijl TD, Bontkes HJ, Stukart MJ, *et al.* (1996) T cell proliferative responses against human papillomavirus type 16 E7 oncoprotein are most prominent in cervical intraepithelial neoplasia patients with persistent viral infection. *J Gen Virol* **77**: 2183–91.

28. de Gruijl TD, Bontkes HJ, Walboomers JM, *et al.* (1996) Analysis of IgG reactivity against human papillomavirus type-16 E7 in patients with cervical intraepithelial neoplasia indicates an association with clearance of viral infection: results of a prospective study. *Int J Cancer* **68**: 731–8.

29. Dillner J. (1990) Mapping of linear epitopes of human papillomavirus type 16: the E1, E2, E4, E5, E6 and E7 open reading frames. *Int J Cancer* **46**: 703–11.

30. Dohring C, Colonna M. (1997) Major histocompatibility complex (MHC) class I recognition by natural killer cells. *Crit Rev Immun* **17**: 295–9.

31. Eisemann C, Fisher SG, Gross G, *et al.* (1996) Antibodies to human papillomavirus type 11 virus-like particles in sera of patients with genital warts and in control groups. *J Gen Virol* **77**: 1799–803.

32. Ellis JR, Keating PJ, Baird J, *et al.* (1995) The association of an HPV16 oncogene variant with HLA B7 has implications for vaccine design in cervical cancer. *Nat Med* **1**: 464–70.

33. Evans C, Bauer S, Grubert T, *et al.* (1996) HLA-A2-restricted peripheral blood cytolytic T lymphocyte response to HPV type 16 proteins E6 and E7 from patients with neoplastic cervical lesions. *Cancer Immunol Immunother* **42**: 151–60.

34. Evans EM, Man S, Evans AS, *et al.* (1997) Infiltration of cervical cancer tissue with human papillomavirus-specific cytotoxic T-lymphocytes. *Cancer Res* **57**: 2943–50.

35. Feltkamp MC, Smits HL, Vierboom MP, *et al.* (1993) Vaccination with cytotoxic T lymphocyte epitope containing peptide protects against a tumor induced by human papillomavirus type 16 transformed cells. *Eur J Immunol* **23**: 2242–9.

36. Ferluga D, Luzar B, Vodovnik A, *et al.* (1997) Langerhans cells in human papillomaviruses types 6/11 associated laryngeal papillomas. *Acta Otolaryngol Stockh* **527** (Suppl.): 87–91.

37. Gao L, Chain B, Sinclair C, *et al.* (1994) Immune response to human papillomavirus type 16 E6 gene in a live vaccinia vector. *J Gen Virol* **75**: 157–64.

38. Ghosh AK, Glenville S, Bartholomew J, *et al.* (1994) Analysis of tumour-infiltrating lymphocytes in cervical carcinoma. In *Immunology of human papillomaviruses*, ed. MA Stanley. New York, Plenum Press, 249–53.

39. Ghosh AK, Moore M. (1992) Tumour infiltrating lymphocytes in cervical carcinoma. *Eur J Cancer* **28A**: 1910–16.

40. Ghosh AK, Smith NK, Stacey SN, *et al.* (1993) Serological response to HPV 16 in cervical dysplasia and neoplasia: correlation of antibodies to E6 with cervical cancer. *Int J Cancer* **53**: 591–6.

41. Glew SS, Connor ME, Snijders PJ, *et al.* (1993) HLA expression in pre invasive cervical neoplasia in relation to human papilloma virus infection. *Eur J Cancer* **29A**: 1963–70.

42. Glew SS, Duggan Keen M, Ghosh AK, *et al.* (1993) Lack of association of HLA polymorphisms with human papillomavirus related cervical cancer. *Hum Immunol* **37**: 157–64.

43. Greer CE, Wheeler CM, Ladner MB, *et al.* (1995) Human papillomavirus (HPV) type distribution and serological response to HPV type 6 virus-like particles in patients with genital warts. *J Clin Microbiol* **33**: 2058–63.

44. Han R, Breitburd F, Marche PN, *et al.* (1992) Linkage of regression and malignant conversion of rabbit viral papillomas to MHC class II genes. *Nature* **356**: 66–8.

45. Hawthorn RJ, Murdoch JB, MacLean AB, *et al.* (1988) Langerhans' cells and subtypes of human papillomavirus in cervical intraepithelial neoplasia. *BMJ* **297**: 643–6.

46. Heim K, Christensen ND, Hoepfl R, *et al.* (1995) Serum IgG, IgM, and IgA reactivity to human papillomavirus types 11 and 6 virus like particles in different gynecologic patient groups. *J Infect Dis* **172**: 395–402.

47. Herd K, Fernando GJ, Dunn LA, *et al.* (1997) E7 oncoprotein of human papillomavirus type 16 expressed constitutively in the epidermis has no effect on E7-specific B- or Th-repertoires or on the immune response induced or sustained after immunization with E7 protein. *Virology* **231**: 155–65.

48. Hilders CGJM, Houbiers JGA, Krul EJT, *et al.* (1994) The expression of histocompatability-related leukocyte antigens in the pathway to cervical carcinoma. *Am J Clin Pathol* **101**: 5–12.

49. Hong K, Greer CE, Ketter N, *et al.* (1997) Isolation and characterization of human papillomavirus type 6-specific T cells infiltrating genital warts. *J Virol* **71**: 6427–32.

50. Jochmus I, Osen W, Altmann A, *et al.* (1997) Specificity of human cytotoxic T lymphocytes induced by a human papillomavirus type 16 E7-derived peptide. *J Gen Virol* **78**: 1689–95.

51. Jochmus-Kudielka I, Schneider A, Braun R, *et al.* (1989) Antibodies against the human papillomavirus type 16 early proteins in human sera: correlation of anti-E7 reactivity with cervical cancer. *J Natl Cancer Inst* **81**: 1698–704.

52. Kast WM, Brandt RM, Sidney J. (1994) Role of HLA-A motifs in identification of potential CTL epitopes in human papillomavirus type 16 E6 and E7 proteins. *J Immunol* **152**: 3904–12.

53. Kirnbauer R, Booy F, Cheng N, *et al.* (1992) Papillomavirus L1 major capsid protein self assembles into virus like particles that are highly immunogenic. *Proc Natl Acad Sci USA* **89**: 12180–4.

54. Lawlor GJ Jr, Ammann AJ, Wright WC Jr, *et al.* (1974) The syndrome of cellular immunodeficiency with immunoglobulins. *J Pediat* **84**: 183–92.

55. Lehtinen M, Dillner J, Knekt P, *et al.* (1996) Serologically diagnosed infection with human papillomavirus type 16 and risk for subsequent development of cervical carcinoma: nested case control study. *BMJ* **312**: 537–9.

55a. Lopez MC, Stanley MA. (2000) Cytokine profile of draining lymph node lymphocytes in mice grafted with syngenic keratinocytes expressing papillomavirus type 16 E7 protein. *J Gen Virol* **81**: 1175–82.

56. Ludmerer SW, Benincasa D, Mark GE 3rd, *et al.* (1997) A neutralizing epitope of human papillomavirus type 11 is principally described by a continuous set of residues which overlap a distinct linear, surface-exposed epitope. *J Virol* **71**: 3834–9.

57. Lutzner MA. (1985) Papillomavirus lesions in immunodepression and immunosuppression. *Clin Dermatol* **3**: 165–9.

58. Luxton JC, Rowe AJ, Cridland JC, *et al.* (1996) Proliferative T cell responses to the human papillomavirus type 16 E7 protein in women with cervical dysplasia and cervical carcinoma and in healthy individuals. *J Gen Virol* **77**: 1585–93.

59. Malejczyk J, Malejczyk M, Majewski S, *et al.* (1993) NK cell activity in patients with HPV16 associated anogenital tumors: defective recognition of HPV16 harboring keratinocytes and restricted unresponsiveness to immunostimulatory cytokines. *Int J Cancer* **54**: 917–21.

60. Mann VM, De Lao SL, Brenes M, *et al.* (1990) Occurrence of IgA and IgG antibodies to select peptides representing human papillomavirus type 16 among cervical cancer cases and controls. *Cancer Res* **50**: 7815–9.

61. McGarvie GM, Grindlay GJ, Chandrachud LM, *et al.* (1995) T-cell responses to BPV-E7 during infection and mapping of T-cell epitopes. *Virology* **206**: 504–10.

62. McKenzie J, King A, Hare J, *et al.* (1991) Immunocytochemical characterization of large granular lymphocytes in normal cervix and HPV associated disease. *J Pathol* **165**: 75–80.

63. McLean CS, Sterling JS, Mowat J, *et al.* (1993) Delayed type hypersensitivity response to the human papillomavirus type 16 E7 protein in a mouse model. *J Gen Virol* **74**: 239–45.

64. Melero I, Singhal MC, McGowan P, *et al.* (1997) Immunological ignorance of an E7-encoded cytolytic T-lymphocyte epitope in transgenic mice expressing the E7 and E6 oncogenes of human papillomavirus type 16. *J Virol* **71**: 3998–4004.

65. Morelli AE, Belardi G, DiPaola G *et al.* (1994) Cellular subsets and epithelial ICAM 1 and HLA DR expression in human papillomavirus infection of the vulva. *Acta Derm Venereol Stockh* **74**: 45–50.

66. Müller M, Viscidi RP, Sun Y, *et al.* (1992) Antibodies to HPV 16 E6 and E7 proteins as markers for HPV 16 associated invasive cervical cancer. *Virology* **187**: 508–14.

67. Murakami M, Gurski KJ, Marincola FM, *et al.* (1999) Induction of specific CD8+ T-lymphocyte responses using a human papillomavirus-16 E6/E7 fusion protein and autologous dendritic cells. *Cancer Res* **59**: 1184–7.

68. Nakagawa M, Stites DP, Farhat S, *et al.* (1997) Cytotoxic T lymphocyte responses to E6 and E7 proteins of human papillomavirus type 16: relationship to cervical intraepithelial neoplasia. *J Infect Dis* **175**: 927–31.

69. Nakagawa M, Stites DP, Palefsky JM, *et al.* (1999) CD4 and CD8 positive cytotoxic T lymphocytes contribute to human papillomavirus 16 E6 and E7 responses. *Clin Diagn Immunol* **6**: 494–8.

70. Nimako M, Fiander AN, Wilkinson GWG, *et al.* (1997) Human papillomavirus-specific cytotoxic T lymphocytes in patients with cervical intraepithelial neoplasia grade III. *Cancer Res* **57**: 4855–61.

71. Nonnenmacher B, Hubbert NL, Kirnbauer R, *et al.* (1995) Serologic response to human papillomavirus type 16 (HPV 16) virus like particles in HPV 16 DNA positive invasive cervical cancer and cervical intraepithelial neoplasia grade III patients and controls from Colombia and Spain. *J Infect Dis* **172**: 19–24.

72. Ressing ME, Sette A, Brandt RM, *et al.* (1995) Human CTL epitopes encoded by human papillomavirus type 16 E6 and E7 identified through *in vivo* and *in vitro* immunogenicity studies of HLA A*0201 binding peptides. *J Immunol* **154**: 5934–43.

73. Ridge JP, Di Rosa F, Matzinger P. (1998) A conditioned dendritic cell can be a temporal bridge between CD4+ helper and a T-killer cell. *Nature* **393**: 474–8.

74. Rocha-Zavaleta L, Jordan D, Pepper S, *et al.* (1997) Differences in serological IgA responses to recombinant baculovirus-derived human papillomavirus E2 protein in the natural history of cervical neoplasia. *Br J Cancer* **75**: 1144–50.

75. Routes JM, Ryan S. (1995) Oncogenicity of human papillomavirus or adenovirus transformed cells correlates with resistance to lysis by natural killer cells. *J Virol* **69**: 7639–47.

76. Sadovnikova E, Stauss HJ. (1994) T cell epitopes in human papilloma virus proteins. *Behring Inst Mitt* **94**: 87–93.

77. Santin AD, Hermonat L, Ravaggi A, *et al.* (1999) Induction of human papillomavirus-specific CD4(+) and CD8(+) lymphocytes by E7-pulsed autologous dendritic cells in patients with human papillomavirus type 16- and 18-positive cervical cancer. *J Virol* **73**: 5402–10.

78. Sasagawa T, Inoue M, Lehtinen M, *et al.* (1996) Serological responses to human papillomavirus type 6 and 16

virus-like particles in patients with cervical neoplastic lesions. *Clin Diagn Lab Immunol* **3**: 403–10.

79. Selvakumar R, Ahmed R, Wettstein FO. (1995) Tumor regression is associated with a specific immune response to the E2 protein of cotton tail rabbit papillomavirus. *Virology* **208**: 298–302.

80. Selvakumar R, Borenstein LA, Lin Y-L, *et al.* (1995) Immunization with nonstructural proteins E1 and E2 of cotton tail rabbit papillomavirus stimulates regression of virus-induced papillomas. *J Virol* **69**: 602–5.

81. Shepherd PS, Rowe AJ, Cridland JC, *et al.* (1996) Proliferative T cell responses to human papillomavirus type 16 L1 peptides in patients with cervical dysplasia. *J Gen Virol* **77**: 593–602.

82. Stacey SN, Bartholomew JS, Ghosh A, *et al.* (1992) Expression of human papillomavirus type 16 E6 protein by recombinant baculovirus and use for detection of anti E6 antibodies in human sera. *J Gen Virol* **73**: 2337–45.

83. Stanley MA, Chambers MA, Coleman N. (1994) Immunology of human papillomavirus infection. In *Genital warts*, ed. A. Mindel. London, Edward Arnold. 252–70.

84. Stanley M, Coleman N, Chambers M. (1994) The host response to lesions induced by human papillomavirus. In Ciba Foundation Symposium, Vol. 187, *Vaccines against virally induced cancers*. Chichester, John Wiley & Sons, 21–46.

85. Steele JC, Gallimore PH. (1990) Humoral assays of human sera to disrupted and nondisrupted epitopes of human papillomavirus type 1. *Virology* **174**: 388–98.

86. Strang G, Hickling JK, McIndoe GA, *et al.* (1990) Human T cell responses to human papillomavirus type 16 L1 and E6 synthetic peptides: identification of T cell determinants, HLA DR restriction and virus type specificity. *J Gen Virol* **71**: 423–31.

87. Tarpey I, Stacey S, Hickling J, *et al.* (1994) Human cytotoxic T lymphocytes stimulated by endogenously processed human papillomavirus type 11 E7 recognize a peptide containing a HLA A2 (A*0201) motif. *Immunology* **81**: 222–7.

88. Tay SK, Jenkins D, Maddox P, *et al.* (1987) Lymphocyte phenotypes in cervical intraepithelial neoplasia and human papillomavirus infection. *Br J Obstet Gynaecol* **94**: 16–21.

89. Thompson S, Davies M, O'Neill T, *et al.* (1997) Immunogenicity and reactogenicity of a recombinant HPV6 fusion protein vaccine adjuvanted with monophosphoryl lipid A. *Biochem Soc Trans* **25**: 274S.

90. Viac J, Guerin Reverchon I, Chardonnet Y, *et al.* (1990) Langerhans cells and epithelial cell modifications in cervical intraepithelial neoplasia: correlation with human papillomavirus infection. *Immunobiology* **180**: 328–38.

91. Wang Z, Hansson BG, Forslund O, *et al.* (1996) Cervical mucus antibodies against human papillomavirus type 16, 18, and 33 capsids in relation to presence of viral DNA. *J Clin Microbiol* **34**: 3056–62.

92. Wank R, Thomssen C. (1991) High risk of squamous cell carcinoma of the cervix for women with HLA-DQw3. *Nature* **352**: 723–5.

93. Warhol MJ, Gee B. (1989) The expression of histocompatibility antigen HLA DR in cervical squamous epithelium infected with human papilloma virus. *Mod Pathol* **2**: 101–4.

94. Wideroff L, Schiffman MH, Nonnenmacher B, *et al.* (1995) Evaluation of seroreactivity to human papillomavirus type 16 virus like particles in an incident case control study of cervical neoplasia. *J Infect Dis* **172**: 1425–30.

95. Wikström A, Van Doornum GJ, Kirnbauer R, *et al.* (1995) Prospective study on the development of antibodies against human papillomavirus type 6 among patients with condyloma acuminata or new asymptomatic infection. *J Med Virol* **46**: 368–74.

96. Youde SJ, Dunbar PRR, Evans EML, *et al.* (2000) Use of fluorogenic histocompatibility leucocyte antigen-A*0201/HPV 16 E7 peptide complexes to isolate rare human cytotoxic T-lymphocyte recognising endogenous human papillomavirus antigens. *Cancer Res* **60**: 365–71.

97. Zhou J, Sun XY, Stenzel DJ, *et al.* (1991) Expression of vaccinia recombinant HPV 16 L1 and L2 ORF proteins in epithelial cells is sufficient for assembly of HPV virion like particles. *Virology* **185**: 251–7.

Part III

Diseases and infections

5

Cutaneous warts

Angela Yen Moore and Stephen K. Tyring

5.1 CLINICAL FORMS

Eight percent of patient visits to dermatologists are for cutaneous warts, despite the fact that half of all patients with warts are evaluated and treated for warts by family practitioners, internists, and pediatricians rather than dermatologists.[32] On the other hand, in one study, 8% of patients referred to dermatologists for wart treatment actually had clinical mimics of warts, with the most common being acrochordons (skin tags) or corns.[31] In this study, the age of patients ranged from 2 to 81 years, with the median age of presentation being 11 years. Children were affected more often, with 84% of patients being under 35 and 65% being between 5 and 20 years old.

Except for an additional genetic predisposition in those with epidermodysplasia verruciformis, cutaneous warts are transmitted by skin-to-skin contact. Predisposing factors include frequent wet work,[31] hyperhidrosis of the feet,[32] nail-biting,[31] and occupation as a butcher or slaughterhouse worker.[15,17]

Classifications of cutaneous warts include verruca vulgaris (common warts), verruca plana (plane warts), verruca plantaris (deep plantar warts), mosaic plantar warts, butcher's warts, condyloma acuminata (genital warts), and epidermodysplasia verruciformis. Each classification of cutaneous warts is associated with characteristic clinical appearances, human papillomavirus (HPV) genotypes, histologic features, and prognostic features. Each category is described in this chapter in detail except for condyloma acuminatum (see Chapter 6) and epidermodysplasia verruciformis (see Chapter 9).

The categorization of warts is usually based on anatomic location, but is somewhat artificial in that 15% of patients in one study exhibited a combination of common warts and one or more of other classifications of warts.[31] In this study, 40% were common warts and 38% were plantar warts, with 3% being filiform, 2% being periungual, and 2% being mosaic plantar warts.

5.1.1 Verruca vulgaris

Verruca vulgaris, or the common wart, appears clinically as a well-defined papule with an irregular cauliflower surface with minute papillary projections. The size varies from 1–2 mm to greater than 2 cm, while the color ranges from flesh-colored to brown to gray. Lesions may be single or multiple, with clustering, development of satellite lesions, and koebnerization (self-inoculation with extension of lesions through trauma). Usually limited to glabrous surfaces, common warts most commonly appear on the extremities (Figure 5.1), especially the dorsa of hands (Figure 5.2) or fingers, but may be on periungual or subungual areas, palmar or plantar surfaces, trunk, face, vermillion border of the lips, and rarely on the mucous membranes of the mouth (Figure 5.3) or nose.

One subtype of common warts is the *periungual wart* (Figures 5.4 and 5.5), which are usually non-painful but are often coalescent, nail deforming, and difficult to eradicate.

Another subtype of common warts is the *endophytic wart*, which appear in palmar or plantar locations and resemble keratoderma punctata. Endophytic warts are small, round, keratotic, usually less than 5 mm in size, and most frequently painless. Often multiple, these endophytic warts

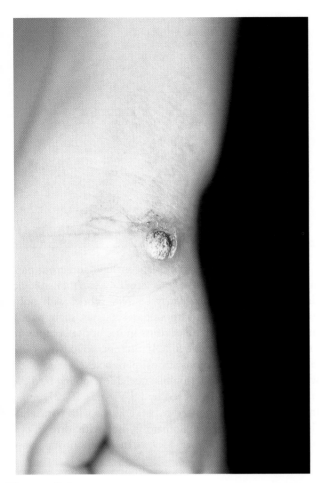

Figure 5.1
Verruca vulgaris on the left ventral wrist.

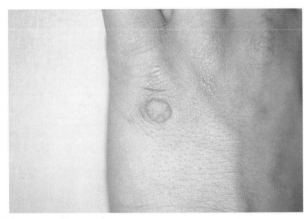

Figure 5.2
Verruca vulgaris on the left dorsal hand.

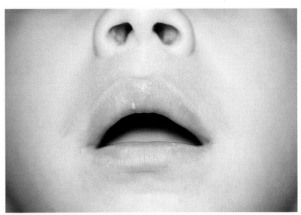

Figure 5.3
Verruca vulgaris on lip mucosa.

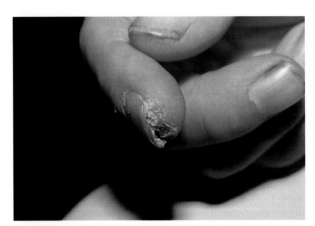

Figure 5.4
Periungual wart on the nailbed deforming the nail.

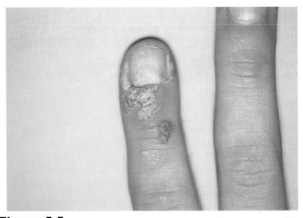

Figure 5.5
Periungual wart and verruca vulgaris.

characteristically display a horny wall around a central depression.

Yet another subtype of verruca vulgaris is the *filiform wart* (Figure 5.6), which are usually multiple but non-clustered, hyperkeratotic, pin-shaped, pedunculated papules with a narrow point of attachment. Filiform warts most commonly present on the head and neck and in body folds.

Although classic verruca vulgaris is easily diagnosed, clinical mimics include other hyperkeratotic or papular lesions (Table 5.1). Periungual warts must additionally be differentiated from fibromas, chondromas, osteomas, and glomus tumors.

Histologic findings are usually diagnostic. In warts induced by HPV 2, prominent, compact hyperkeratosis with focal parakeratotic tiers, hypergranulosis, acanthosis, papillomatosis, and dilated papillary capillaries are present (Figure 5.7). The characteristic koilocytosis consists of vacuolization of granular cells with eccentric, pyknotic nuclei surrounded by a perinuclear halo and prominent condensed keratohyaline granules of numerous shapes, sizes, and stainability (Table 5.2). In warts induced by HPV 4, koilocytes resemble signet rings, with large, vacuolized cells with peripheral crescentic nuclei and no keratohyaline granules.

HPV types associated with verruca vulgaris most commonly include HPV 2 but may include multiple other types,

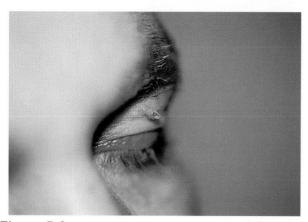

Figure 5.6
Filiform wart on the eyelid.

including HPV types 1–4 and 7 (Table 5.3). Endophytic warts are induced primarily by HPV 4, whereas periungual warts and filiform warts are induced by HPV 2.

5.1.2 Verruca plana

Verruca plana, also known as flat warts, juvenile warts, or plane warts, clinically appear as flat-topped, round or polygonal, smooth or slightly hyperkeratotic papules (Figure 5.8). Often multiple and asymmetrically disseminated, verruca plana may be grouped, confluent, and often linear through koebnerization. Plane warts are often distributed preferentially on the dorsa of the hands or the cheeks, chin, or forehead of the face. Facial lesions are usually flatter and often pigmented, whereas lesions on the dorsal hands are usually elevated, coalescent, and more hyperkeratotic.

Table 5.1
Clinical differential diagnosis of cutaneous warts

Verruca vulgaris
Acrochordons
Acrokeratosis verruciformis of Hopf
Actinic keratosis
Cutaneous horns
Darier's disease
Dermatomyositis – Gottron's papules
Epidermolytic hyperkeratosis
Granuloma annulare, perforating
Lichen nitidus
Lichen planus
Molluscum contagiosum
Naevi
Seborrheic keratosis
Squamous cell carcinoma
Veruca plana
Acrokeratosis verruciformis of Hopf
Arsenical keratosis
Basal cell carcinoma
Benign adnexal tumors (tricholemmoma, trichoepithelioma, syringoma, etc.)
Confluent reticulated and pigmented papillomatosis of Gougerot and Carteaud
Dowling–Degos disease
Darier's disease
Ephelides (freckles)
Lentigo simplex or lentigo solaris
Lichen planus
Naevi
Seborrheic keratosis, early
Syphilis, secondary
Tinea versicolor

Myrmecia
Acquired digital fibrokeratoma
Clavus
Corn
Foreign body
Mycetoma
Pyogenic granuloma
Squamous cell carcinoma
Mosaic wart
Clavus
Foreign body
Keratoderma, punctate
Squamous cell carcinoma
Tuberculosis cutis
Butchers' wart
Same as **verruca vulgaris**

Clinical mimics of verruca plana include numerous papular as well as pigmented lesions (see Table 5.1). Histological findings in verruca plana may be very subtle, with only a loose stratum corneum without parakeratosis, slight papillomatosis, and minimal koilocytosis in the upper spinous and granular layers (see Table 5.2). If present, koilocytosis associated with HPV 3 consists of perinuclear vacuolization with centrally located basophilic nuclei resembling bird eyes. In comparison, warts caused by HPV types 10, 27, and 28 manifest more pronounced hyperkeratosis with parakeratosis, acanthosis, and papillomatosis, but with similar cytopathic changes (Figure 5.9). In immunosuppressed

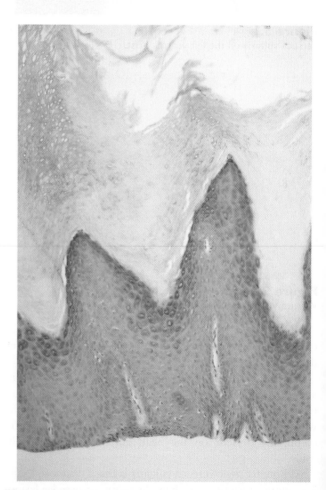

Figure 5.7
Histology of verruca vulgaris with compact hyperkeratosis with focal parakeratotic tiers, hypergranulosis, acanthosis, papillomatosis, and dilated papillary capillaries.

Table 5.2
History of cutaneous warts

Clinical manifestation	HPV[a]	Epidermal changes[b]	Koilocytosis features
Verruca vulgaris	2	Prominent (granular)	Eccentric nucleus; large, uneven keratohyaline granules
	4	Prominent (granular)	Signet ring nuclei; no keratohyaline granules
Verruca plana	3	Subtle; no parakeratosis (upper spinous and granular)	Bird eyes with central nuclei
	5	(Upper spinous and granular)	Swollen basophilic keratinocytes with vesicular nuclei
Myrmecia	I	Prominent; endophytic	(Malpighii) Sickle-like, ring-like keratohyaline granules
Mosaic wart	2	Prominent (granular)	Eccentric nucleus; large, uneven keratohyaline granules
Butchers' wart	7	Prominent (granular)	Central small, shrunken nuclei

[a] Most common associated HPV genotype.
[b] Papillomatosis, compact hyperkeratosis with focal parakeratosis, hypergranulosis, and acanthosis (epidermal layer affected by koilocytosis).

individuals, HPV 5 may induce verruca plana; in these warts, keratinocytes in the granular and upper spinous layers resemble 'swollen keratinocytes,' with abundant pale, basophilic cytoplasm and enlarged vesicular nuclei.[1]

Verruca plana may affect individuals of all ages, but are more prevalent in the immunosuppressed and in those with epidermodysplasia verruciformis. Plane warts are induced primarily by HPV 3, but are also associated with HPV types 10, 26, 27, and 28 (Table 5.3).

5.1.3 Verruca plantaris

Verruca plantaris, also known as myrmecia warts or deep plantar warts, usually arise on the pressure points of feet but may also occur on the palms or subungual areas. Endophytic and deep, verruca plantaris often are single, painful nodules that possess a hyperkeratotic surface overlying soft keratinous debris and circumscribed by a hyperkeratotic ring. When the surface is pared away, punctate bleeding or black dots appear (Figure 5.10). These punctate points are created from thrombosed capillaries in the papillae.

The clinical differential includes other hyperkeratotic or fungating lesions (see Table 5.1). Histologically, myrmecia

Table 5.3
Cutaneous warts and associated human papillomavirus (HPV) genotypes

Clinical manifestation	HPV genotypes
Verruca vulgaris	I, **2**, 3, 4, 7
Verruca plana	**3**, 10, 26, 27, 28
Myrmecia	I
Mosaic wart	2
Butchers' wart	7

Most common HPV genotype is in **bold**.

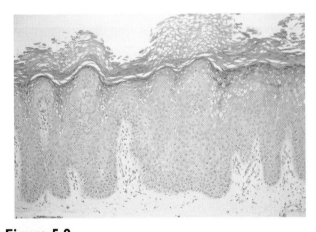

Figure 5.9
Histology of verruca plana with centrally located basophilic nuclei resembling bird eyes.

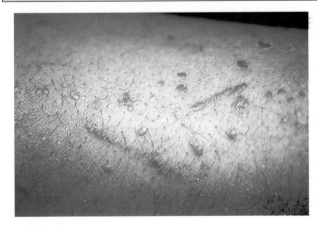

Figure 5.8
Veruca plana.

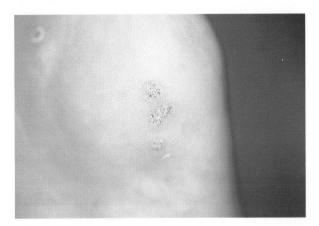

Figure 5.10
Verruca plantaris, after paring, with punctuate black dots.

warts exhibit broad endophytic acanthosis with inward bending of the rete ridges, compact hyperkeratosis, prominently disorganized hypergranulosis, and koilocytosis in the stratum malpighii (see Table 5.2). Koilocytotic cells contain large, irregular, sickle-like or ring-like eosinophilic cytoplasmic inclusions that represent clumped keratin filaments as well as eosinophilic nuclear inclusions (Figure 5.11).

Most commonly occurring in patients between 12 and 15 years of age, myrmecia rarely recur because neutralizing antibodies develop in the host.[19,23] The HPV genotype that classically induces plantar warts is HPV 1, although HPV 2 is also very common.

5.1.4 Mosaic plantar warts

Usually plantar, mosaic warts differ from myrmecia by being painless, multiple, confluent, and more superficial (Figure 5.12). In addition, mosaic plantar warts often recur and are difficult to eradicate. Also hyperkeratotic, mosaic warts often coexist with myrmecia.

The clinical differential consists primarily of hyperkeratotic lesions (see Table 5.1). Histologically, mosaic warts resemble verruca vulgaris because HPV 2 induces most mosaic warts as well (see Tables 5.2, and 5.3).

5.1.5 Butchers' warts

Butchers' warts, as suggested by their nomenclature, affect primarily the hands of meat handlers, including butchers,

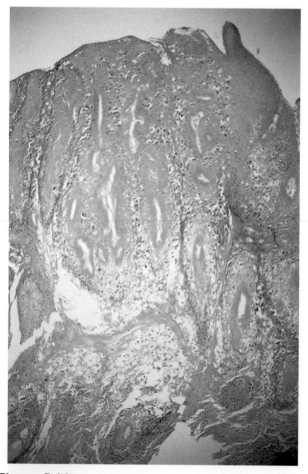

Figure 5.11
Histology of verruca plantaris with large, irregular cytoplasmic inclusions as well as eosinophilic nuclear inclusions.

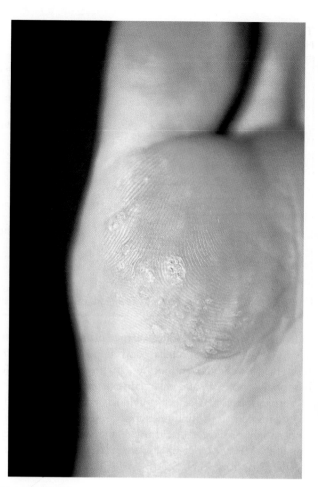

Figure 5.12
Mosaic plantar warts on the left sole.

slaughterhouse workers, and fish handlers.[25] Clinically, lesions appear cauliflower-like, hypertrophic, and sometimes confluent.

As the clinical appearance resembles that of verruca vulgaris, the same clinical mimics exist (see Table 5.1). Histologic findings in butchers' warts, however, are unique, with koilocytosis occurring primarily in the granular layer as small, shrunken, centrally located nuclei in vacuolated keratinocytes (see Table 5.2). HPV 7 most commonly induces butchers' warts.

5.2 NATURAL HISTORY

Studies of warts in children show that two-thirds will spontaneously regress within 2 years, with continuing regression of the remaining third.[20] New warts, however, may continue to appear while others are regressing. In fact, in this study of 1000 institutionalized children, the 18% of patients with at least one verruca at initial evaluation were three times more likely to develop new warts. Of the remaining 82% without a verruca at baseline, 12% developed new warts.

Immunosuppression after renal transplantation, malignancies such as Hodgkin's disease, other lymphomas, or chronic lymphatic leukemia, and/or infection with the human immunodeficiency virus (HIV) increases the reported incidences of verruca to those ranging from 24% to 100%.[1,21] Each year after immunosuppression the number of warts increases. In addition to the HPV genotypes associated with the previously described verruca, however, immunocompromised patients are also infected by HPV genotypes usually present in patients with epidermodysplasia verruciformis.[9] These include HPV types 5, 8, 9, 12, 14, 15, 17, 19–27, 36, 46, 47, 49, and 50, and also more recently isolated, closely related types.

If a cutaneous wart is persistent despite therapy, and especially if continued growth is observed, biopsy to evaluate for possible malignant degeneration is warranted. HPV 16 has been reported in association with periungual 'warts' that histologically were diagnosed as squamous cell carcinoma *in situ* (Bowen's disease).[26] Verrucae in immunocompromised patients also progress to squamous cell carcinomas with a greater incidence. Although verrucae in immunocompromised patients are often more recalcitrant to treatment, biopsies should be performed on any persistent verruca. In one study of clinically diagnosed verruca vulgaris, biopsy specimens only confirmed the clinical diagnosis in 27% of cases.[4] Indeed, 31% of 'warts' were actually squamous cell carcinomas and 32% were warts with dysplasia.

5.3 TREATMENT

The algorithm for the management of cutaneous warts is based on the age of the patient, presence and degree of symptoms, the extent and duration of lesions, the patient's immunological status, and the patient's desire for therapy. Most currently approved treatment modalities for cutaneous warts are destructive in nature, but few rigorous, well-controlled clinical trials exist. Destructive therapies include liquid nitrogen,[24] topical cantharidin, topical retinoic acid, topical salicylic plaster,[7] and topical salicylic acid and lactic acid (Duofilm, Duoplant, Occlusol HP).

Cryosurgery with liquid nitrogen ($-195\,^\circ$C) with either a cotton tip or cryospray unit usually involves application for 10–60 seconds to the center of the wart until a 1–2 mm halo appears. After thawing, a second application of liquid nitrogen is applied. Immediate side-effects include erythema and a sensation of burning followed by throbbing and swelling (Figure 5.13). Blistering followed by crusting may occur in 24 hours to 1 week later and be followed by possible hyperpigmentation, hypopigmentation, or hypoesthesia. In one study of 72 patients with warts on the hands prospectively

treated with cryotherapy at 2-week, 3-week, and 4-week intervals for a total of 12 weeks, 70–80% of patients in the 2-week and 3-week interval groups were successfully treated with three treatments.[5] In contrast, only 40% of patients in the 4-week interval group were successfully treated. No significant difference was found in cure rates for cryotherapy alone, topical salicylic acid and acetic acids, and a combination of cryotherapy with topical salicylic and acetic acids. In another study, the cure rate was inversely related both to the duration of wart infection and to the diameter of the largest lesion.[3] Paring prior to cryotherapy and keratolytics improved the cure rate for plantar warts but not for hand warts.

Because it is obtained from the blister fluid of green blister beetles, cantharidin is not currently approved by the Federal Drug Administration in the USA for warts due to the inability to regulate the exact concentration of the cantharidin. Application of topical cantharidin diluted in acetone to a 0.7% solution should occur after paring of warts. After the cantharidin dries, adhesive tape is applied and left on for 24 hours. Afterwards, the wart is debrided. Side-effects include pain, tenderness, and blistering, especially when the tape is removed after 24 hours.

Topical retinoic acid at 0.05% concentration is applied daily to flat warts. Topical adhesive plasters with 20–40% salicylic acid concentrations can be applied 1 day prior to cryosurgery. Topical salicylic acid and lactic acid are applied nightly and occluded with adhesive tape. The tape is removed every morning.

Immunomodulating treatments include induction with dinitrochlorobenzene (DNCB)[8] or diphenciprone,[22] intralesional bleomycin,[28] topical 5-fluorouracil,[11,14] and intralesional recombinant interferon alpha.[33]

Contact immunotherapy consists of initial sensitization of patients to DNCB[8] or diphenciprone[22] and subsequent application of progressively more concentrated solutions of the sensitizer from 0.01% to 0.5% to 1% to the warts. This treatment resolves 60% of warts in 3–4 months.

Intralesional bleomycin[28] applied at up to 2 mg divided into two or three injections is an alternative therapy for large warts recalcitrant to other treatment modalities. This may be repeated after 4 weeks, but the total dose of bleomycin should not exceed 5 mg. Because of the painful nature of the injections, premedication with 2% lidocaine should be used in the periungual areas and palms or soles. Side-effects include possible distortion of the nail matrix and pain.

Topical 5-fluorouracil as an ointment or solution applied twice daily for several days is yet another possible treatment.[11] One side-effect is pain. Another treatment alternative is intralesional interferon alpha two to three times a week for 8 weeks. Such topical agents as podophyllin, podophyllotoxin, and trichloroacetic acid are not effective for non-genital, cutaneous warts.

Other reported treatments for cutaneous warts include hypnosis[29] and oral cimetidine.[2,10] Hypnosis may be particularly effective in children with recalcitrant warts. Previously shown to possess immunomodulatory activity when high dosages (30–40 mg kg^{-1} day^{-1}) are employed, oral cimetidine therapy at 30–40 mg kg^{-1}day^{-1} in three divided doses (maximum dose, 3.5 g day^{-1}) for 3 months was shown in one open label study to resolve 84% of warts without any reported adverse effects. Recent randomized, placebo-controlled studies, however, have not been so promising.[16,34]

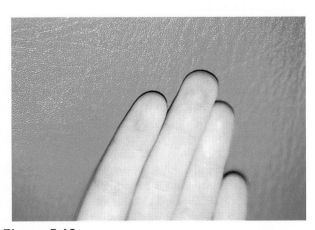

Figure 5.13
Erythema and swelling present immediately after liquid nitrogen application.

Other medical treatments currently being studied for cutaneous warts include imiquimod,[12] antisense oligonucleotides,[6] cidofovir,[18,35] and recombinant HPV protein vaccines. Although not approved for cutaneous warts, imiquimod, an immunomodulatory heterocyclic amine, was approved by the Federal Drug Administration in the USA in 1997 for condyloma accuminata as a topical 5% cream for use overnight three times per week for up to 16 weeks.[30] Imiquimod stimulates human peripheral blood mononuclear cells to produce and release such cytokines as tumor necrosis factor and interleukins 1, 6, 8, 10, and 12 as well as interleukin-1 receptor antagonist.[13] Similarly, cidofovir 3% gel, a nucleotide analog with a broad spectrum of activity against a variety of DNA viruses, is not approved for cutaneous warts but has been proven effective against condyloma accuminata in acquired immune deficiency syndrome (AIDS) patients.[35]

Although employed less often, surgical modalities may be used for large or recalcitrant warts. These surgical alternatives include excision, electrodesiccation and curettage, and laser surgery. Scissor excision with sharp iris scissors effectively treats filiform warts. Excision of large, pedunculated warts may be effective through debulking. All of the surgical alternatives can result in atrophic scarring, hypertrophic scarring, or nail dystrophy. Unfortunately, curettage and desiccation as well as carbon dioxide laser therapy can also vaporize HPV and hypothetically transmit aerosolized HPV.[27] Recently, the pulsed-dye laser at 585 mm was reported to clear 72% of warts in 39 patients after 1.68 treatments by selectively targeting the dilated blood vessels present in warts.

Thus, multiple treatment alternatives, each with potential benefits but possible hazards, have been reported for cutaneous warts, but no definitive therapy exists. Therefore, management of warts is empiric and should be individualized for each patient.

REFERENCES

1. Androphy EJ, Beutner K, Olbricht S. (1996) Human papillomavirus infection. In *Cutaneous medicine and surgery: an integrated program in dermatology*, eds KA Arndt, PE LeBoit, JK Robinson, BU Wintroub. Philadelphia, W.B. Saunders, 1100–22.
2. Bauman C, Francis JS, Vanderhooft S, Sybert VP. (1996) Cimetidine therapy for multiple viral warts in children. *J Am Acad Dermatol* **35**(2): 271–2.
3. Berth-Jones J, Hutchinson P. (1992) Modern treatment of warts: cure rates at 3 and 6 months. *Br J Dermatol* **127**: 262–5.
4. Blessing K, McLaren K, Benton E, *et al.* (1989) Histopathology of skin lesions in renal allograft recipients: an assessment of viral features and dysplasia. *Histopathology* **14**: 129–39.
5. Bunney M, Nolan M, Williams D. (1976) An assessment of methods treating viral warts by comparative treatment trials based on a standard design. *Br J Dermatol* **94**: 667–79.
6. Cowsert LM, Fox MC, Zone G, *et al.* (1993) In vitro evaluation of phosphorothioate oligonucleotides targeted to the E2 mRNA of papillomavirus: potential treatment for genital warts. *Antimicrob Agents Chemother* **37**: 171.
7. Dachow-Siwiec E. (1985) Technique of cryotherapy. *Clin Dermatol* **3**: 185–98.
8. Dunagin W, Millikan L. (1982) Dinitrochlorobenzene immunotherapy for verrucae resistant to standard treatment modalities. *J Am Acad Dermatol* **6**: 40–5.
9. Gassenmaier A, Fuchs P, Schell H, *et al.* (1986) Papillomavirus DNA in warts of immunosuppressed renal allograft recipients. *Arch Dermatol Res* **278**: 219–23.
10. Glass AT, Solomon BA. (1996) Cimetidine therapy for recalcitrant warts in adults. *Arch Dermatol* **132**: 680–2.
11. Goette DK. (1981) Topical chemotherapy with 5-fluorouracil. *J Am Acad Dermatol* **6**: 633.
12. Hengge UR, Arndt R. (2000) Topical treatment of warts and mollusca with imiquimod. *Ann Int Med* **132**: 95.
13. Herne K, Cirelli R, Lee P, *et al.* (1996) Advances in antiviral therapy. *Curr Opin Dermatol* **3**: 195–201
14. Hursthouse MW. (1975) A controlled trial on the use of topical 5-fluorouracil on viral warts. *Br J Dermatol* **92**: 93–6.
15. Jablonska S, Obalek S, Golebiowska A, *et al.* (1988) Epidemiology of butchers' warts. *Arch Dermatol Res* **280** (Suppl): S24–8.
16. Karabulut AA, Sahin S, Eksioglu M. (1997) Is cimetidine effective for nongenital warts? A double-blind, placebo-controlled study. *Arch Dermatol* **133**(4): 533–4.
17. Keefe M, Al-Ghamdi A, Coggon D, *et al.* (1994) Cutaneous warts in butchers. *Br J Dermatol* **130**: 15–17.
18. Lalezari JP, Stagg RJ, Jaffe MS, *et al.* (1996) A preclinical and clinical overview of the nucleotide-based antiviral agent cidofovir (HPMPC). In *Antiviral chemotherapy 4. New directions for clinical application and research*, eds JA Mills, PA Volberding, L Corey. New York, Plenum Press, 105–15.
19. Laurent R, Kienzler JL, Croissant O, Orth G. (1982) Two anatomicoclinical types of warts with plantar localization: specific cytopathogenic effects of papillomavirus type 1 (HPV-1) and type 2 (HPV-2). *Arch Dermatol Res* **274**: 101–11.
20. Massing AM, Epstein WL. (1963) Natural history of warts: a two year study. *Arch Dermatol* **87**: 306.
21. Morison W. (1975) Viral warts, herpes simplex and herpes zoster in patients with secondary immune deficiencies and neoplasms. *Br J Dermatol* **92**: 625.
22. Naylor M, Neldner K, Yarborough G, *et al.* (1988) Contact immunotherapy of resistant warts. *J Am Acad Dermatol* **19**: 679–83.
23. Pfister H, zur Hausen H. (1978) Seroepidemiological studies of human papillomavirus (HPV 1) infections. *Int J Cancer* **21**: 161–5.
24. Rademaker M, Meyrick Thomas RH, Munro DD. (1987) The treatment of resistant mosaic plantar warts with aggressive cryotherapy under general anaesthetic. *Br J Dermatol* **116**: 557–60.
25. Rudlinger R, Bunney MH, Grob R, *et al.* (1989) Warts in fish handlers. *Br J Dermatol* **120**: 375–81.
26. Sau P, McMarlin SL. (1994) Bowen's disease of the nail bed and periungual area. A clinicopathologic analysis of seven cases. *Arch Dermatol* **130**: 204–9.
27. Sawchuk WS, Weber P, Lowy D, *et al.* (1989) Infectious papillomavirus in the vapor of warts treated with carbon dioxide laser or electrocoagulation: detection and protection. *J Am Acad Dermatol* **21**: 41–49.

28. Shelley W, Shelley E. (1991) Intralesional bleomycin sulphate therapy for warts. *Arch Dermatol* **127**: 234–7.

29. Spanos NP, Williams V, Gwynn MI. (1990) Effects of hypnotic, placebo, and salicylic acid treatments on wart regression. *Psychosom Med* **52**: 109–14.

30. Spruance S, Douglas J, Hougham A, *et al.* (1993) Multicenter trial of 5% imiquimod (IQ) cream for treatment of genital and perianal warts (abstract 1432). New Orleans, Louisiana, American Society for Microbiology, 33rd ICAAC meeting.

31. Steele K, Irwin W, Merrett J. (1989) Warts in general practice. *Ir Med J* **82**: 122–4.

32. Stern R, Johnson M, DeLozier J. (1987) Utilization of physician services for dermatologic complaints. *Arch Dermatol* **113**: 1062–6.

33. Steinberg BM, Topp WC, Schneider PS, *et al.* (1988) Persistence and expression of human papillomavirus during interferon therapy. *Arch Otolaryngol Head Neck Surg* **144**: 27.

34. Yilmaz E, Alpsoy E, Basaran E. (1996) Cimetidine therapy for warts: a placebo-controlled, double-blind study. *J Am Acad Dermatol* **34**: 1005–7.

35. Zabawski EF, Cockerell CJ. (1998) Topical and intralesional cidofovir: a review of pharmacology and therapeutic effects. *J Am Acad Dermatol* **39**: 741–5.

6

Genital warts

Humphrey D.L. Birley and Charles J.N. Lacey

6.1 INTRODUCTION

Genital warts are one of the commonest sexually transmitted diseases (STDs) worldwide. In the developed world they have been recorded as occurring at an incidence rate of 2.4 cases per 1000 per year in the whole population with a peak attack rate of 1.2% in men and women aged 20–24 years.[48] To the physician they represent a clinical condition, whereas to a virologist they are a manifestation of infection with certain genital strains of human papillomavirus (HPV). Because of their very ubiquity, genital warts are usually treated without any specific diagnostic investigation and certainly without HPV typing, which still remains a research tool. Undoubtedly, therefore, many a 'wart' is diagnosed and treated which does *not* contain HPV, let alone HPV 6 or 11, the commonest types found in genital warts. Equally, many infections with HPV types 6 or 11 remain subclinical. Furthermore, such subclinical HPV infection may persist for months and perhaps years. Although persistence and recurrence after treatment may seem to mirror the virus's persistence or reactivation, the natural history of warts is only a dim reflection of the virus/host interaction. This chapter seeks to bridge the gap between the clinician's view of the disease and the new information about HPV infection provided by virological studies. What factors underlie the conversion of subclinical infection into overt disease? How does transmission take place? How can an understanding of the pathogenesis of this common STD be used to improve treatments (which are currently rudimentary and fairly ineffective)? Our understanding of these questions is still developing but we try, in this chapter, to flesh out the main areas.

6.2 THE NATURAL HISTORY OF GENITAL WARTS SUGGESTS TREATMENT OPTIONS

The biology of HPVs is discussed in chapter 2. Using nucleotide sequence analysis, Van Ranst and his colleagues compared the genetic relatedness of the E6 gene amongst 48 HPV types whose sequences were known.[69] This places all the low-risk mucosal HPVs in one genetically related group. This group contains almost all the types that are commonly found in genital warts, the most common by far being HPV 6 and the closely related type HPV 11 (see Figure 2.3, p. 14). It is suggestive that the E6 protein of HPV 6/11 does not bind to or degrade the important anti-oncoprotein, p53, unlike that of HPV 16, the main cause of cervical cancer worldwide.[26] Some high-risk genital types (especially HPV 16 and 18) are also found occasionally in genital warts, sometimes as mixtures with more typical types, e.g., 6 and 11. The biological significance of this is not clear, although HPV 16 and other high-risk types are certainly found in other anogenital malignancies (besides cervical cancer) as well as in intraepithelial neoplastic lesions such as bowenoid papulosis.[62] A very small number of genital warts, in particular a proportion of those found in children, may also contain 'cutaneous/mucosal' types such as HPV 2a/27/57, which are more commonly found on non-anogenital sites such as the hands and buccal cavity.[34] Thus the 'classification' produced by this genetic analysis, while it corresponds closely to the types of HPV most commonly found in genital warts, is not entirely comprehensive. Most crucially, for the clinician, it leaves a very slight degree of doubt whether there is absolutely *no* risk of malignant transformation of genital warts and whether warts may be non-sexually transmitted or even transferred to a genital from a non-genital site.

Population-based epidemiological studies which have identified HPV DNA from genital sites have repeatedly provided evidence of the high prevalence of the virus relative to the disease. Thus, although genital warts are a very common disease in western populations, the virus types which cause them, HPV 6 and 11, are twice as common.[5,68] Perhaps approximately the same order of relative frequencies applies to the high-risk HPV types, which generally have a much higher prevalence than that of anogenital intra-epithelial neoplasia. Using vulval and cervical samples taken from American college students, Bauer and her colleagues found HPV DNA in 46% of subjects.[5] Somewhat lower prevalences have been found in other population-based surveys.[42] Estimates of HPV prevalence from single samples taken at one site only may considerably underestimate the true prevalence of these viruses, which are distributed in the anogenital mucosa in a regional rather than a localized manner. HPV 6/11 in particular can be found at all anogenital sites.[52,68] As well as the genital tract, HPV 6/11 clearly infects and causes macroscopic lesions in the oropharynx and larynx (see Chapter 8). Several studies have documented the frequency of oral lesions in patients with genital warts.[46,72] It is very likely that HPV carriage in this site also exceeds macroscopic disease and that transmission of the virus occurs by orogenital as well as by genito-genital contact.

Even low-risk HPVs such as type 6 have occasionally been found in tumors such as penile carcinomas.[62] Furthermore, infected keratinocytes found in genital warts are clearly abnormal and are growing excessively although not invasively. Thus, although the low-risk HPVs are less oncogenic than the high-risk ones, it would be wrong to suggest that they have absolutely no tumorigenic potential. On the contrary, one reason to study genital warts is precisely as a model of disordered keratinocyte growth. Much of the morbidity of benign genital warts lies in the cosmetic effect of ugly hypertrophic epidermal masses (Figure 6.1). Such masses may be considerably worse than cosmetic nuisances when they obstruct the anus or introitus. Keratinocyte excess may also fail to provide a flexible outer integument and contribute to the irritation and fissuring which also characterizes genital warts (Figure 6.2). Many of the tissue-destructive processes that are currently used to treat warts may contribute to this process by promoting the growth of inelastic fibrous tissue subcutaneously.

Another histological abnormality associated with warts is the promotion of host vascular beds in order to support them – analogous to the neovascularization in cervical neoplasia.[56] Because the epidermis has no vasculature, these must be induced in the dermis for excessive epidermal growth to be metabolically supported. The release of angiogenic factors by HPV-infected cells is a possible target of therapeutic agents. Treatment of HPV lesions could also be developed from agents which specifically interfere with viral metabolism. However, the relatively small and thrifty papillomaviruses only code for an E1 helicase and are generally highly dependent upon host machinery. In general, antiviral agents for papillomaviruses are at an early stage of development, although there are case reports of

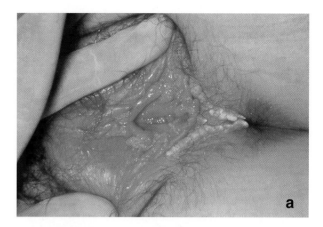
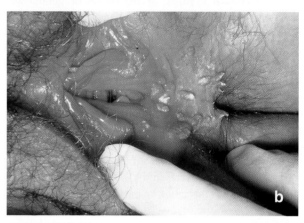

Figure 6.1
Vulval warts. (a) Extensive genital warts around introitus and extending in a linear arrangement toward the anterior anal margin. (b) Same patient, six weeks later, without any treatment. Warts are present but regressing.

the use of intralesional nucleotide analogs in upper aero-digestive tract papillomatosis[67] and anogenital disease in immunodeficient subjects.[57]

Both genital and cutaneous warts are very common in immunosuppressed individuals such as organ transplant recipients and those infected with human immunodeficiency virus (HIV). Such patients are also at high risk of intra-epithelial neoplastic and even malignant change within such lesions.[21,39] Cutaneous malignancies are a substantial cause of morbidity and death in organ transplant recipients (see Chapter 10). Furthermore, the types of HPV found, especially in the cutaneous warts of these patients, tend to be those of

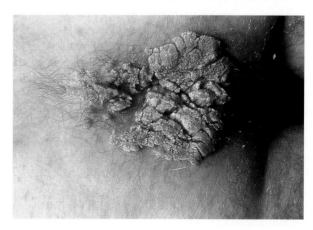

Figure 6.2
Perianal warts. A large mass of perianal warts extending into the natal cleft. Deep fissures develop between the protruberances.

the epidermodysplasia verruciformis group, i.e., types that are characteristically found in individuals with a specific genetic susceptibility to disseminated warts (see Chapter 9). Taken as a whole, these facts point to an immune basis for infection with papillomaviruses in these patients such that the conversion of subclinical to overt clinical infection and the development of neoplasia depend on the degree of immunological deficit and other cofactors. Perhaps even the spectrum of latent infection with HPV 6/11 versus the clinical manifestations of genital warts may itself have an immunological basis in immunocompetent subjects.

Regression of genital warts is a well-attested clinical phenomenon (as is that of certain cutaneous warts, Chapter 5). The most familiar example of regression of genital warts occurs in, or more usually immediately after, pregnancy. During pregnancy, massive growth of genital warts is not uncommon[45] – rarely, this can lead to obstetric problems. Characteristically, such warts regress in the puerperium. The factors underlying such manifestations are poorly understood, but could include the relative immunological tolerance of pregnancy enhancing HPV replication, growth factors, including hormones acting as promoters of viral transcription of HPV 6/11 as of other HPV types,[47] and the altered vascular environment of the lower genital tract. Regression of genital warts in the *absence* of such physiological perturbation is rarer, but we have observed regression to less than 50% of the original size of some individual warts in 22% of untreated patients over a 4-week period in both non-pregnant female and male patients (see Figure 6.1).[13] Similar observations had previously been made by others.[8]

A comparison of biopsies taken from regressing and from non-regressing warts of our patients showed striking differences. Whereas non-regressing warts showed no infiltrate of inflammatory cells, warts which were clinically regressing almost uniformly showed a striking lymphocytic infiltrate, both in the subepidermal stroma and in the epidermis itself (where normally very few such cells are found). Immunohistochemical staining of these lymphocytes revealed that they were largely CD4+ve cells and showed evidence of activation (expressing CD25). Evidence of activation was also suggested by the expression of accessory molecules, e.g., intercellular adhesion molecule (ICAM) and human leukocyte antigen (HLA) class II molecules, on the epithelial keratinocytes of regressing warts (but not in non-regressing warts). Such expression could be induced by cytokines e.g., interferon-α (IFN-α) released by infiltrating CD4+ve lymphocytes.[13] Bishop and colleagues did not observe this striking infiltrate in their regressing wart biopsies – possibly because these were taken before regression had begun.[8] The lymphocytic infiltrates we observed are very similar to those seen by Tagami and colleagues in regressing flat warts of the skin.[2,27] The primary immunological mechanism which precipitates the CD4-cell-dominated, delayed-type hypersensitivity mechanism of wart regression found in our study remains under investigation. The mechanisms appear distinct from those mediated by CD8+ve lymphocytes, which respond to endogenous peptides presented with class I molecules.[73] Recent data suggest that interleukin-12 is acting as the key cytokine in this CD4+ T helper 1(Th1) lymphocyte-mediated phenomenon.[53]

Mechanism apart, histochemical analysis of regressing genital (and other) warts supports an immunological mechanism for the abrogation of viral infection. This is not surprising as most viral infection resolves in this way. There are several mechanisms whereby papillomaviruses may evade immune surveillance, one being their tropism to epithelial cell layers where immunocompetent cells are rare. While this may contribute both to their chronicity and to their evolutionary success, it does not imply that papillomavirus infection must be resolved in a non-immunological way. It is possible that some current therapies may succeed precisely by stimulating a local inflammatory response and local cellular immunity. Similarly, there is optimism that the success of vaccines in animal models of papillomavirus infection may lead to better treatment for anogenital warts (and other human papillomavirus diseases).

6.3 TRANSMISSION OF GENITAL WARTS

Epidemics of genital warts that have occurred following sexual exposure in humans confirm the long-held theory that this condition is sexually transmissible.[4] How efficient is such transmission is very much less clear. Oriel's pioneering study of the natural history of genital warts looked at this question by trying to follow all sexual contacts of patients with warts in the 9 months before the diagnosis was made and new contacts in the 9 months after diagnosis.[45] Oriel commented that this was 'the most difficult part of this study;' his valiant effort has never been repeated. Out of a population of 332 patients with warts, 97 secondary contacts were examined, of whom 62 (64%) developed warts themselves (after an interval of 3 weeks to 8 months, average 2.8 months). These figures seem to be an accurate reflection of the infectivity and incubation periods of genital warts.[33]

6.4 ANOGENITAL WARTS IN CHILDREN: IMPLICATIONS FOR ADULTS

Anogenital warts are rare in children below the age of sexual consent but can present from birth onwards.[34,63] Viral transmission in such cases may take place vertically, horizontally (through inoculation from a cutaneous wart either of the child or from a contact), or through sexual abuse. Vertical transmission is well described, HPV DNA having been detected in amniotic fluid and in samples taken from neonates.[55] Vertical transmission may be the cause of upper aero-digestive tract papillomata of juveniles (see Chapter 7). HPV types 2a/27/57 are found in approximately a sixth of cases of genital warts in children and are usually associated with cutaneous warts in either the mother or the child.[34] Also, anogenital warts are found in some children who have been sexually abused. Such cases cannot be identified by HPV typing alone. (For a more detailed discussion of this subject, see references 15 and 34.)

The observations of pediatric genital warts raise important implications for adult genital warts. If horizontal transmission can take place in children, then non-sexual acquisition of genital warts should be considered in adults too. If vertical transmission can result in disease years later, how long could the incubation time for adult warts be? A familiar situation in STD practice involves the patient with newly presenting genital warts who denies exogamous sexual contact (or sometimes *any* sexual contact) for several years previously. Such cases are anecdotal and lacking of proof, but the accepted course of HPV-related malignancy (i.e., clinical disease occurring *years* after infection) furnishes an instance of a spectacularly long 'incubation period'.

6.5 OTHER SHIBBOLETHS ABOUT GENITAL WARTS

To the folly of excluding a prolonged incubation period for genital warts is commonly added the stigma of prolonged or even permanent infectivity. This unproven prejudice is widespread and causes enormous anxiety to patients. There are data showing that the standard treatments currently used do not clear HPV.[19] However, this is unsurprising in view of the regional nature of the infection and the lack of antiviral effect of most current treatments (see above). Regional infection also predicts that barrier methods may not reduce transmission. Studies of HPV acquisition in young women have supported this view (Koutsky LA, personal communication). The common prescription of condoms to long-standing monogamous couples when one develops warts seems particularly unwarranted because viral transmission is likely to have taken place already. Cohort studies strongly suggest that older populations do acquire greater resistance to the virus and there is no reason to doubt that this generally occurs in the infected individual also. Possibly a majority of the population have had 'common' warts of the hands or 'verruca vulgaris' of the feet at some stage in their lives. Both these entities can be stubborn. Yet years later, most people are unafraid to shake hands or to walk barefoot. There is no evidence to suggest long-term infectivity of genital warts.

Of all the fears prevalent and perpetuated among patients with genital warts, that of an increased risk of genital malignancy is most widespread. A significant rate of cervical intraepithelial neoplasia is certainly common amongst female patients with genital warts and, as well, a small number of genital warts contain and may be caused by high-risk HPV types of the kind found in anogenital malignancies.

Indeed, a number of case-control studies of women with invasive cervical cancer and pre-cancer documented an increased frequency of a history of condylomata acuminata compared with controls. This evidence was summarized by Muñoz and Bosch.[43] As 95% of genital wart biopsies contain HPV 6 and 11,[10] which in turn are only found in 0.2% of cervical cancer tissues, they proposed that the observed association between genital warts and cervical cancer might be explained if genital warts were markers of infection with other HPV types that were causally associated with cervical cancer. This hypothesis was explored by Lacey *et al.*,[35] who studied 470 women attending a STD clinic. The study population comprised 268 women with genital warts, 151 women with abnormal cytology, and 51 control women. All subjects had cytology, an HPV-DNA assay, colposcopy and biopsies of any aceto-white area. In multivariate analysis

only the presence of HPV 16 (odds ratio (OR) 3.8, 95% confidence interval 2.3–6.3) and abnormal cytology (OR 3.0, 95% confidence interval 2.0–4.5 for mild dyskaryosis or worse) were independently associated with cervical intraepithelial neoplasia (CIN) 2/3. Therefore, in women with genital warts, the risk of high-grade cervical intraepithelial neoplasia is related to concurrent HPV 16 infection, rather than to the presence of genital warts themselves. This evidence also supports cervical cytology as a valid screening test for cervical neoplasia in women with genital warts.

We would therefore propose that proper and sufficient management of women with genital warts should include cervical cytology, unless this has been performed recently. If this is negative, the women should be returned to routine screening as defined by local practice. However, if cervical warts or a macroscopic abnormality of the cervix is identified by speculum examination a colposcopic examination should be performed.

Several other studies have shown that patients with warts are at risk of other STDs and should be screened for them. Twenty-eight percent of male and 23% of female patients with warts had other STDs diagnosed at the time of presentation with warts.[7] However, there was no significant relation between outcome and past or present STD. An exception to this would be HIV infection, which has been shown to worsen the outcome of treatment for warts (an effect probably mediated by immunosuppression). Thus, in areas of high HIV prevalence, warts are becoming an increasing therapeutic problem and are often associated with intraepithelial neoplasia (see Chapter 10).

6.6 TREATMENT

Current therapies and some of those under development are summarized in Table 6.1. None of the compounds discussed under antiviral agents is licensed for treatment at the current time. None of the other categories of treatment is known directly to target viral components in replication, although the antimitotic agents affect replication via cellular targets. HPV is not cytopathic and is poorly recognized by the immune system. It is possible that any of the first four categories of therapy may be associated with induction of an immune response, although evidence is lacking.

6.6.1 Antimitotic agents

Podophyllin/podophyllotoxin
Podophyllin is a crude resin extract prepared from the roots of different species of *Berberidacae* (May apple). *Podophyllum peltatum* is the Northern American species and *Podophyllum emodi* is native to the Far East. In Europe podophyllin resin is imported as a dry powder from China and is prepared

Table 6.1
Medical therapy for genital warts

Antimitotic agents
Antiviral agents
Destructive/excision therapies
Cryotherapy
Immunomodulators/vaccines

from *P. emodi*, whereas in North America it may be derived from *P. peltatum*.

Although Kaplan first recorded the efficacy of podophyllin resin (25% in mineral oil) for the treatment of genital warts,[29] its usage in this condition probably substantially predates this.[61] Podophyllin is not a uniform substance and contains a number of active constituents, although podophyllotoxin has been shown to be the most active of these in animal models.[44] Both podophyllin and podophyllotoxin may cause local adverse effects such as inflammation, edema, and ulceration. Severe systemic toxicity may arise after topical use of podophyllin, most commonly when it is applied in large volumes. Death, intrauterine death, teratogenicity, and a variety of neurological and other complications have all been described.[20]

Unsatisfactory response rates and side-effects with podophyllin led to further study of podophyllotoxin as a primary therapy. In a mouse model, it was shown to cause both epidermal and dermal necrosis, as well as dermal microcirculatory injury.[70] A regimen of patient-applied podophyllotoxin 0.5% solution twice a day for 3 days in weekly cycles was developed and shown to be effective, and this regimen was also shown to be free of systemic absorption and toxicity.[44]

Until recently, podophyllotoxin had only been formulated as an alcoholic solution. However, this was not ideal for application by women, nor by men perianally. Therefore, stable cream preparations of podophyllotoxin were developed. There are a number of studies which have reported direct comparisons of the efficacy of podophyllin and podophyllotoxin solution or cream in the treatment of genital warts (Table 6.2),[17,25,30,36,38] as well as two comparative studies of podophyllotoxin 0.5% solution versus 0.3% cream versus 0.15% cream (Table 6.3).[12,59] Certainly the last three studies in Table 6.2 were able to demonstrate superior efficacy of podophyllotoxin formulations compared to podophyllin. The studies, which included direct comparisons of podophyllotoxin solution versus cream (Table 6.3),[36] essentially showed equivalence of the two preparations, with some marginal superiority of podophyllotoxin solution in some analyses. Podophyllotoxin cream is only currently available in the UK, Ireland, and other European countries, whilst a podophyllotoxin gel preparation is available in the USA.

Fluorouracil

5-Fluorouracil in the form of a 5% cream has been available for a number of years. Its use on the external genitalia is limited by the marked degree of inflammation it produces. It is occasionally useful for intrameatal lesions if used on a twice weekly schedule.

6.6.2 Antiviral agents

Idoxuridine

Two small trials have studied the use of idoxuridine as treatment for genital warts. Hasumi compared 0.25% idoxuridine ointment with placebo in a randomized double-blind trial in 24 women.[24] Twice-daily application for 2 weeks resulted in 11/14 complete regressions in the active group and none in the placebo group. Happonen *et al.* compared 0.25% with 0.5% idoxuridine cream in a randomized double-blind trial involving 50 men.[23] Twice-daily application for 4 weeks resulted in 19/25 and 13/25 complete clearances in the 0.25% and 0.5% groups respectively.

Table 6.2
Podophyllin versus podophyllotoxin b.d. for 3 days in the treatment of genital warts

Study	Treatments	Maximum duration (weeks)	Initial complete clearance Males (%)	Females (%)
Lassus (1987)[38]	Podophyllin 20%, × 1/week	4	37/52 (71)	–
	Podophyllotoxin solution 0.5%	4	48/48 (100)	–
Edwards et al. (1988)[17]	Podophyllin 20%, × 1/week	6	12/19 (63)	–
	Podophyllotoxin solution 0.5%	6	28/32 (88)	–
Kinghorn et al. (1993)[30]	Podophyllin 25%, × 2/week	5	26/36 (72)	16/26 (62)
	Podophyllotoxin solution 0.5%	5	83/97 (86)	32/41 (78)
Hellberg et al. (1995)[25]	Podophyllin 20%, × 1/week	4	–	16/27 (59)
	Podophyllotoxin cream 0.5%	4	–	23/28 (82)
Lacey et al.[36]	Podophyllin 25%, × 2/week	4	–	–
	Podophyllotoxin solution 0.5%	4	–	–
	Podophyllotoxin cream 0.5%	4	–	–

Table 6.3
Comparative studies of podophyllotoxin solution and cream, b.d. for 3 days in four cycles of 1 week each for the treatment of genital warts

		Initial complete clearance 0.5% solution	0.3% cream	0.15% cream
Strand et al. (1995)[59]	Males	24/29 (83%)	25/31 (81%)	21/30 (70%)
Claesson et al. (1996)[12]	Males	20/30 (67%)	19/30 (63%)	13/30 (43%)
	Females	23/30 (77%)	22/30 (73%)	19/30 (63%)

However, caution is necessary when considering further development of this agent as there are two case reports of squamous carcinoma of the lip[31] and penis[65] following its use for herpes simplex.

Cidofovir

Cidofovir is one agent in a class of compounds termed phosphonomethyl ethers. It is a nucleotide analog, related to, but chemically distinct from, nucleoside analogs such as aciclovir and ganciclovir. It is phosphorylated by cellular enzymes to metabolites with a long intracellular half-life (24 hours) and has potent activity against a spectrum of viruses including HIV, herpesviruses, and HPVs. There are individual case reports of its activity in a topical formulation as treatment for genital warts in HIV-infected subjects[57] and also in an injectable form for upper respiratory tract papillomatosis.[67]

6.6.3 Destructive/excision therapies

Trichloroacetic acid

Trichloroacetic acid (TCA) is another topical therapy commonly used in the treatment of genital warts. It is a clinic-based treatment in which a 90% solution is applied directly to the warts. Burning at the site of application is common and usually subsides after 10–15 minutes. TCA has no specific therapeutic properties other than being a locally destructive therapy. One of the problems of TCA is in controlling the depth of tissue destruction. If dermal injury occurs, healing will take longer and scarring is more likely. The local side-effects are therefore potentially unpleasant if it is applied without appropriate care. However, TCA does benefit from a complete lack of systemic side-effects and can be used in pregnancy. There are surprisingly few data regarding efficacy. One study comparing TCA to cryotherapy found no significant difference, with 81% clearance and a 36% recurrence rate for those treated with TCA, compared with 88% clearance and 39% recurrence for the cryotherapy.[22] Another study comparing TCA to cryotherapy with liquid nitrogen documented 70% clearance after six applications of TCA versus 86% after six applications of liquid nitrogen.[1] TCA is probably of similar therapeutic efficacy to podophyllin, but has a greater tendency to cause ulceration and scarring if not used cautiously. It remains an alternative topical therapy which can be used in pregnancy.

Laser therapy

Carbon dioxide laser therapy remains a useful treatment modality, especially for extensive warts or where there is vaginal, vulval, or anal intraepithelia neoplasia. There is, however, a high recurrence rate of genital warts after laser therapy.

Scissor excision

Scissor excision as a specific therapy for perianal and anal condylomata was first described by Thompson and Grace.[66] The technique clearly requires local anesthesia and operator technique, but has a number of advantages. A randomized comparison with once-weekly podophyllin showed initial complete clearance of 93% versus 77% for excision versus podophyllin and recurrence rates at 6 months of 22% versus 56%. Although published descriptions usually only refer to its use in the anal region it is equally applicable to other external genital sites.

Electrosurgical techniques

These can be divided into electrocautery, in which direct current flows only through the instrument to produce heat, and not through the patient, and into those more modern systems in which alternating current is used.[54] The alternating current systems can produce differing types of waveforms which produce cutting, coagulation, or a blend of the two. These systems should only use isolated circuitry, but can use monopolar or bipolar instruments. Patient return electrodes should always be used. The principal development in this field in recent years was the modification by Prendiville of Cartier's original technique with his description of large loop excision of the transformation zone.[49] The same equipment, with minor modifications to technique can be used for the treatment of external genital lesions.[58]

6.6.4 Cryotherapy

Freezing of external genital warts causes epidermal and dermal cellular necrosis. Shortly after freezing, dermal vascular damage and edema are also seen. Two methods of freezing can be employed. First, liquid nitrogen can be applied by cotton swab or spray gun. Second, a cryoprobe with a closed system using either gaseous nitrous oxide or carbon dioxide or liquid nitrogen can be utilized. Freezing is applied to each wart for a variable time so that the wart and 1–2 mm of the surrounding margin of normal skin are frozen. This can be done for one or two freeze/thaw cycles. Discomfort is mild to moderate, so that anesthesia is rarely required. A 'burning' sensation is produced at the time of freezing, with the discomfort lasting a variable time afterwards, usually 10–15 minutes but occasionally longer. Freezing can lead to erythema, edema, and blister formation. Occasionally, necrosis and ulceration may occur. Typically, the freeze time required to obtain a good cure rate does not lead to scarring.

Efficacy from 79% to 88% with recurrences in 21–39% using multiple treatments have been documented.[22,58] Although the number of treatment sessions needed to clear clinically apparent warts is variable, the majority experience a resolution with three treatments or fewer. Although cryotherapy requires special equipment and can be uncomfortable, it offers a relatively inexpensive treatment option which does not require local anesthesia and does not lead to scarring if properly used. Cryotherapy offers a further, safe method of treatment which can be used to good effect throughout pregnancy.

6.6.5 Immunomodulators/vaccines

Interferons

Interferons (IFNs) are a group of glycoproteins with antiviral, immunoregulatory, and antiproliferative properties. They have been used successfully in other viral infections and have been evaluated in the context of HPV-related disease. IFNs have been administered topically, intralesionally, subcutaneously, and intramuscularly, with recombinant IFN-α most extensively studied. The results have, however, been variable. Most patients who receive systemic therapy experience dose-related adverse reactions similar to non-specific viral symptoms (e.g., fever, headache, fatigue, myalgia, etc). Intralesional therapy can achieve higher local concentrations without or with minimal systemic reactions. Several randomized, placebo-controlled trials of patients with genital warts have demonstrated a degree of efficacy of intralesional IFN-α and IFN-β compared to placebo,[32] and intralesional IFN-α, when combined with podophyllin, was superior to podophyllin alone.[16] However, the modest efficacy, inconvenience, and cost have precluded its use by this route. IFN has also been evaluated as an adjunct to more conventional therapies. However, IFN-α has been shown not to affect outcome compared to placebo following carbon dioxide laser ablation.[64] Similarly, a recent study comparing IFN-α, IFN-β, IFN-γ, or placebo in combination with cryotherapy found no difference in response.[9] IFN therapy has never really gained a therapeutic niche. It is expensive, with a potential for adverse effects and no real advantage in terms of efficacy. It is, therefore, not recommended for routine clinical practice.

Inosine pranobex

This is a synthetic immunomodulatory agent that has secondary antiviral effects. Rigorous evaluation of the agent has been limited, and the only published double-blind, placebo-controlled study of inosine pranobex as treatment for genital warts does not convincingly document efficacy.[14] The agent is certainly safe, including when used in HIV-infected individuals.

Imiquimod

Imiquimod is a member of a new class of imidazoquinolines and has shown potent immunomodulating, antiviral, and antitumor activities in animal models. In human peripheral blood mononuclear cells, it induces a wide array of cytokines, including IFN-α, IL-1, IL-6, IL-8, granulocyte/macrophage colony-stimulating factor (GM-CSF) and macrophage inflammatory protein-1α (MIP-1α). Topical application of 5% cream to mouse skin resulted in increased IFN-α mRNA.[3] In a pivotal phase III trial using 5% imiquimod cream for up to 16 weeks, 77% of women and 40% of men in an on-treatment analysis completely cleared their genital warts.[18] In imiquimod-cleared patients, a recurrence rate of only 13% was observed. Imiquimod 5% cream is now licensed for the treatment of anogenital warts.

Vaccines

The concept of using antigens found in HPV-infected tissue to stimulate an infected subjects's immune response is not new, and Biberstein reported the use of autogenous wart vaccines in 1925.[6] There was some renewed interest in the technique in the 1970s, but a properly designed study failed to show benefit.[41]

However, in recent years, experiments in a number of animal papillomavirus systems have demonstrated that either protection from infection or regression of established infection can be induced by administration of various early and late proteins, or peptides, or DNA, or virus-like particles.[11,40] These findings have stimulated a number of groups to establish development programs for HPV vaccines. Recently, the results of phase I/II trials of an HPV 6 L2E7 fusion protein vaccine as a therapeutic agent for genital warts have been presented.[37] These showed safety, immuno-genicity *in vitro*, and encouraging clinical responses. The prospects for prophylactic and therapeutic vaccines are discussed more fully in Chapter 12.

6.7 MANAGEMENT STRATEGIES

Having screened for other STDs in the patient presenting with genital warts, the physician may be uncomfortably aware that they were rather easier to treat than the warts themselves! In our series examining male and female patients undergoing a standard treatment regime at a UK STD clinic, relapse after the first course of treatment occurred in 75% of the men and 37% of the women. Thirty-nine percent of men (and 22% of women) were still undergoing treatment 6 months after presentation with warts.[7]

The wide variety of commonly used treatments is a reflection of the problems of the treatment of genital warts. However, at least as much of a problem is discouragement (of both patient and doctor!) and inappropriate or repetitive treatments. Von Krogh and Wikstrom achieved wart clearance for at least 3 months after only four courses of treatment in 77% of men who had 'resistant' warts which had persisted for at least a year despite treatment.[71] Each course consisted either of topical podophyllotoxin or scissor excision. Choosing an appropriate treatment is a key factor in the successful management of warts. In an audit of wart treatment,[51] it was noted that 96% of men and 84% of women were treated with podophyllin 25%. Only 1% of male patients were prescribed podophyllotoxin as primary treatment. Forty-four percent of men and 38% of women still had warts at 3 months. A treatment algorithm was introduced by Reynolds *et al.*[50] Essentially, this prescribed more cryotherapy or trichloroacetic acid and podophyllotoxin as primary treatment but also encouraged treatment *change* in the event of partial or non-response. After these guidelines had been in place for 6 months, the number of men and women still receiving treatment at 3 months had fallen to 8% and 3% respectively.[50] Further support for the place of patient-applied therapy emerged from pharmaco-economic analyses of treatments for genital warts, which suggested that self-applied therapy, such as podophyllotoxin, results in overall lowest treatment costs.[36,60]

6.8 SUMMARY

At present, management of the patient with genital warts usually involves two broad phases – pre-treatment and treatment. Before embarking on any treatment it is important to a) be sure of the diagnosis, b) screen for and treat any other sexually-transmitted diseases and c) explain to the patient the available therapies and the likelihood or otherwise of a successful response. Treatment will be based on a number of considerations, especially cost, convenience, patient acceptability and effectiveness. In most cases, podophyllotoxin is the first treatment of choice, but for some, and for those in whom the initial approach is unsuccessful, other therapies such as topical trichloroacetic acid, imiquimod, freezing or surgery will often be considered. However, if the development of immunotherapy and anti-viral agents proves to be very successful, a treatment algorithm for these patients could look very different in a few decades.

REFERENCES

1. Abdullah AN, Walzman M, Wade A. (1993) Treatment of external genital warts comparing cryotherapy (liquid nitrogen) and trichloroacetic acid. *Sex Transm Dis* **20**: 344–5.

2. Aiba S, Rokugo M, Tagami H. (1986) Immunohistologic analysis of the phenomenon of spontaneous regression of numerous flat warts. *Cancer* **58**: 1246–51.

3. Arany I, Tyring SK, Stanley MA, *et al.* (1999) Enhancement of the innate cellular immune response in patients with genital warts treated with topical Imiquimod cream 5%. *Antiviral Res* **43**: 55–63.

4. Barrett TJ, Silbar JD, McGinlay JP.(1954) Genital warts – a venereal disease. *J Am Med Assoc* **154**: 333–4.

5. Bauer HM, Ting Y, Greer CE, *et al.* (1991) Genital human papillomavirus infection in female university students as determined by a PCR-based method. *J Am Med Assoc* **265**: 472–7.

6. Biberstein J. (1925) Versuche über immunotherapie der warzen und kondylome. *Klin Wochenschr* **4**: 638–41.

7. Birley HDL, Kupek E, Byrne M, Whitaker L, Renton AM. (1994) Clinical features and outcome of anogenital warts in men and women. *J Eur Acad Dermatol Venereol* **3**: 198–205.

8. Bishop PE, McMillan A, Fletcher S. (1990) An immunohistological study of spontaneous regression of condylomata acuminata. *Genitourin Med* **66**: 79–81.

9. Bonnez W, Oakes D, Bailey-Farchione A, *et al.* (1995) A randomised, double-blind, placebo-controlled trial of systemically administered interferon-α, -β or -γ in combination with cryotherapy for treatment of condylomata acuminata. *J Infect Dis* 171: 1081–9.

10. Bosch FX, Manos MM, Muñoz N, *et al.* (1995) Prevalence of human papillomavirus in cervical cancer: a worldwide perspective. *J Natl Cancer Inst* **87**: 796–802.

11. Campo MS. (1994) Towards vaccines against papillomavirus. In *Human papillomaviruses and cervical cancer. Biology and immunology*, eds PL Stern, MA Stanley. Oxford: Oxford University Press, 177–91.

12. Claesson U, Lassus A, Happonen H, Hogstrom L, Siboulet A. (1996) Topical treatment of venereal warts: a comparative open study of podophyllotoxin cream versus solution. *Int J STD AIDS* **7**: 429–34.

13. Coleman N, Birley HDL, Renton AM, *et al.* (1994) Immunological events in regressing genital warts. *Am J Clin Pathol* **102**: 768–74.

14. Davidson-Parker J, Dinsmore W, Khan MH, Hicks DA, Morris CA, Morris DF. (1988) Immunotherapy of genital warts with inosine pranobex and conventional treatment: double blind placebo controlled study. *Genitourin Med* **64**: 383–6.

15. de Villiers E-M. (1995) Importance of human papillomavirus DNA typing in the diagnosis of ano-genital warts in children. *Arch Dermatol* **131**: 366–7.

16. Douglas JM, Eron LJ, Judson FN, *et al.* (1990) A randomised trial of combination therapy with intralesional interferon-α$_{2b}$ and podophyllin versus podophyllin alone for the therapy of anogenital warts. *J Infect Dis* **162**: 52–9.

17. Edwards A, Atma-Ram A, Thin RN. (1988) Podophyllotoxin 0.5% *v* podophyllin 20% to treat penile warts. *Genitourin Med* **64**: 263–5.

18. Edwards L, Ferenczy A, Eron L, and the HPV Study Group. (1998) Self administered topical 5% Imiquimod cream for external anogenital warts. *Arch Dermatol* **134**: 25–30.

19. Ferenczy A, Mitao M, Nagai N, Silverstein S, Crum C. (1985) Latent papillomavirus and recurring genital warts. *N Engl J Med* **313**: 784–8.

20. Fraser PA, Lacey CJN, Maw RD. (1993) Motion: podophyllotoxin is superior to podophyllin in the treatment of genital warts. *J Eur Acad Dermatol Venereol* **2**: 328–34.

21. Fruchter RG, Maiman M, Sedlis A, Bartley L, Camilien L, Arrastia CD. (1996) Multiple recurrences of cervical intraepithelial neoplasia in women with the human immunodeficiency virus. *Obstet Gynecol* **87**: 338–44.

22. Godley MJ, Bradbeer CS, Gellan M, Thin RNT. (1987) Cryotherapy compared with trichloroacetic acid in treating genital warts. *Genitourin Med* **63**: 390–2.

23. Happonen H, Lassus A, Santalahti J, Forsstrom S, Lassus J. (1990) Topical idoxuridine for treatment of genital warts in males. A double-blind comparative study of 0.25% and 0.5% cream. *Genitourin Med* **66**: 254–6.

24. Hasumi K. (1987) A trial of topical idoxuridine for vulvar condylomatum. *Br J Obstet Gynaecol* **94**: 366–8.

25. Hellberg D, Svarrer T, Nilsson S, Valentin J. (1995) Self-treatment of female external genital warts with 0.5% podophyllotoxin cream (Condyline®) *vs* weekly applications of 20% podophyllin solution. *Int J STD AIDS* **6**: 257–61.

26. Inman GJ, Cook ID, Lau RKW. (1993) Human papillomaviruses, tumour suppressor genes and cervical cancer. *Int J STD AIDS* **4**: 128–34.

27. Iwatsuki K, Tagami H, Takigawa M, Yamada M. (1986) Plane warts under spontaneous regression: immunopathologic study on cellular constituents leading to the inflammatory reaction. *Arch Dermatol* **122**: 655–9.

28. Jensen SL. (1985) Comparison of podophyllin application with simple surgical excision in clearance and recurrence of perianal condylomata acuminata. *Lancet*, **ii**: 1146–8.

29. Kaplan IW. (1942) Condylomata acuminata. *New Orleans Med Surg J* **94**: 388–90.

30. Kinghorn GR, McMillan A, Mulcahy F, Drake S, Lacey C, Bingham JS. (1993) An open, comparative study of the efficacy of 0.5% podophyllotoxin lotion and 25% podophyllin solution in the treatment of condyloma acuminata in males and females. *Int J STD AIDS* **4**: 194–9.

31. Koppang HS, Aas E. (1983) Squamous carcinoma induced by topical idoxuridine therapy? *Br J Dermatol* **108**: 501–3.

32. Kraus SJ, Stone KM. (1990) Management of genital infections caused by human papillomavirus. *Rev Infect Dis* **12**: 5620–32.

33. Krebs HB, Helmkamp BF. (1991) Treatment failure of

genital condyloma acuminata in women: role of the male sexual partner. *Am J Obstet Gynecol* **165**: 337–40.

34. Lacey CJN. ed. (1996) Genital warts in children. In Lacey *Papillomavirus reviews – current research on papillomaviruses*. Leeds, Leeds Medical Information, 291–6.

35. Lacey CJN, Monteiro EF, Macdermott RIJ, Andrew A, Gibson P. (1996) High grade CIN: associations and screening strategies. *Genitourin Med* **72**: 304.

36. Lacey CJN, Tennvall GR, and the Perstorp Pharma Clinical Trial Group (submitted) Randomised controlled trial and economic evaluation of patient-applied podophyllotoxin solution or cream, or clinic-applied podophyllin in the treatment of genital warts.

37. Lacey CJ, Thompson HS, Monteiro EF, *et al.* (1999) Phase IIa safety and immugenicity of a therapeutic vaccine, TA-GW, in persons with genital warts. *J Infect Dis* **179**: 612–18.

38. Lassus A. (1987) Comparison of podophyllotoxin and podophyllin in the treatment of genital warts. *Lancet* **ii**: 512–13.

39. London NJ, Farmerty SM, Will EJ, Davison AM, Lodge PA. (1995) Risk of neoplasia in renal transplant patients. *Lancet* **346**: 403–6.

40. Ludmerer SM, McClements WL, Wang XM, Ling JC, Jansen KU, Christensen ND. (2000) HPV11 mutant virus-like particles elicit immune responses that neutralize virus and delineate a novel neutralizing domain. *Virology* **266**: 237–45.

41. Malison MD, Morris R, Jones LW. (1982) Autogenous vaccine therapy for condyloma acuminatum. A double-blind controlled study. *Br J Vener Dis* **58**: 62–7.

42. Melkert PWJ, Hopman E, van den Brule AJC, *et al.* (1993) Prevalence of HPV in cytomorphologically normal cervical smears, as determined by the polymerase chain reaction. *Int J Cancer* **53**: 919–23.

43. Muñoz N, Bosch FX. (1992) HPV and cervical neoplasia, review of case-control and cohort studies. In *The epidemiology of cervical cancer and human papillomavirus*, eds Muñoz N, Bosch FX, Shah KV, Meheus A. *IARC Scientific Publications* **No. 119**. Lyon, IARC, 251–61.

44. Murphy ME, Lacey CJN. (1996) Podophyllin or podophyllotoxin as treatment for condylomata acuminata? In *Papillomavirus reviews – current research on papillomaviruses*, ed. CJN Lacey. Leeds, Leeds Medical Information, 309–15.

45. Oriel, JD. (1971) Natural history of genital warts. *Br J Vener Dis* **467**: 1–13.

46. Panici PB, Scambia G, Perrone L, *et al.* (1992) Oral condyloma lesions in patients with extensive genital human papillomavirus infection. *Am J Obstet Gynecol* **167**: 451–8.

47. Pater A, Bayatpour M, Pater MM. (1990) Oncogenic transformation by human papillomavirus type 16 deoxyribonucleic acid in the presence of progesterone or progestins from oral contraceptives. *Am J Obstet Gynecol* **162**: 1099–103.

48. Persson G, Andersson K, Krantz I. (1996) Symptomatic genital papillomavirus infection in a community. Incidence and clinical picture. *Acta Obstet Gynecol Scand* **75**: 287–90.

49. Prendiville W, Cullimore J, Norman S. (1989) Large loop excision of transformation zone (LLETZ). A new method of management for women with cervical intraepithelial neoplasia. *Br J Obstet Gynaecol* **96**: 105–460.

50. Reynolds M, Fraser PA, Lacey CJN. (1996) Audit of the treatment of genital warts: closing the feedback loop. *Int J STD AIDS* **7**: 347–52.

51. Reynolds M, Murphy M., Waugh MA, Lacey CJN. (1993) An audit of treatment of genital warts: opening the feedback loop. *Int J STD AIDS* **4**: 226–31.

52. Rymark P, Forsland O, Hansson BG, Lindholm K. (1993) Genital HPV infection not a local but a regional infection: experience from a female teenage group. *Genitourin Med* **69**: 18–23.

53. Scarpini CG, Coleman N, Hanna N, *et al.* (1996). Interleukin-12, a key cytokine in the regression of genital warts, is produced by the infected keratinocytes. *15th International Papillomavirus Workshop*, Queensland, Abstract 246.

54. Scoular A. (1991) Choosing equipment for treating genital warts in genitourinary medicine clinics. *Genitourin Med* **67**: 413–19.

55. Sedlacek TV, Lindheim S, Elder C, *et al.* (1989) Mechanism for human papillomavirus transmission at birth. *Am J Obstet Gynecol* **161**: 55–9.

56. Smith-McCune KK, Weidner N. (1994) Demonstration and characterization of the angiogenic properties of cervical dysplasia. *Cancer Res* **54**: 800–64.

57. Snoeck R, van Ranst M, Andrei G, *et al.* (1995) Treatment of anogenital papillomavirus infections with an acyclic nucleoside phosphonate analogue. *N Engl J Med* **333**: 943–4.

58. Stone K, Becker T, Hadgu A, Kraus S. (1990) Treatment of external genital warts: a randomised clinical trial comparing podophyllin, cryotherapy, and electrodesiccation. *Genitourin Med* **66**: 16–19.

59. Strand A, Brinkeborn RM, Siboulet A. (1995) Topical treatment of genital warts in men, an open study of podophyllotoxin cream compared with solution. *Genitourin Med* **71**: 387–90.

60. Strauss MJ, Khanna V, Koenig JD, *et al.* (1996) The cost of treating genital warts. *Int J Dermatol* **35**: 340–8.

61. Sullivan M, King IS. (1947) Effects of resin of podophyllum on normal skin, condylomata acuminata and verrucae vulgares. *Arch Dermatol Syph* **56**: 30–45.

62. Syrjänen KJ. (1995) Association of human papillomavirus with penile cancer. In *Genital warts – human papillomavirus infection*, ed. A Mindel. London, Edward Arnold, 163–97.

63. Tang CK, Shermeta DW, Wood C. (1978) Congenital condylomata acuminatum. *Am J Obstet Gynecol* **131**: 912–13.

64. The Condyloma International Collaborative Study Group. (1993). Randomised placebo-controlled double-blind combined therapy with laser surgery and systemic interferon-α_{2a} in the treatment of anogenital condylomata acuminata. *J Infect Dis* **167**: 824–9.

65. Thompson J, O'Neill SM. (1976) Idoxuridine in dimethyl sulfoxide: is it carcinogenic in man? *J Cutan Pathol* **3**: 269.

66. Thompson JPS, Grace RH. (1978) The treatment of perianal and anal condylomata: a new operative technique. *J R Soc Med* **71**: 180–5.

67. van Cutsem E, Snoeck R, van Ranst M. (1995) Successful

treatment of a squamous papilloma of the hypopharynx–esophagus by local injections of (S)-1-(3-hydroxy-2-phosphonyl methoxypropyl) cytosine. *J Med Virol* **45**: 230–5.

68. Van Doornum GJJ, Prins M, Juffermans LHJ, *et al.* (1994) Regional distribution and incidence of human papillomavirus infections among heterosexual men and women with multiple sexual partners: a prospective study. *Genitourin Med* **70**: 240–6.

69. van Ranst M, Kaplan JB, Burk RD. (1992) Phylogenetic classification of human papillomaviruses: correlation with clinical manifestations. *J Gen Virol* **73**: 2653–60.

70. von Krogh G, Maibach HI. (1982) Cutaneous cytodestructive potency of lignans. I. A comparative evalua-

tion of influence on epidermal and dermal DNA synthesis and on dermal microcirculation in the hairless mouse. *Arch Dermatol Res* **274**: 9–20.

71. von Krogh G, Wikström A. (1991) Efficacy of chemical and/or surgical therapy against condylomata acuminata: retrospective evaluation. *Int J STD AIDS* **2**: 333–8.

72. Yeudall WA, Campo MS. (1991) Human papillomavirus in biopsies of oral tissues. *J Gen Virol* **72**: 173–6.

73. Zinkernagel RM, Doherty, PC. (1979) MHC-restricted cytotoxic T-cells: studies on the biological role of polymorphic major transplantation antigens determining T-cell restriction-specificity, function and responsiveness. *Ad Immunol* **27**: 51–177.

7

Human papillomavirus and oral disease

Catherine M. Flaitz and Sandra Felefli

7.1 INTRODUCTION

Human papillomaviruses (HPVs) have been identified in normal oral mucosa and in a variety of proliferative lesions involving the oral cavity. To date, over 25 HPV DNA genotypes have been identified and isolated in the oral cavity, including types 1, 2, 3, 4, 6, 7, 10, 11, 13, 16, 18, 30, 31, 32, 33, 35, 45, 51, 52, 55, 57, 59, 61, 69, 72, and 73 (Table 7.1).[13,17,28,82,83,86] Similar to other mucocutaneous sites, the most common oral manifestations associated with HPV infection are benign papillary surface lesions. However, the detection of this virus in normal oral mucosa and in a diverse group of benign, pre-malignant, and malignant lesions of the oral cavity makes it difficult to interpret the exact role, if any, that HPV plays in these other mucosal disorders.

7.2 SQUAMOUS PAPILLOMA

7.2.1 Natural history and clinical features

The squamous papilloma is the most common benign epithelial neoplasm affecting the oral mucosa. It makes up

Table 7.1
HPV types in oral lesions

	Common HPV types	Other HPV types	Common oral sites
Normal oral mucosa	6/11, 16/18	7, 31/33, 59, 61	
Squamous papilloma	6, 11	2, 13, 16, 32, 31/33/35	Soft palate, tongue
Verruca vulgaris	2, 4, 57	1, 6, 7, 11, 16	Vermilion border, labial mucosa
Condyloma acuminatum	6, 11	2, 16/18, 31/33/35	Labial mucosa, tongue, floor of mouth, gingiva
Focal epithelial hyperplasia	13, 32	6, 11, 16, 24	Labial mucosa, buccal mucosa, tongue
Koilocytic dysplasia	16/18, 31/33/35	6/11	Tongue, lips, buccal mucosa
Oral warts in human immunodeficiency virus	7, 32	2, 6, 11, 13, 16, 18, 55, 59, 69, 72, 73	Vermilion border, labial and buccal mucosa, gingiva, palate
Oral epithelial dysplasia	16/18	2, 6, 11, 31/33/35	Tongue, vermilion border, floor of mouth
Leukoplakia	6/11	2, 16/18	Vermilion border, buccal mucosa, gingiva
Proliferative verrucous leukoplakia	16	18	Buccal mucosa, tongue, gingiva
Verrucous carcinoma	6/11	2, 16/18	Mandibular vestibule, buccal mucosa, hard palate
Papillary squamous cell carcinoma	16/18	6/11	Tonsillar region, oropharynx
Squamous cell carcinoma	16/18	2, 3, 13, 31/33/35, 52, 57	Lateral and ventral tongue, floor of mouth, soft palate, gingiva

approximately 2% of all oral lesions submitted to surgical oral and maxillofacial pathology services,[1] with adult prevalence rates varying from 1/1000 to 4/1000 persons.[4,10] Although somewhat controversial, it is generally accepted that the squamous papilloma is a viral-induced lesion, and is primarily associated with HPV types 6, 11, and 16.[63] Infrequently, other HPV types have been identified in the squamous papilloma, including 2, 13, 16, 32, and 31/33/35.[45,55,68,79] HPV detection rates in squamous papilloma are quite variable but in most studies that strictly define squamous papilloma, they range from 13% to 80%.[17,63,77] The exact mode of transmission is not clearly understood, although direct contact is favored. In addition, the viruses in this lesion appear to have a very low virulence and infectivity rate, with a latency period for infection of 3–12 months.

The peak age of occurrence for the oral squamous papilloma is the third through the fifth decades, with a mean age of 36 years and with no significant gender predilection.[1] Although any oral mucosal site can be affected, the palatal complex and tongue are the most common sites. Clinically, these lesions present as solitary, soft, pedunculated enlargements with either numerous finger-like projections or a pebbly surface (Figure 7.1). The coloration may vary from white to pink to red, depending on the amount of surface keratinization and degree of secondary inflammation. Typically, these asymptomatic papillary lesions grow rapidly until reaching a maximum size of 0.2–1.0 cm and then remain static.

7.2.2 Histopathologic features

The squamous papilloma is characterized by a papillary proliferation of keratinized stratified squamous epithelium with thin fibrovascular connective tissue cores on a pedunculated base. Most lesions are hyperorthokeratinized, hyperparakeratinized, or both, and demonstrate a normal maturation pattern of the surface epithelium. However, occasional lesions exhibit mild atypia, including basilar hyperplasia, increased mitotic activity, individual cell keratinization, increased nuclear/cytoplasmic ratio and multinucleated giant epithelial cells.[1,77] Koilocytes are not a prominent finding and may not be identified at all. An inflammatory infiltrate within the underlying connective tissue stroma is a frequent finding due to secondary lesional trauma, which is usually chronic in nature. A candidal superinfection of the superficial epithelium may be detected among the papillary fronds.

7.2.3 Treatment and prognosis

Conservative surgical removal by excision, electrocautery, or laser ablation is the treatment of choice for the squamous papilloma. The recurrence rate of this lesion is low, with the largest series studied reporting that 4% recurred.[1] Although mild epithelial atypia may be observed in up to 25% of the lesions,[1,77] no malignant transformation, progressive enlargement, or dissemination to other oral mucosal sites has been documented, even when the lesions are present for many years.[56]

7.3 VERRUCA VULGARIS (COMMON WART)

7.3.1 Natural history and clinical features

The oral verruca vulgaris or common wart is analogous to the cutaneous counterpart but is infrequently observed in the oral cavity. In marked contrast to skin infections, the overall prevalence rate of oral verruca vulgaris in schoolchildren is estimated to be only 0.03%.[41] Because the skin of the hands is a common site of infection, it is speculated that many oral lesions develop from direct orocutaneous transmission, especially from autoinoculation. Recently, increased rates of oral warts have been described in immunocompromised populations, especially in human immunodeficiency virus (HIV)-positive individuals, transplant patients, and immunosuppressed cancer patients.[6,20,69,92] The development of oral warts in patients with an immune dysfunction may result from autoinoculation or may represent a latent HPV infection with the oral mucosa acting as a reservoir for new or recurring infections.[13,59]

Oral verrucae are associated with HPV types 1, 2, 4, 7, and 57,[3,21,32,59,94] with a detection rate of 55–75% in biopsied samples.[17,21,59] Although types 6, 11, and 16 have also been detected,[55,94] it has been suggested that lesions with mucosal HPV types actually represent squamous papillomas or oral condylomata, implicating another source of infection, such as an orogenital transmission.[72]

Significant clinical overlap exists between the common oral wart and the squamous papilloma. Similar to the squamous papilloma, the mean age at diagnosis in large studies is 35 years, with a wide age distribution spanning from the first through the eighth decades.[31] However, several limited investigations favor a younger age group, with most lesions observed in the second and third decades.[3,59,64] A male predilection is observed. The majority of oral verrucae occur on the vermilion and labial mucosa of the lips, followed by the palate, anterior tongue and gingiva. They are generally asymptomatic and present as white, rough, firm papules or nodules with a papillary, conical, or heavily stippled surface (Figure 7.2). Lesions on the vermilion border of the lip or perioral skin tend to be tan in color and scaly (Figure 7.3). The typical base of the lesion is sessile but, infrequently, a pedunculated appearance is detected. The usual finding is few to numerous orocutaneous warts that are often clustered; however, a single, discrete intraoral lesion

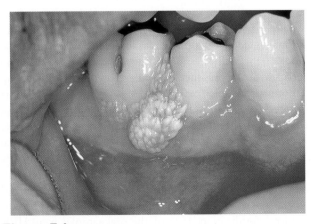

Figure 7.1
White nodule with multiple, finger-like projections of the gingiva, characteristic of a squamous papilloma.

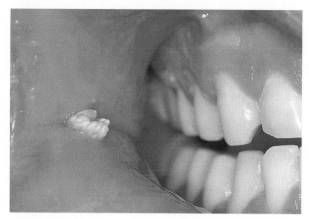

Figure 7.2
Verruca vulgaris of the buccal mucosa in an individual with perioral lesions.

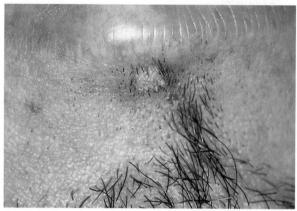

Figure 7.3
Verruca vulgaris of the perioral skin in the same individual as in Figure 7.2.

may be observed. The oral verruca develops suddenly, usually reaching a maximum size of 0.5–1.0 cm, and, unless traumatized, remains unchanged for several months to years.

7.3.2 Histopathology

The verruca vulgaris is characterized by a papillomatous proliferation of hyperkeratotic stratified squamous epithelium exhibiting acanthosis and hypergranulosis with prominent keratohyaline granules. The surface architecture is characterized by numerous blunted and/or acutely angulated hyperkeratotic projections with an underlying connective tissue core. The hyperkeratotic surface is usually a combination of orthokeratinization and parakeratinization, although a single type may be seen.[31] When the surface lining is parakeratotic, vertical tiers of nucleated cells, often displaying a smudgy effect, overlie the papillary crests. The elongated rete ridges tend to radiate toward the center of the lesion, producing a 'cupping' effect and discrete margins.[56] The supporting connective tissue usually contains a diffuse chronic inflammatory infiltrate. Abundant koilocytes may be observed in the upper spinous cell layer and granular cell layer, although this feature may not be as obvious in more mature lesions. Eosinophilic intranuclear viral inclusions may be found occasionally within the cells of the granular layer. In a few cases, the papillary projections are minimally exophytic and exhibit acanthotic bulbous rete ridges, which

tend to bend toward the center of the lesion. Mild epithelial atypia may be observed and is most prominent during the early proliferative phase.[30] Ultrastructural examination of oral verruca vulgaris demonstrates numerous viral particles within the nuclei, which often assumes a paracrystalline configuration.[90]

7.3.3 Treatment and prognosis

Oral verrucae are usually managed by surgical excision, laser ablation, electrocautery, or cryotherapy. Although conservative therapy is recommended, the treatment should extend to the base of the lesion to prevent recurrences. It is prudent to manage cutaneous lesions, especially those involving the hands, prior to the removal of oral or labial lesions to decrease the risk of re-infection. Occasionally, oral verrucae will resolve spontaneously, especially when the cutaneous lesions have been treated. This phenomenon of spontaneous resolution is more frequently observed in children. Recurrences are uncommon and there is no evidence of malignant transformation of oral verrucae.[56]

7.4 CONDYLOMA ACUMINATUM

7.4.1 Natural history and clinical features

Condyloma acuminatum is a sexually transmitted wart that is commonly associated with mucosa of the anogenital region but is rarely reported intraorally. Oral transmission of this infection probably results from direct contact due to orogenital sex or self-inoculation from hand-to-mouth exposure. Another route of exposure is perinatal transmission from infected mother to newborn.[11,39,66,81] Because cases of HPV infection have been identified in infants delivered by cesarean section, transplacental infection[84] and transmission from the amniotic fluid[81] are additional proposed modes of infection. Although the precise period of incubation is not known, the time between HPV infection and the appearance of condyloma acuminatum is quite variable, and usually ranges from 1 to 3 months[56] but may be as long as 20 months.[15] The most common HPV types associated with oral condyloma acuminatum are 6 and 11, which have been isolated in up to 85% of the oral lesions analysed.[22] Other HPV types, including 2, 16, 18, and 31/33/35, have been identified in oral condyloma acuminatum.[22,40,51,79]

Several large-scale studies have evaluated the concomitant presence of oral and anogenital HPV infection with and without evidence of clinically detectable mucosal lesions.[40,51,62] Melbye and co-investigators[51] observed no overlap with the presence of oral and anal warts in a group of homosexual men. Although 4% of the study cohort exhibited oral HPV infection, these lesions were not detected concurrently with the 15% of men who had anal warts. Interestingly, the HPV types associated with the oral lesions included 31/33/35 and 16/18, raising the possibility of orogenital transmission. Similarly, Kellokoski and others[40] evaluated the presence of oral HPV infection in normal and lesional mucosa in women with genital warts. Using Southern blot hybridization, 15% of the oral samples were HPV positive, whereas polymerase chain reaction (PCR) results were positive in almost 30% of the cases. The HPV types dentified included 6/11 and 16/18, with only two patients demonstrating similar types for both oral and genital lesions.

In marked contrast, using both clinical and colposcopic evaluation of the oral mucosa in females and males with extensive genital HPV infection, Panici and co-workers[62] observed a high incidence of concurrent oral infection. In 50% of the study group who practiced orogenital sex, histopathologic confirmation of HPV lesions was obtained. Interestingly, only 9% of this study cohort had clinically obvious oral warts, while an additional 83% of the patients required colposcopic examination for the detection of suspicious lesions. In the same study, a subset of patients was evaluated for HPV types in cytologic specimens and an 80% concordance rate was obtained for cervical and oral smears. As opposed to other studies,[39,40,51] this investigation supports a high incidence of oral HPV infection in patients with genital lesions.[62]

Most oral condyloma acuminatum occur in white males, most frequently in the third and fourth decades.[22,95] The most common sites of involvement include the labial mucosa, tongue, floor of the mouth, and gingiva, with multiple lesions diagnosed in over one-third of the patients.[95] The typical condyloma acuminatum of the oral cavity presents as a sessile, pink, well-demarcated enlargement, which is asymptomatic. The surface consists of multiple, short, blunted projections, which resemble cauliflower, mulberries, or cockscombs (Figures 7.4 and 7.5). Early lesions may have a flat-topped papular or nodular presentation with a stippled surface. It is not unusual for these warts to enlarge rapidly, proliferate, and coalesce. Because of this behavior, condylomata acuminatum tend to be larger than squamous papillomas, ranging in size from 1 cm to 3 cm.[56]

7.4.2 Histopathology

The classic histopathologic features of condyloma acuminatum include a broadly papillomatous proliferation of squamous epithelium with prominent acanthosis. Typically, mild parakeratosis, creating the appearance of deep parakeratin crypts, is found, although the surface may be non-keratinized. Both the keratinized and spinous cell layer contain varying numbers of koilocytes, whereas mitotic figures are often numerous, involving both the basal cell and lower spinous cell layers. A thin fibrovascular core supports the papillary projections, which are more blunted and broader

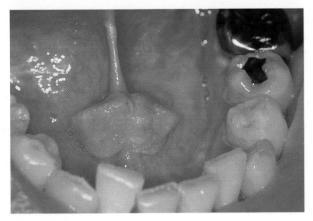

Figure 7.4
Pink papillary nodule involving the midline floor of the mouth, consistent with condyloma acuminatum.

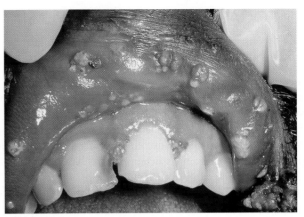

Figure 7.5
Multiple condyloma acuminata of the maxillary labial mucosa.

than in the squamous papilloma and verruca vulgaris. The bulbous rete ridges impart a vertical anastomosis appearance, in contrast to the horizontal branching pattern that is observed in focal epithelial hyperplasia. In addition to koilocytic cells, dyskeratotic cells may be found either singly or in clusters, and binucleation and multinucleation are common. The lamina propria contains dilated capillaries and a variably dense inflammatory infiltrate of lymphocytes and plasma cells. The base of the lesion is usually sessile, but may be pedunculated. Typically, the margin between epithelial proliferation and normal mucosa is abrupt. Mild to moderate epithelial atypia has been identified in approximately 30% of biopsied lesions.[77] Ultrastructural examination reveals complete virus within the koilocytes in both the cytoplasm and nucleus, while viral genome can also be detected in the basal cell layers.[22]

7.4.3 Treatment and prognosis

Oral condylomata are usually managed by conservative surgical excision. When multiple lesions are present, removal, using electrocautery, laser ablation, and cryotherapy, may be preferred. Isolated case reports and limited studies have evaluated the effect of topical podophyllin resin for intraoral condyloma acuminatum treatment, with mixed results.[27,49] Interferon may be indicated when surgery is not an alternative or for some refractory cases, and retinoids may be effective in some cases.[72]

Recurrences are common for these oral lesions and, similar to their genital counterpart, they may be refractory to multiple modalities of treatment. Diagnosis and management of anogenital condyloma acuminatum in both infected individuals and their sexual partners are necessary to prevent re-inoculation. Furthermore, spontaneous regression of oral lesions has been reported.[22,76] Although condylomata of the anogenital, cervical, and laryngeal regions exhibit a low malignant transformation rate, there have been no documented cases in the oral cavity.[56]

7.5 FOCAL EPITHELIAL HYPERPLASIA

7.5.1 Natural history and clinical features

Focal epithelial hyperplasia, also known as Heck's disease, is a benign condition of the oral cavity that has a predilection for Native Indians from North and South America, Eskimos,[12] and South Africans of Khoi-Shan extraction.[35] It has also been reported sporadically in many other populations and ethnic groups. There is a strong association with HPV types 13 and 32, which are found in over 90% of biopsied lesions.[29,36,60] These two HPV types have only occasionally been detected in other oral lesions and, except for an isolated case report of perianal Bowenoid papulosis, have not been identified in lesions outside the oral cavity.[68] In addition, a genetic predisposition and an immunocompromised host status, due to malnutrition and crowded living conditions, are speculated to be contributing factors.[12,35] Although several reports have demonstrated a familial tendency,[12,15] which would favor an infectious disease transmission, an epidemiologic study failed to demonstrate a statistical difference between household infections and general community infections.[85]

Focal epithelial hyperplasia shows a female predilection and is typically observed in the first two decades of life.[12,35] However, an increasing number of focal epithelial hyperplasia lesions are being documented in adults over a wide age range.[14,36] Clinically, this disease is characterized by multiple, non-tender, sessile, soft papules, plaques, and nodules with a flat-topped, pink to pale, grainy surface (Figures 7.6 and 7.7). Diffuse, multifocal mucosal involvement of the labial and buccal mucosa and lateral tongue is the classic presentation. Occasionally, palatal and gingival lesions have been diagnosed. The lesional margins may be discrete or indistinct due to coalescing sheets of papules and nodules resulting in a cobblestone or fissured surface. Although the papulonodular eruption is the most common presentation, a papillomatous pattern with a pale or white surface may be observed on the lateral tongue and buccal mucosa. Repeated occlusal trauma to the clustered lesions is the suspected cause for this papillary architecture, which mimics the condyloma acuminatum.

7.5.2 Histopathology

Focal epithelial hyperplasia exhibits an abrupt acanthosis of the epithelium, irregular elongation and horizontal anastomosis of the rete ridges, and mild parakeratosis. The rete ridges are widened, often confluent, and occasionally are club-shaped. Vacuolated cells vary in number from abundant to sparse and are typically located in the upper spinous cell or superficial keratinocyte layers. Random cells of the spinous cell layer demonstrate mitosis-like nuclear degeneration and are referred to as mitosoid figures. These mitosoid cells apparently result from viral alteration of the squamous cells. Binucleated and multinucleated epithelial cells may be found scattered within the spinous cell layer. The underlying lamina propria usually contains a scant inflammatory infiltrate with a predominance of lymphocytes. Although most lesions have an elevated smooth surface, a papillary architecture is occasionally observed. Ultrastructurally, virus-like particles have been observed within both the cytoplasm and nuclei of affected cells in the spinous cell layer.[56]

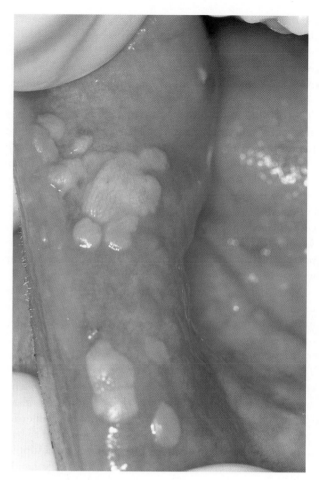

Figure 7.6
Clustered, flat-topped papules and nodules of the buccal mucosa, consistent with focal epithelial hyperplasia.

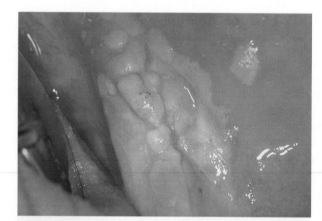

Figure 7.7
Diffuse plaques with a cobblestone appearance of the alveolar mucosa, consistent with focal epithelial hyperplasia, in the same individual as in Figure 7.6.

7.5.3 Treatment and prognosis

Other than confirmation of this viral infection by surgical biopsy, management is often limited. The lesions of focal epithelial hyperplasia spontaneously resolve in some patients within a few months to several years. Conservative surgical excision may be performed for aesthetic or functional purposes. Other treatment modalities with variable effectiveness have included cryotherapy, carbon dioxide laser ablation, topical application of 25% podophyllin resin, and vitamin therapy.[15] Recurrence of these oral lesions, even following spontaneous regression, is not uncommon. It is uncertain whether these lesions recur due to latent infection, new infection, or fluctuation of the immune response to this viral disease.[35] An isolated case of malignant transformation has been reported in a patient with long-standing focal epithelial hyperplasia.[58]

7.6 HPV-ASSOCIATED ORAL EPITHELIAL DYSPLASIA (KOILOCYTIC DYSPLASIA)

7.6.1 Natural history and clinical features

Papillary lesions referred to as HPV-associated oral epithelial dysplasia or koilocytic dysplasia have been described, with microscopic features resembling those of intraepithelial neoplasia of the female genital tract.[28] This disease primarily affects adult males, with a mean age of 39 years. Either a solitary or multiple lesion distribution may be observed, with a predilection for the tongue, lips, and buccal mucosa. Clinically, most lesions appear as flat or slightly elevated white lesions, which may have a cobblestone or papillary surface (Figure 7.8).

Interestingly, over 20% of koilocytic dysplasia lesions are diagnosed in patients who are HIV positive or at risk for infection, while the immune status of the remaining patients is unknown.[28] Likewise, epithelial dysplasia has been reported in another study evaluating oral warts excised from adult HIV-positive patients with a similar age, gender, and site predilection.[67]

Whether koilocytic dysplasia lesions are related to the rare case reports of Bowenoid papulosis of the oral cavity is unclear.[42,46,52] In contrast to the white papillary lesions associated with koilocytic dysplasia, multifocal, red, velvety papules and plaques (Figure 7.9) of the oral mucosa are described in patients with Bowenoid papulosis. However, similar to koilocytic dysplasia, these red, dysplastic, oral lesions are found in immunocompromised patients.

7.6.2 Histopathology

Koilocytic dysplasia lesions are characterized by acanthotic epithelium covered by orthokeratin or parakeratin, with a flat or papillary surface architecture. The rete pegs are broad-

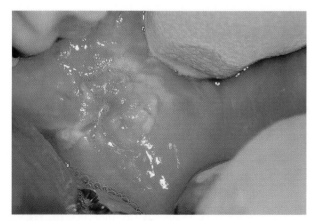

Figure 7.8
Cobblestone plaque with a depressed center in an HIV-infected man with koilocytic dysplasia.

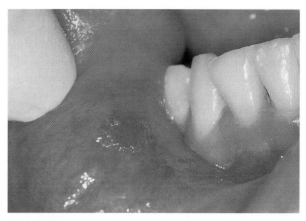

Figure 7.9
Red, velvety patch of the mandibular, labial mucosa in a liver transplant patient, characteristic of Bowenoid papulosis.

based or tear-drop shaped and commonly exhibit anastomosis. HPV-induced features consist of koilocytosis, binucleated or multinucleated keratinocytes, mitosoid figures, and dyskeratosis. A 'wind-blown' or swirling disorganization of the cells that involves partial or full thickness of the epithelium may be seen in some dysplastic lesions.[24] All grades of epithelial dysplasia may be observed in these lesions.[24,28,67]

The majority of koilocytic dysplasia lesions are positive for either high-risk HPV types 16/18 or intermediate-risk types 31/33/35. Dual infections with HPV types 6/11 and the above types are also observed.[28] Similarly, all cases of Bowenoid papulosis of the oral cavity are positive for HPV type 16,[42,46] and ultrastructural examination of the tissue supports an HPV infection.[42]

7.6.3 Treatment and prognosis

Due to the limited number of recently described cases, the appropriate management and prognosis of koilocytic dysplasia lesions are speculative. Because the biologic potential of these oral lesions is unknown, it is recommended that residual lesions be excised.[28] To date, one patient with multifocal Bowenoid papulosis of the oral mucosa, penis, and scrotum developed invasive squamous cell carcinoma of the tongue which was positive for HPV type 16.[46] Further studies are needed to evaluate whether koilocytic dysplasia and Bowenoid papulosis are the same lesions and if these oral mucosal lesions have similar treatment responses and biologic behavior as their genital counterparts.

7.7 ORAL WARTS ASSOCIATED WITH HUMAN IMMUNODEFICIENCY VIRUS INFECTION

7.7.1 Natural history and clinical features

Opportunistic infections of the oral cavity in HIV-infected individuals are a common complication and associated with immunosuppression. HPV-induced oral lesions in HIV disease include the verruca vulgaris, condyloma acuminatum, focal epithelial hyperplasia, and koilocytic dysplasia. All of these lesions, with the exception of the last mentioned, fall into the category of lesions less commonly associated with

HIV infection.[19] Their prevalence ranges from 1% to 4%, depending on the study population.[7,70,74,89] These oral lesions have been diagnosed in adults of both genders, with a mean age in the fourth decade.[74,89] HPV-related oral lesions in HIV infection have been reported mainly in homosexual/bisexual men and among heterosexual injecting drug users.[7,57,74] Several distinct patterns have been described, including cauliflower-like, spiky/conical, and flat, stippled or corrugated warts (Figures 7.10 and 7.11), which have a predilection for different mucosal sites.[32,57] The labial and buccal mucosa, lip vermilion, tongue, and gingiva are the most frequently affected sites. Usually, there is a multifocal presentation, with many individuals reporting a concurrent or recent history of cutaneous warts, especially involving facial and digital sites, and/or anogenital warts.[57,74]

The most common HPV types identified in these oral warts are 7 and 32, although 2, 6, 11, 13, 16, 18, 55, 59, 69, 72, and 73 have all been documented.[24,32,86] In addition, multiple HPV types in these oral mucosal infections have been identified.[28,80,86] HPV 7 papillomas, usually found on the hands of butchers or meat handlers, have been observed in both the oral and facial cutaneous warts of HIV-positive individuals.[18,86] In contrast, the flat oral warts and papules, which resemble focal epithelial hyperplasia or flat condylomata, tend to harbor 13 and 32 and, to a lesser extent, 6/11 and 16/18.[24,32] The presence of these latter types, which are more commonly associated with anogenital lesions, raises

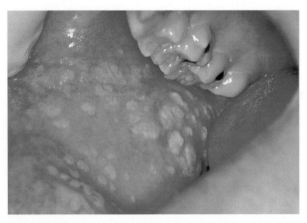

Figure 7.10
Florid, flat-topped nodules of the buccal mucosa in an HIV-infected man, consistent with focal epithelial hyperplasia.

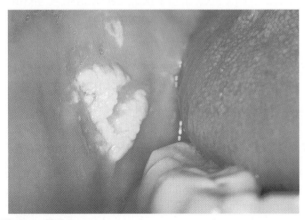

Figure 7.11
Solitary corrugated plaque of the posterior buccal mucosa in an HIV-infected man, exhibiting an atypical appearance for an oral wart.

the possibility of sexual transmission of oral warts in this patient population.

7.7.2 Histopathology

The histopathologic features correspond to the specific type of lesion, as previously discussed. The primary differences between oral warts in HIV-infected and immunocompetent individuals appear to be the novel types of HPV found in these lesions and the presence of epithelial atypia in some cases.[24,28,32,67,86]

Epithelial atypia, ranging from mild to severe dysplasia, has been observed in a number of oral warts from this immunocompromised population, which contain intermediate-risk (31/33/51), high-risk (16/18), and novel (72, 73) HPV types.[28,86] The significance of these HPV types in dysplastic lesions is not known because they have also been identified in unrelated oral lesions, such as hairy leukoplakia and hyperkeratosis, and in normal mucosa of HIV-infected individuals.[2,23,33,80] In fact, mucosatropic HPV 16 has been found in 60% of specimens from clinically normal oral mucosa in this immunosuppressed population.[2]

7.7.3 Treatment and Prognosis

As with other HPV-induced oral lesions, the most common management approach is surgical removal by scalpel, laser ablation, electrocautery and cryotherapy. Topical podophyllin resin has been applied before surgery to decrease the size of the lesions and, theoretically, lessen the viral load and minimize recurrences.[57]

Oral and perioral recurrences of these warts in this immunocompromised population are common, especially when multiple, widespread lesions exist.[57] For recalcitrant lesions, surgical excision and the use of intralesional or systemic interferon have been recommended.[8] An isolated case report describes the effectiveness of the histamine H2 antagonist, cimetidine, for the management of refractory oral warts in an HIV-positive patient.[87] Additional therapeutic modalities include intralesional cidofovir injections. Even with multimodality treatment, a 35% recurrence rate has been reported.[57]

Although the potential for malignant transformation is a valid concern because of the detection of intermediate-risk or high-risk HPV types, this disease progression has not been confirmed at oropharyngeal sites. To date, only a limited number of studies have identified HIV infection as a risk factor for oral squamous cell carcinoma.[26,43,74] Only one investigation has identified high-risk and intermediate-risk HPV types 16/18 and 31/33/35 in these oral malignancies.[26]

7.8 OVERVIEW OF HPV EXPRESSION IN THE ORAL CAVITY

7.8.1 Oral normal mucosa and HPV expression

Multiple studies have evaluated the presence of HPV in cytologic and surgical samples of normal oral mucosa. Widely variable detection rates have been reported, ranging from 0% to 81%.[53,63,83] In general, HPV DNA is present in normal oral mucosa in more than one-third of the population.[72] A higher number of immunocompromised individuals tend to harbor HPV in the oral mucosa with up to 60% of HIV-infected adults demonstrating positivity.[2] This wide variation in detection rates may be attributed to different tissue sampling and preparation techniques and to the wide sensitivity range of the various detection methods used.

The distribution of HPV in normal mucosa in healthy young adults is similar at various oral mucosal sites, including the buccal mucosa, dorsal tongue, and hard palate.[38] In decreasing order of frequency, the HPV types identified in normal mucosa are 16/18, 6/11, 31/33, and 7.[53] Recently, types 59, 61, and an unknown type have been identified.[84] These studies suggest that the oral mucosa is a common site for HPV and may act as a reservoir for new or recurrent infections.[13]

7.8.2 Oral leukoplakia and HPV expression

By definition, leukoplakia is a white patch or plaque that cannot be characterized clinically or pathologically as any other disease, and is therefore a diagnosis of exclusion.[5] Leukoplakia has an estimated lifetime risk for malignant transformation of 3–6%.[5] Because of the plethora of lesions loosely defined as leukoplakia, studies evaluating the significance of HPV in these lesions are difficult to interpret. Investigations evaluating the presence of HPV in leukoplakia show the mean detection rate to be 15%, and as high as 80%.[48,53,78] Use of frozen or fresh tissues significantly increases the rate of viral detection to 43%, in contrast to an average of 12% in paraffin-embedded samples.[53]

Most keratotic lesions evaluated are in adults, with a mean age of 41 years. Leukoplakias of the buccal/labial mucosa, tongue, and palate most often contain HPV, with types 6/11 accounting for the majority of cases (56%), followed by 16/18 (29%), and 2 (15%).[53] Although one study reported a high progression to carcinoma when the leukoplakias contained HPV,[44] its etiologic role in the pathogenesis or malignant transformation of this oral lesion is still uncertain.

7.8.3 Oral epithelial dysplasia and HPV expression

Studies evaluating HPV expression in all grades of oral epithelial dysplasia have shown an average detection rate of 18.5%.[53] As expected, higher detection rates are observed with PCR (42%) and when fresh or frozen tissues are studied (30%). Based on lesion site, it appears that dysplastic lesions from the tongue are more likely to express the virus. HPV types 2, 6, 11, 16, 18, and 31/33/35 have been identified in over 11% of these dysplastic lesions. Significantly, high-risk types 16 and 18 are found in the majority of the HPV-positive samples studied (75%).[53]

Included in the group of oral lesions is the aggressive clinical entity proliferative verrucous leukoplakia. This lesion is characterized by spreading white plaques that initially begin as focal keratosis and eventually become multifocal, exophytic, and verrucoid in appearance (Figure 7.12).[34] Proliferative verrucous leukoplakia is extremely resistant to therapy and has a high rate of malignant transformation. Over an extended follow-up period, 70–100% of

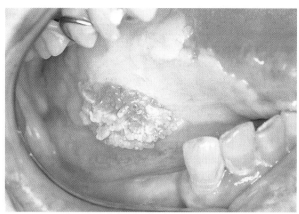

Figure 7.12
Diffuse white plaque with an exophytic, red and white, papillary focus of the lateral tongue, representing malignant transformation of proliferative verrucous hyperplasia.

individuals with proliferative verrucous leukoplakia develop invasive squamous cell carcinoma and 40% die from their disease.[73,93] From an epidemiologic standpoint, proliferative verrucous leukoplakia is unusual because it has a predilection for elderly women without a history of tobacco use, which is in distinct contrast to most cases of oral cancer.[34,56]

The role of HPV in this poorly understood disease remains controversial. Whereas one study has demonstrated HPV 16 and 18 by PCR in 89% of proliferative verrucous leukoplakia lesions,[61] a more recent study also using PCR showed an HPV detection rate of only 20%.[30]

7.8.4 Oral verrucous carcinoma and HPV expression

Oral verrucous carcinoma, a rare variant of squamous cell carcinoma with low aggressiveness, has been linked to tobacco use, especially smokeless tobacco products and betel nut chewing.[13] Due to the papillary morphology of verrucous carcinoma with dyskeratosis and koilocytosis, HPV has been suspected as an etiologic factor. The mean prevalence of HPV in multiple studies of verrucous carcinoma is 27%, with a greater detection rate (67%) with PCR.[53,63] HPV-positive verrucous carcinoma occurs 5 years earlier than HPV-negative cases and displays a female predilection of 2:1. The buccal/labial mucosa, palate, and alveolus are the tumor sites most likely to harbor HPV, accounting for 75% of the positive cases. The HPV types expressed in these cancers include 2, 6, 11, 16, and 18, with HPV 6/11 identified in 47% and HPV 16/18 in 35%.[53]

7.8.5 Oral papillary squamous cell carcinoma and HPV expression

Papillary squamous cell carcinoma is another uncommon variant of squamous cell carcinoma, which has a predilection for the head and neck. Confusion regarding the histologic criteria for defining this lesion, complicating any accurate assessment of its prevalence, anatomic distribution, and biologic behavior, is evident in the literature.[9] A strict clinicopathologic definition of papillary squamous cell carcinoma has been proposed in order to limit the ambiguity surrounding it. Included in this definition is an exophytic papillary architecture with minimal keratinization, full-thickness epithelial dysplasia, and minimal or focal stromal microinvasion. Although papillary squamous cell carcinoma occurs in the oral cavity, there is a site predilection for the larynx and sinonasal tract.

When it occurs in the head and neck region, a wide age range, with a mean age at diagnosis of 66 years, and a 2:1 male to female ratio are observed. The oral cavity and oropharynx are affected in 13% of the head and neck cases.[75] HPV is demonstrated in 29% and 43% of cases, respectively, utilizing *in-situ* hybridization and PCR. In the same study, HPV types detected in these lesions by PCR include 6/11 and 16/18.

7.8.6 Oral squamous cell carcinoma and HPV expression

HPV is widely implicated in the pathogenesis of squamous cell carcinoma of the anogenital region, in contrast to its more speculative role in oral squamous cell carcinoma, which has been strongly associated with tobacco and/or alcohol use.[56] The proposed role of HPV in oral carcinogenesis involves the interaction between HPV oncogenes and the proteins of the host cell that regulate cellular growth and proliferation. The protein product of the HPV E6 gene binds to and results in the degradation of host cell p53 tumor suppressor protein. Similarly, HPV E7 protein complexes with the protein products of the retinoblastoma (*Rb*) gene family, which are negative cell-cycle regulators.[50] The resultant disruption of cell-cycle control by these mechanisms supports the notion that high-risk HPV types may be important cofactors in the initiation and progression of oral squamous cell carcinoma.

After collectively summarizing the results of numerous studies, the mean prevalence for HPV in oral malignancies is 26%.[53] Higher detection rates are observed with fresh or frozen tissue (50%), when PCR is utilized (37%), and when HPV early gene primers are used (43%).

The tongue and floor of the mouth, the most common sites for oral squamous cell carcinoma, are the anatomic sites most often positive for HPV.[53] Although HPV types 16 and 18 account for 80% of the positive cases, other types include 2, 3, 13, 31/33/35, 52, and 57. In addition, dual HPV infections have been observed, and it appears that patients with dual high-risk HPV types develop an oral cancer one decade earlier than those patients who harbor either no or one high-risk type.[54,90] HPV DNA sequences have also been found in leukocytes from patients with oral carcinoma[37] and in the majority of metastatic lymph nodes.[53] Detection of the same HPV type in the primary and metastatic disease supports the oncogenic role of this virus as opposed to being a passenger that coincidentally infects an oral carcinoma.

Numerous studies have examined HPV infection as a risk factor for oral cancer. When evaluating oral cancer risk in relation to sexual history and HPV infection, a positive correlation is demonstrated between oral squamous cell carcinoma and risk factors for HPV infection among males.[47,71] Oral cancer risk is increased in men with 30 or more sexual partners and in those with oral HPV 6 infection.[47] In women with oral squamous cell carcinoma evaluated for cervicovaginal HPV infection, the same HPV types are frequently found in the oral carcinomas and the genital tract.[65] Overall,

when multiple studies are analysed, HPV is identified as the only risk factor for oral cancer in 7% of the cases.[53]

A significant association has been firmly established between tobacco and alcohol use and the development of oral cancer, irrespective of the HPV infection. However, the availability of more sensitive methods for HPV detection may further implicate this virus as an important cofactor in oral carcinogenesis.[54,88,90] In the future, additional interactions between HPV and other carcinogenic agents and viruses, such as herpes simplex virus, Epstein–Barr virus and the human immunodeficiency virus, may be identified which participate with HPV in oral cancer development.[25]

7.9 SUMMARY

Clinically manifest HPV lesions of the oral cavity include squamous papilloma, verruca vulgaris, condyloma acuminatum, focal epithelial hyperplasia, and possibly koilocytic dysplasia, and various pre-malignant and malignant epithelial lesions. Excluding the squamous papilloma, most of these HPV-induced oral lesions are uncommon at this mucosal site. Interestingly, the HIV-infected population appears to be most vulnerable to the development of oral warts, but to a lesser degree than anogenital and cervical infection. Typically, diagnosis of these lesions depends on clinical presentation and histopathologic features, and less frequently on the HPV type isolated. Within the past decade, numerous HPV types have been identified in normal oral mucosa and several oral diseases with a questionable causal relationship. Although the exact role of HPV in the malignant transformation of oral epithelium is still not fully understood, it appears to be an important cofactor for the development of oral squamous cell carcinoma that requires further investigations.

REFERENCES

1. Abbey LM, Page DG, Sawyer DR. (1980) The clinical and histopathologic features of a series of 464 oral squamous cell papillomas. *Oral Surg Oral Med Oral Pathol* **49**: 419–28.
2. Adler-Storthz K, Ficarra G, Woods KV, *et al.* (1992) Prevalence of Epstein–Barr virus and human papillomavirus in oral mucosa of HIV-infected patients. *J Oral Pathol Med* **21**: 164–70.
3. Adler-Storthz K., Newland JR, Tessin BA, *et al.* (1986) Identification of human papillomavirus types in oral verruca vulgaris. *J Oral Pathol* **15**: 230–3.
4. Axell T. (1976) A prevalence study of oral mucosal lesions in an adult Swedish population. *Odontologisk Rev* **27**: 1–103.
5. Axell T, Holmstrup P, Kramer I, *et al.* (1984) International seminar on oral leukoplakia and associated lesions related to tobacco habits. *Community Dent Oral Epidemiol* **12**: 145–54.
6. Barasch A, Eisenberg E, D'Ambrosio JA, *et al.* (1996) Oral verruca vulgaris in a bone marrow transplant patient: a case report and review of literature. *Eur J Cancer Part B, Oral Oncol* **32B**: 137–9.
7. Barone R, Ficarra G, Gaglioti D, *et al.* (1990) Prevalence

of oral lesions among HIV-infected intravenous drug abusers and other risk groups. *Oral Surg Oral Med Oral Path* **69**: 169–73.

8. Barr CE. (1994) Practical considerations in the treatment of the HIV-infected patient. *Dent Clin North Am* **38**: 403–23.

9. Batsakis JG, Suarez P. (2000) Papillary squamous carcinoma: will the real one please stand up? *Adv Anatom Path* **7**: 2–8.

10. Bouquot JE, Gundlach KK (1986) Oral exophytic lesions in 23,616 white Americans over 35 years of age. *Oral Surg Oral Med Oral Pathol* **62**: 284–91.

11. Boyd AS. (1990) Condylomata acuminata in the pediatric population. *Am J Dis Child* **144**: 817–24.

12. Carlos R, Sedano HO. (1994) Multifocal papilloma virus epithelial hyperplasia. *Oral Surg Oral Med Oral Pathol* **77**: 631–5.

13. Chang F, Syrjanen S, Kellokoski J, *et al.* (1991) Human papillomavirus (HPV) infections and their associations with oral disease. *J Oral Pathol Med* **20**: 305–17.

14. Clausen FP, Mogeltoft M, Roed-Petersen B, *et al.* (1970) Focal epithelial hyperplasia of the oral mucosa in a south-west Greenlandic population. *Scand J Dent Res* **78**: 287–94.

15. Cohen PR, Herbert AA, Adler-Storthz K. (1993) Focal epithelial hyperplasia: Heck disease. *Pediatr Dermatol* **10**: 245–51.

16. De Jong AR, Weiss J, Brent R, *et al.* (1982) Condylomata acuminata in children. *Am J Dis Child* **136**: 704–6.

17. de Villiers E-M. (1989) Papilloma viruses in cancers and papillomas of the aerodigestive tract. *Biomed Pharmacother* **43**: 31–6.

18. de Villiers E-M. (1989) Prevalence of HPV 7 papillomas in the oral mucosa and facial skin of patients with human immunodeficiency virus [letter]. *Arch Dermatol* **125**: 1590.

19. EEC-Clearinghouse on Oral Problems Related to HIV Infection and WHO Collaborating Centre on Oral Manifestations of the Human Immunodeficiency Virus. (1991) An update of the classification and diagnostic criteria of oral lesions in HIV-infection. *J Oral Pathol Med* **20**: 97–100.

20. Eversole RL. (1992) Viral infections of the head and neck among HIV-seropositive patients. *Oral Surg Oral Med Oral Path* **73**: 155–63.

21. Eversole LR, Laipis PJ, Green TL. (1987) Human papillomavirus type 2 DNA in oral and labial verruca vulgaris. *J Cutan Pathol* **14**: 319–25.

22. Eversole LR, Laipis PL, Merrell P, *et al.* (1987b) Demonstration of human papillomavirus DNA in oral condyloma acuminatum. *J Oral Pathol* **16**: 266–72.

23. Eversole LR, Stone CE, Beckmann AM. (1988) Detection of EBV and HPV DNA sequences in oral 'hairy' leukoplakia by in situ hybridization. *J Med Virol* **26**: 271–7.

24. Felefli S, Flaitz CM, Nichols CM, *et al.* (2000) Multifocal human papillomavirus infection of the oral cavity in HIV-positive individuals (abstract). *Oral Surg Oral Med Oral Pathol Oral Radiol Endod* **90**: 496.

25. Flaitz CM, Hicks MJ. (1998) Molecular piracy: the viral link to carcinogenesis. *Eur J Cancer* **34**: 448–53.

26. Flaitz CM, Nichols CM, Adler-Storthz K, *et al.* (1995) Intraoral squamous cell carcinoma in human immunodeficiency virus infection. A clinicopathologic study. *Oral Surg, Oral Med Oral Pathol Oral Radiol Endod* **80**: 55–62.

27. Flaitz CM, Nichols CM, Hicks MJ, Adler-Storthz K. (1993) Oral human papillomavirus infection in HIV-seropositive males: diagnostic and therapeutic management (abstract). *Oral Surg Oral Med Oral Pathol* **76**: 598.

28. Fornatora M, Jones AC, Kerpel S, *et al.* (1996) Human papillomavirus-associated oral epithelial dysplasia (koilocytic dysplasia). An entity of unknown biologic potential. *Oral Surg Oral Med Oral Pathol Oral Radiol Endod* **82**: 47–56.

29. Garlick JA, Calderon S, Buchner A, *et al.* (1989) Detection of human papillomavirus (HPV) DNA in focal epithelial hyperplasia. *J Oral Pathol Med* **18**: 172–7.

30. Gopalakrishnan R, Weghorst CM, Lehman TA, *et al.* (1997) Mutated and wild-type p53 expression and HPV integration in proliferative verrucous leukoplakia and oral squamous cell carcinoma. *Oral Surg Oral Med Oral Pathol, Oral Radiol Endod* **83**: 471–7.

31. Green TL, Eversole LR, Leider AS. (1986) Oral and labial verruca vulgaris: clinical, histologic and immunohistochemical evaluation. *Oral Surg Oral Med Oral Pathol* **62**: 410–6.

32. Greenspan D, de Villiers E-M, Greenspan JS. (1988) Unusual HPV types in oral warts in association with HIV infection. *J Oral Pathol* **17**: 482–8.

33. Greenspan D, Greenspan JS, Conant M, *et al.* (1984) Oral 'hairy' leucoplakia in male homosexuals: evidence of association with both papillomavirus and a herpes-group virus. *Lancet* **2**: 831–4.

34. Hansen LS, Olson JA, Silverman S Jr. (1985) Proliferative verrucous leukoplakia. A long-term study of thirty patients. *Oral Surg Oral Med Oral Pathol* **60**: 285–98.

35. Harris AM, van Wyk CW. (1993) Heck's disease (focal epithelial hyperplasia): a longitudinal study. *Community Dent Oral Epidemiol* **21**: 82–5.

36. Henke R-P, Guerin-Reverchon I, Milde-Langosch K, *et al.* (1989) In situ detection of human papillomavirus types 13 and 32 in focal epithelial hyperplasia of the oral mucosa. *J Oral Pathol Med* **18**: 419–21.

37. Honig JF, Becker MJ, Brinck Y, *et al.* (1995) Detection of human papillomavirus DNA sequences in leucocytes: a new approach to identify hematological markers of HPV infection in patients with oral SCC. *Bull Group Int Rech Sci Stomatol Odontol* **38**: 25–31.

38. Jalal H, Sanders CM, Prime SS, *et al.* (1992) Detection of human papillomavirus type 16 DNA in oral squames from normal young adults. *J Oral Pathol Med* **21**: 465–70.

39. Kaye JN, Starkey WG, Kell B, *et al.* (1996) Human papillomavirus type 16 in infants: use of DNA sequence analyses to determine the source of infection. *J Gen Virol* **77**: 1139–43.

40. Kellokoski JK, Syrjänen SM, Chang F, *et al.* (1992) Southern blot hybridization and PCR in detection of oral human papillomavirus (HPV) infections in women with genital HPV infections. *J Oral Pathol Medi* **21**: 459–64.

41. Kleinman DV, Swango PA, Pindborg JJ. (1994) Epidemiology of oral mucosal lesions in United States

schoolchildren: 1986–87. *Community Dent Oral Epidemiol* **22**: 243–53.

42. Kratochvil FJ, Cioffi GA, Auclair PL, *et al.* (1989) Virus-associated dysplasia (bowenoid papulosis?) of the oral cavity. *Oral Surg Oral Med Oral Pathol* **68**: 312–16.

43. Langford A, Langer R, Lobeck H, *et al.* (1995) Human immunodeficiency virus-associated squamous cell carcinomas of the head and neck presenting as oral and primary intraosseous squamous cell carcinomas. *Quint Int* **26**: 635–54.

44. Lind PO, Syrjanen SM, Syrjanen KJ, *et al.* (1986) Local immunoreactivity and human papillomavirus (HPV) in oral precancer and cancer lesions. *Scand J Dent Res* **94**: 419–26.

45. Loning T, Ikenberg H, Becker J, *et al.* (1985) Analysis of oral papillomas, leukoplakias, and invasive carcinomas for human papillomavirus type related DNA. *J Invest Dermatol* **84**: 417–20.

46. Lookingbill DP, Kreider JW, Howett MK, *et al.* (1987) Human papillomavirus type 16 in bowenoid papulosis, intraoral papillomas, and squamous cell carcinoma of the tongue. *Arch Dermatol* **123**: 363–8.

47. Maden C, Beckmann AM, Thomas DB, *et al.* (1992) Human papillomaviruses, herpes simplex viruses, and the risk of oral cancer in men. *Am J Epidemiol* **135**: 1093–102.

48. Maitland N J, Bromidge T, Cox MF, *et al.* (1989) Detection of human papillomavirus genes in human oral tissue biopsies and cultures by polymerase chain reaction. *Br J Cancer* **59**: 698–703.

49. Marquard JV, Racey GL. (1981) Combined medical and surgical management of intraoral condyloma acuminata. *J Oral Surg* **39**: 459–61.

50. McKaig RG, Baric RS, Olshan AF. (1998) Human papillomavirus and head and neck cancer: epidemiology and molecular biology. *Head Neck* **20**: 250–65.

51. Melbye M, Palefsky J, Gonzales J, *et al.* (1990) Immune status as a determinant of human papillomavirus detection and its association with anal epithelial abnormalities. *Int J Cancer* **46**: 203–6.

52. Miller CS. (1994) Herpes simplex virus and human papillomavirus infections of the oral cavity. *Semin Dermatol* **13**: 108–17.

53. Miller CS, White DK. (1996) Human papillomavirus expression in oral mucosa, premalignant conditions, and squamous cell carcinoma. A retrospective review of the literature. *Oral Surg Oral Med Oral Pathol Oral Radiol Endod* **82**: 57–68.

54. Miller CS, Zeuss MS, White DK. (1994) Detection of HPV DNA in oral carcinoma using polymerase chain reaction together with in situ hybridization. *Oral Surg, Oral Med Oral Pathol* **77**: 480–6.

55. Naghashfar Z, Sawada E, Kutcher M,. *et al.* (1985) Identification of genital tract papillomaviruses HPV-6 and HPV-16 in warts of the oral cavity. *J Medical Virol,* **17**: 313–24.

56. Neville BW, Damm DD, Allen CM, *et al.* (eds) (1995) Epithelial Pathology. In *Oral and maxillofacial pathology.* Philadelphia, WB Saunders, 259–321.

57. Nichols CM, Flaitz CM, Allen KH, *et al.* (1998) Human papillomavirus-induced oral warts in HIV infection: assessment of treatment outcomes. *Oral Surg Oral Med Oral Pathol Oral Radiol Endod* **85**: 416–17(A).

58. Niebrugge B, Villiers E, Gerlach K, *et al.* (1999) Demonstration of HPV 24 in long-standing Heck's disease with malignant transformation. *Euro J Dermatol* **9**: 477–9.

59. Padayachee A. (1994) Human papillomavirus (HPV) types 2 and 57 in oral verrucae demonstrated by *in situ* hybridization. *J Oral Pathol Med* **23**: 413–17.

60. Padayachee A, van Wyk CW. (1991) Human papillomavirus (HPV) DNA in focal epithelial hyperplasia by in situ hybridization. *J Oral Pathol Med* **20**: 210–4.

61. Palefsky JM, Silverman S Jr, Abdel-Salaam M, *et al.* (1995) Association between proliferative verrucous leukoplakia and infection with human papillomavirus type 16. *J Oral Pathol Med* **24**: 193–7.

62. Panici PB, Scambia G, Perrone L, *et al.* (1992) Oral condyloma lesions in patients with extensive genital human papillomavirus infection. *Am J Obstet Gyneco.* **167**: 451–8.

63. Praetorius F. (1997) HPV-associated diseases of oral mucosa. *Clin Dermatol* **15**: 399–413.

64. Premoli-de-Percoco G, Galindo I, Ramirez JL, *et al.* (1993) Detection of human papillomavirus-related oral verruca vulgaris among Venezuelans. *J Oral Pathol Med* **22**: 113–6.

65. Premoli-de-Percoco G, Ramirez JL, Galindo I. (1998) Correlation between HPV types associated with oral squamous cell carcinoma and cervicovaginal cytology. *Oral Surg Oral Med Oral Pathol Oral Radiol Endod* **86**: 77–81.

66. Puranen M, Yliskoski M, Saarikoski S, *et al.* (1996) Vertical transmission of human papillomavirus from infected mothers to their newborn babies and persistence of the virus in childhood. *Am J Obstet Gynecol* **174**: 694–9.

67. Regezi JA, Greenspan D, Greenspan JS, *et al.* (1994) HPV-associated epithelial atypia in oral warts in HIV+ patients. *J Cutan Pathol* **21**: 217–23.

68. Rolighed J, Sorensen IM, Jacobsen NO, Lindeberg H. (1991) The presence of HPV types 6/11, 13, 16 and 33 in bowenoid papulosis in an HIV-positive male, demonstrated by DNA in situ hybridisation. *APMIS* **99**: 583–5.

69. Schubert MM. (1991) Oral manifestations of viral infections in immunocompromised patients. *Curr Opin Dent* **1**: 384–97.

70. Schulten EA, ten Kate RW, van der Waal I. (1989) Oral manifestations of HIV infection in 75 Dutch patients. *J Oral Pathol Med* **18**: 42–6.

71. Schwartz SM, Daling JR, Doody DR, *et al.* (1998) Oral cancer risk in relation to sexual history and evidence of human papillomavirus infection. *J Nat Cancer Ins* **90**: 1626–36.

72. Scully C. (1996) New aspects of oral viral diseases. In *Oral pathology. Actual diagnostic and prognostic aspects,* ed. G. Seifert, *Current Topics in Pathology*, Vol. 90. Berlin, Springer, 29–96.

73. Silverman S, Gorsky M. (1997) Proliferative verrucous leukoplakia: a follow-up study of 54 cases. *Oral Surg, Oral Med Oral Pathol Oral Radiol Endod* **84**: 154–7.

74. Silverman S Jr, Migliorati CA, Lozada-Nur F, *et al.* (1986) Oral findings in people with or at high risk for

AIDS: a study of 375 homosexual males. *J Am Dent Assoc* **112**: 187–92.

75. Suarez PA, Adler-Storthz K, Luna MA, *et al.* (2000) Papillary squamous cell carcinomas of the upper aerodigestive tract: a clinicopathologic and molecular study. *Head Neck* **22**: 360–8.

76. Swan RH, McDaniel RK, Dreiman BB, *et al.* (1981) Condyloma acuminatum involving the oral mucosa. *Oral Surg Oral Med Oral Pathol* **51**: 503–8.

77. Syrjänen K, Happonen R-P, Syrjänen S, *et al.* (1984) Human papilloma virus (HPV) antigens and local immunologic reactivity in oral squamous cell tumors and hyperplasias. *Scand J Dent Res* **92**: 358–70.

78. Syrjänen SM, Syrjänen KJ, Happonen R-P. (1988) Human papillomavirus (HPV) DNA sequences in oral precancerous lesions and squamous cell carcinoma demonstrated by in situ hybridization. *J Oral Pathol* **17**: 273–8.

79. Syrjänen SM, Syrjänen KJ, Happonen R-P, *et al.* (1987) In situ DNA hybridization analysis of human papillomavirus (HPV) sequences in benign oral mucosal lesions. *Arch Dermatol Res* **279**: 543–9.

80. Syrjänen S, von Krogh G, Kellokoski J, *et al.* (1989) Two different human papillomavirus (HPV) types associated with oral mucosal lesions in an HIV-seropositive man. *J Oral Pathol Med* **18**: 366–70.

81. Tenti P, Zappatore R, Migliora P, *et al.* (1999) Perinatal transmission of human papillomavirus from gravidas with latent infections. *Obstet Gynecol* **93**: 475–9.

82. Terai M, Hashimoto K, Yoda K, *et al.* (1999) High prevalence of human papillomaviruses in the normal oral cavity of adults. *Oral Microbiol Immunol* **14**: 201–5.

83. Terai M, Takagi M, Matsukura T, *et al.* (1999) Oral wart associated with human papillomavirus type 2. *J Oral Pathol Med* **28**: 137–40.

84. Tseng CJ, Lin CY, Wang RL, *et al.* (1992) Possible transplacental transmission of human papillomaviruses. *Am J Obstet Gynecol* **166**: 35–40.

85. van Wyk W, Harris A. (1987) Focal epithelial hyperplasia: a survey of two isolated communities in the Cape Province of South Africa. *Community Dent Oral Epidemiol* **15**: 161–3.

86. Volter C, He Y, Delius H, *et al.* (1996) Novel HPV types present in oral papillomatous lesions from patients with HIV infection. *Int J Cancer* **66**: 453–6.

87. Wargon O. (1996) Cimetidine for mucosal warts in an HIV positive adult. *Australas J Dermatol* **37**: 149–50.

88. Watts SL, Brewer EE, Fry TL. (1991) Human papillomavirus DNA types in squamous cell carcinomas of the head and neck. *Oral Surg Oral Med Oral Pathol* **71**: 701–7.

89. Wiltshire A, Flaitz C, Nichols M, *et al.* (1996) Prevalence of HIV-associated oral disease in women. *J Dent Res* **75**(Special Issue): 239(A).

90. Woods KV, Shillitoe EJ, Spitz MR, *et al.* (1993) Analysis of human papillomavirus DNA in oral squamous cell carcinoma. *J Oral Pathol Med* **22**: 101–8.

91. Wysocki GP, Hardie J. (1979) Ultrastructural studies of intraoral verruca vulgaris. *Oral Surg Oral Med Oral Pathol* **47**: 58–62.

92. Zaia JA. (1990) Viral infections associated with bone marrow transplantation. *Hematol Oncol Clin North Am* **4**: 603–23.

93. Zakrzewska JM, Lopes V, Speight P, *et al.* (1996) Proliferative verrucous leukoplakia: a report of ten cases. *Oral Surg Oral Med Oral Pathol Oral Radiol Endod* **82**: 396–401.

94. Zeuss MS, Miller CS, White DK. (1991) In situ hybridization analysis of human papillomavirus DNA in oral mucosal lesions. *Oral Surg Oral Med Oral Pathol* **71**: 714–20.

95. Zunt SL, Tomich CE. (1989) Oral condyloma acuminatum. *J Dermatol Surg Oncol* **15**: 591–4.

8

Respiratory papillomatosis

Zoltan Trizna and Stephen K. Tyring

8.1 INTRODUCTION

Papillomatosis of the upper aero-digestive tract was originally described as juvenile laryngeal papillomatosis by MacKenzie in 1880. Later, laryngeal papillomatosis was reported in all age groups and it became apparent that papillomatosis can occur at other sites of the aero-digestive tract, including the oral cavity, hypopharynx, esophagus, and bronchial system.

Papilloma is one of the most common benign laryngeal tumors, but its prevalence is difficult to estimate. Approximately four to seven cases of laryngeal papillomatosis per million person-years occur in the USA and in Europe.[10,42,69] The incidence of recurrent respiratory papillomas among children is estimated at 4.3 per 100 000 and among adults 1.8 per 100 000.[18] Approximately 50% of laryngeal papillomas occur by the early teens. The presentation of the adult type of laryngeal papillomatosis peaks in the thirties and forties.

Human papillomaviruses (HPVs) are the causative agents of a variety of benign epidermal tumors such as common warts, flat warts, condylomas, and papillomas. The viral etiology of laryngeal papillomatosis is well established, with several types of HPVs, especially types 6, 11, 16, and 18, being significant etiologic factors. Even though the lesions are histologically benign, their recurrence or dissemination can impair the patency of the airways and necessitate multiple surgical treatments. The clinical behavior is variable: the lesions most often regress, occasionally persist, and, in the presence of certain environmental factors (e.g., smoking), can progress to cancer.

8.2 EPIDEMIOLOGY AND PATHOGENESIS OF HPV INFECTION

The prevalence of HPV infection varies widely, depending on the disease entities, anatomical site and ethnicity. In non-tumorous tissues from head and neck organs, the prevalence is typically between 8.7%[25] and 25%.[51] Fifty-nine percent of benign laryngeal papillomas in Hong Kong Chinese showed the presence of HPV 6, 11,16, or 18, with HPV 11 being the predominant infection.[20] Another study described a 95% prevalence of HPV in solitary laryngeal papillomas.[44]

Multiple HPV infections can occur in the same lesion, and the integration of viral DNA may contribute to the development of severe dysplasias and neoplasias.[41] An endogenous p53 genetic mutation was found to be associated with integration of HPV 11 in histologically malignant lesions.[58] Such associations may lead to a genetic instability and the development and clonal expansion of malignancies.

HPV infections are common among sexually active adolescent and young people, with genital HPV being the most common sexually transmitted viral disease. There is a chance for the transmission of HPV at the time of vaginal delivery. Nurse-midwives find venereal warts in 1–35% of their pregnant clients, depending upon the subpopulation under consideration.[73] Transmission is supposed to be enhanced by vaginal delivery, with the risk of transmission from a mother with HPV infection to her infant being between 1:80 and 1:1500.[63] In a group of 28 children with juvenile laryngeal papillomatosis, 15 (54%) had a maternal history of vulvar condyloma at the time of delivery or pregnancy.[27] HPV type 6/11 was identified in 2% of 45 pregnant women who were predominantly asymptomatic and had normal Papanicolaou smears and normal clinical examinations.[54] In a study of 77 mothers with condylomata at delivery, nine children were found with juvenile laryngeal papillomatosis.[38] Other studies found no correlation between the HPV types detected in mothers and their children.[52,68]

The route of transmission may be different in juvenile-onset and adult-onset recurrent respiratory papillomatosis, as suggested by a case-control study. Patients with the juvenile form of the disease were more often born vaginally to a teenage mother and were more likely to be first-born children than their controls, whereas patients with adult-onset disease had more sexual partners and a higher frequency of oral sex than their controls.[36]

On the other hand, in a survey of 53 adults with genital warts, 70% of whom participated in oral sex, two (3.8%) had lesions attributable to HPV infection, one with laryngeal keratosis, one with papilloma of the pharynx. No other specific risk factors were identified. This is a surprisingly low prevalence as genital warts are generally highly infectious.[15]

8.3 PATHOLOGY

The papillomatous lesions occur at anatomic sites in which ciliated and squamous epithelia are juxtaposed. The predominant sites of recurrent disease are the limen vestibuli, the nasopharyngeal surface of the soft palate, the midzone of the laryngeal surface of the epiglottis, the upper and lower margins of the ventricle, the undersurface of the vocal folds, the carina, and bronchial spurs. Papillomata also occur at the tracheostomy tract and at the mid-thoracic trachea in patients with tracheostomies.[33]

The gross appearance of papilloma is that of a multinodular growth (Figures 8.1 and 8.2). The lesions can be solitary or multiple. A solitary exophytic papilloma usually has a stalk. The sessile stalk shows a confluent spread to involve the mucosal membrane.

Microscopically, the vascularized connective tissue stroma of the lesion is covered with stratified squamous epithelium. The epithelial cells proliferate and abnormal differentiation is seen. The koilocytes (cells with hyperchromatic nuclei surrounded with a wide clear halo) are considered the landmark histologic feature of viral infection.

8.4 CLINICAL PRESENTATION AND COURSE

The symptoms and signs of respiratory papillomatosis are not specific and may mimic a variety of other diseases, with the differential diagnosis including croup, asthma, and common upper airway infections; therefore, the diagnosis may be delayed.

The diagnosis in children is suggested by hoarseness, poor cry, progressive dyspnea, or stridor.[29] Hoarseness is usually noted first. The obstruction of the relatively narrow airways of children caused by papillomas frequently worsens

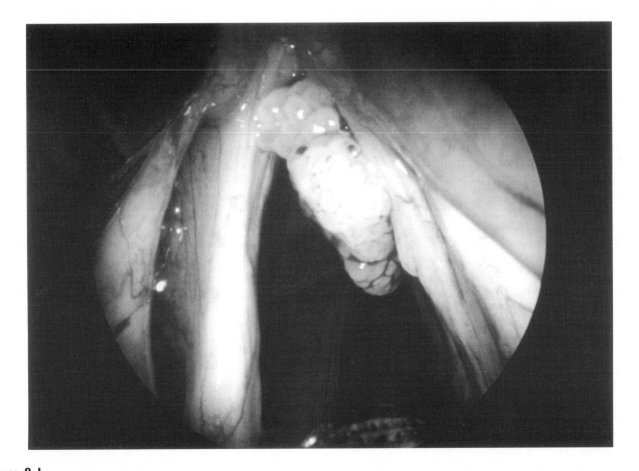

Figure 8.1
The papilloma affects the anterior half of one vocal cord, with its posterior part extending toward the subglottic area. The opposite vocal cord shows an anterior defect caused by the bulk of the tumor. (Courtesy of Brian P. Driscoll, MD, Department of Otolaryngology, UTMB Galveston, Texas.)

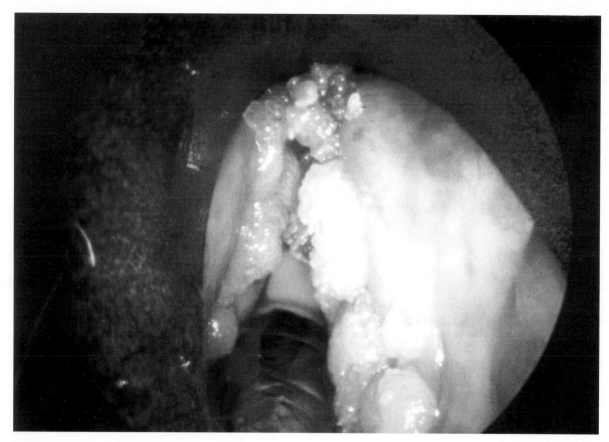

Figure 8.2
Extensive laryngeal papillomatosis. Note how the endotracheal tube is protected by foil to prevent accidental puncturing by laser. (Courtesy of Brian P. Driscoll, MD, Department of Otolaryngology, UTMB Galveston, Texas.)

during upper respiratory infections. This can lead to a clinical presentation as an acute respiratory emergency. In underserved areas, immediate tracheostomy was needed in 25% of cases for treating life-threatening complications of neglected cases of laryngeal papillomatosis.[39] In rare cases, laryngeal papillomas caused sudden death by mechanically blocking the airways.[7]

In adults, the growth of the papillomas is usually slower and, as the airways are wider than in children, the clinical presentation is less dramatic. Hoarseness is the primary complaint.

The radiological features of the primary pulmonary papillomatosis include papillomata in the distal airway and multiple, nodular lung lesions, both solid and cavitated. Changes secondary to pulmonary papillomatosis include atelectasis, infection, and bronchiectasis.[72]

The course of respiratory papillomatosis is unpredictable. The adult-onset disease is usually less severe than its juvenile form with regard to symptomatology, disease extent, and number of recurrences. Malignant transformation is not uncommon in the presence of environmental factors such as smoking and irradiation and these agents may enhance the integration of viral DNA into the genome of the host cells.[5] *In vitro* experiments also support some of these observations. When human laryngeal epithelial cells were first transfected *in vitro* with HPV 16 DNA, the cell line did not proliferate well in culture medium and was not tumorigenic in nude mice. After exposing the cells to a potent chemical carcinogen, N-methyl-N′-nitro-N-nitrosoguanidine, several proliferating colonies were isolated and one exhibited enhanced proliferation in nude mice.[29]

Non-irradiated patients may develop cancer after 30 years, and some develop papilloma in the hypopharynx and trachea, but most patients survive.[34] Bronchogenic squamous cell carcinoma has been reported in patients with recurrent respiratory papillomatosis extending into the tracheobronchial tree, even in the absence of a history of radiation therapy or smoking.[71] The role of smoking as a cofactor in the development of carcinoma origination from a papilloma is still not clear;[59] however, respiratory papilloma converting into carcinoma in the absence of smoking and irradiation is rare, with only about 20 documented cases presented in the literature.[30] In a particularly aggressive form of juvenile laryngeal papillomatosis, the lungs, intrapulmonary lymph nodes, and arteries were invaded by neoplastic tissue. The patient also developed a metastasizing squamous carcinoma of the lung.[62] Other less likely factors, such as drugs given for treatment and radiography performed throughout the illness, should be considered, together with repeated pulmonary infections and the immune status of the host.[26]

The prognosis of respiratory papillomatosis in newborns is less favorable than in infants and older children. In a series of four patients who developed the disease within the first 6 months of life, the mortality was 100% despite laser surgery and medical and immunologic therapy.[14]

HPV may act as a promoter in the multistep process of carcinogenesis in squamous cells of the larynx,[61] but this may be significant only in a minority of cases.[24] A report of two cases of recurrent laryngeal papillomatosis in women who subsequently developed squamous cell cancer when approaching menopause may suggest a relation between HPV and estrogen metabolism.[16]

Patients with multiple confluent lesions with florid koilocytosis and strongly positive reactivity for HPV 6 or 11 had a poor prognosis, requiring multiple endoscopies to control their disease.[57] The presence of HPV 6 conferred a clinically more aggressive behavior than infection with HPV type 11.[53] HPV type and the presence of viral co-infections with Epstein–Barr virus (EBV), cytomegalovirus (CMV) or herpes simplex virus (HSV) may be predictive of an aggressive clinical course.[56]

8.5 IMPACT

The impact of respiratory papillomatosis is significant. In a recent study, 1000 otolaryngologists were surveyed with regard to their current patient load of children and adults with recurrent respiratory papillomas, their surgical and anesthetic management of the disease, and their clinical experiences with risk factors for developing recurrent respiratory papillomas. There were 2354 new cases and 5970 active cases of recurrent respiratory papillomas among children, requiring 16 597 surgical procedures at a cost of $109 million for March 1, 1993 to March 31, 1994. Projected totals for adult recurrent respiratory papillomas were 3623 new cases and 9015 active cases requiring 9284 surgical procedures at a cost of $42 million for the same time period.[18]

8.6 CLASSIFICATION

Based on clinical characteristics, a widely utilized classification method distinguishes between juvenile-onset and adult-onset laryngeal papillomatosis. Another important consideration is the solitary or multiple nature of the lesions.

It was suggested that the preferred term should rather be 'recurrent respiratory papillomatosis,' because this describes the clinically significant features (widespread extent and tendency for rapid regrowth) more accurately. This group can be further divided into juvenile-onset and adult-onset subgroups to reflect the bimodal distribution of the disease.[36] The aggressive form of recurrent respiratory papillomatosis typically occurs in the very youngest of patients (average of 2 years old), whereas the less aggressive form is observed in patients of an average age of 17 years.[21] Others stated that the two most important risk factors for lesions requiring frequent laryngeal procedures were young age at the onset of papilloma and a lesion extending to the anterior third of the vocal folds. However, clinical findings (such as symptoms, size or number of primary papilloma lesions) did not predict the course of the disease, and the classic division of adult-onset laryngeal papilloma into solitary and multiple types was not clinically relevant.[1]

8.7 THERAPY

Papillomatosis presents two principal challenges to the clinician: (i) multiple recurrences, and (ii) widespread localization of the lesions. As a result, patients usually need multiple and often more extensive surgical interventions. Even though adjuvant therapeutic modalities can improve the clinical outcome, surgery is the primary treatment option.

8.7.1 Surgery

The current gold standard of papilloma treatment is endoscopic excision under magnified visualization. Carbon dioxide laser excision is the most widely used for disease elimination,[18] while preserving the normal mucosa to the greatest possible extent. Complete removal of papillomas is not necessarily possible or advisable with one surgical intervention. Following excision of the papillomata, HPV DNA persists in adjacent, normal-appearing mucosa and may serve as a source of viral reseeding.

Surgical excision is considered safe. Local complications include laryngeal scarring, formation of webs, laryngeal edema, or introduction of papillomata into previously unaffected sites. The endotracheal tube should be protected to avoid combustion, and damage to surrounding tissues should also be prevented. Suctioning of the laser plume minimizes the chance to generate airborne transmission of the infection by HPV DNA particles.

Early results with flash pump dye (FPD) laser treatment of laryngeal papillomas showed that FPD was relatively safe and feasible; however, its long-term results are pending. This type of laser coagulates rather than vaporizes tissue; therefore, it may cause less scarring than carbon dioxide laser treatment. Additional advantages are improved patient and operator safety.[11]

Respiratory papillomatosis can be removed by argon plasma coagulation via a flexible endoscope. This method offers precise, circumscribed tissue penetration without carbonization.[9]

Patients with recurrent respiratory papillomatosis often require tracheotomies. These patients usually present at a younger age with more widespread disease, which often involves the distal airway prior to tracheotomy. Distal spread occurs in 50% of patients, but it is generally limited to the tracheotomy site and the authors considered tracheotomy an appropriate option for patients with significant airway compromise resulting from papillomatosis.[64]

The seeding of viral DNA in laryngeal papillomatosis to other sites in the respiratory tract during treatment is a well-perceived possibility, with instrumentation and anesthetic maneuvers being strongly implicated. Injury to the mucosal surface can create a locus susceptible to papillomavirus infection. For instance, at tracheostomy sites, abrasion injury to ciliated epithelium heals with metaplastic squamous epithelium and creates a squamociliary junction. Therefore, avoiding injury to non-diseased squamous and ciliated epithelia is important in the prevention of iatrogenic seeding of papillomatosis.[33]

Concerns were raised regarding potential risks from exposure to the laser plume containing HPV DNA.[35] It was suggested that HPV DNA can be detected in the plume only if direct suction contact is made with the papillomatous tissue during surgery.[2] In the case of laryngeal papillomatosis of a surgeon, who treated his patients with anogenital condylomas, the disease may have been caused by inhaled virus particles present in the laser plume. The causal relationship was implied because HPV 6 and 11, which are harbored in anogenital condylomas, were detected in his laryngeal lesions.[28]

8.7.2 Photodynamic therapy

Photodynamic therapy employs hematoporphyrin derivatives, administered intravenously 48–72 h prior to laser surgery. These agents are activated by an argon pump dye laser system. In 33 patients with recurrent laryngeal papillomatosis, there was a significant (about 50%) decrease in the average rate of papilloma growth following laser surgery. Photosensitivity was the only side-effect.[3] Subsequently, 28 patients with moderate to severe recurrent laryngeal papillomatosis were treated with photodynamic therapy as an alternative treatment modality. Although photodynamic therapy had a beneficial effect on the growth rate of laryngeal papillomatosis, no significant change in response was obtained by increasing the light dose from 50 to 80 J/cm^2.[4] Photodynamic therapy with dihematoporphyrin ether (DHE), either alone or in combination with radiation therapy, may have a role in the treatment of juvenile laryngotracheobronchial papillomatosis.[37] The effects of DHE were dose dependent in laryngeal papillomatosis: patients treated with larger doses of DHE experienced a significantly larger decrease in papilloma growth rate but there was no impact on the persistence of HPV DNA.[65]

8.7.3 Immunotherapy and pharmacotherapy

The role of interferons (IFNs) seems to be promising and safe, with patients having complete or partial remission[6,40] or the growth of papillomas slowing down.[31] During a 3-year follow-up of 16 patients with recurrent respiratory papilloma treated IFN–α, 50% of the patients cleared, 25% improved, and 25% developed severe disease.[46]

In conjunction with laser surgery, adjuvant intralesional IFN–α is effective and safe and extends the therapeutical possibilities available in laryngotracheal papillomatosis.[70] IFN as adjuvant therapy to laser surgery resulted in 16/34 complete responses (for at least 6 months) and 12/34 partial responses in recurrent respiratory papillomatosis.[6] In another study, 3/5 children, treated with daily doses of IFN were disease free up to 22–68 months thereafter; in another patient, the frequency of relapses was reduced.[47] In a randomized cross-over study of IFN–α as an adjuvant to carbon dioxide laser surgical excision, 66 patients with clinically severe juvenile-onset recurrent respiratory papillomatosis were followed over a period of 12 months. Patients received either IFN (5×10^6 units/m^2) daily for 28 days and three times weekly for 5 months or were only observed. Endoscopic excisions were performed every 2 months and clinical courses were compared on a basis of composite scores determined at each endoscopy. Statistically significant improvement occurred in the patient group which received IFN.[32]

In a larger study of 125 patients with laryngeal papillomatosis, employing intramuscular leukocyte IFN–α (102 cases), recombinant IFN–α 2b (12 cases), or both preparations (11 cases) after surgical debulking, 89 cases (71%) had complete response. Sixty of them have been followed for more than 3 years and, even in cases where relapses were noted, the frequency of recurrence generally decreased. This

therapeutic regimen was more effective if it was initiated in less than 3 months after the disease onset.[19]

Side-effects of IFN therapy include flu-like disease, fever, febrile seizures, headache, nausea, vomiting, anorexia, and mild rise in liver enzymes. These side-effects are usually mild and resolve upon discontinuation of the drug. For relieving pain or fever, acetaminophen is the drug of choice because aspirin and non-steroidal anti-inflammatory drugs diminish the effectiveness of IFN.[6]

An *in vitro* system of growing human laryngeal papillomatosis cells showed that retinoic acid modulates the differentiation of human laryngeal papillomatosis cells. The HPV DNA content was in inverse correlation with the concentration of retinoic acid.[60] Isotretinoin was suggested to be an effective adjuvant therapy for aggressive respiratory papillomatosis, based on a single case of an extensive tracheoesophageal and bronchoalveolar papillomatosis that degenerated into squamous cell cancer. Multiple endoscopic laser excisions and prolonged use of IFN both failed to control the progression of the disease. Isotretinoin therapy (1mg/kg/day) resulted in dramatic clinical, radiographic, and functional improvement without significant toxic effects, and no endoscopic procedures were necessary over the ensuing 6-month period.[22] Isotretinoin did not produce any clinical response in patients with recurrent respiratory papillomatosis.[6] In another pilot study, 13-cis-retinoic acid proved to be too toxic for chronic application.[8]

The acyclic nucleoside phosphonate (S)-1-(3-hydroxy-2-phosphonylmethoxypropyl)-cytosine (HPMPC, cidofovir, Vistide) has a broad-spectrum activity against a wide variety of DNA viruses including HPV in different cell culture systems and/or animal models. The diphosphorylated HPMPC derivative HPMPCpp is the active intracellular metabolite, which interacts with the viral DNA polymerase and confers a prolonged antiviral action, which allows infrequent (weekly or biweekly) dosing.[17] Intratumoral cidofovir injections led to complete resolution of the lesions in 14 out of 17 patients with severe laryngeal papillomatosis. The treatment was well tolerated, without significant side-effects.[67] In a case report of laryngeal papillomatosis, for which the patient underwent surgery on more than 80 occasions during 30 years, intralesional cidofovir showed some clinical effect, although only on the superficial tumor growth[55]

Aciclovir is not recommended in the treatment of juvenile respiratory papillomatosis because its activity depends upon the presence of viral thymidine kinase, which is not encoded by papillomaviruses.[49] Therefore, it was surprising that acyclovir decreased the extent of respiratory papillomatosis in patients with recalcitrant disease. However, its limited beneficial effect was insufficient to counteract the rebound of disease in patients in whom IFN was stopped abruptly.[23] In another study of three children with laryngeal papillomatosis, aciclovir was used after surgical removal of the papillomas. No recurrences were seen 18–42 months following therapy.[45]

Local chemotherapy with 5-fluorouracil, methotrexate, and cis-platinum was also tested in laryngeal papillomatosis. Aerosolized 5-fluorouracil resulted in moderate clinical response with significant clinical toxicity.[66] Methotrexate yielded improvement of severity of disease and treatment interval in all three patients to whom it was administered after these patients had a failure of laser surgery followed by adjuvant IFN therapy.[6]

Ribavirin as an adjuvant therapy resulted in significant reduction in the frequency of therapeutic endoscopies in a tracheotomized child with extensive tracheobronchial papillomatosis.[50] In an uncontrolled trial, two of four adults achieved complete remission for 2 months, and both developed only minimal recurrent disease in 4 months. The two other patients had a partial response and an increased interval between the required surgeries. Ribavirin caused only a mild, reversible reduction in hemoglobin and reticulocytosis.[48]

8.7.4 Irradiation

For several decades, irradiation was extensively used in the treatment of laryngeal papillomatosis, especially in children. The role of radiation therapy in the treatment of recurrent adult laryngeal papillomatosis has been controversial, with several reports of malignant transformation following treatment.[12] Irradiated papilloma can become cancerous at about 10 years and these patients rarely survive.[34] This treatment modality increased the risk of laryngeal and even bronchial carcinomas by 16-fold.[43]

8.7.5 Vaccination

Successful results with vaccinating animals (e.g., prophylaxis and rejection of epidermal and alimentary canal tumors in cattle) have important implications for the management of HPV-associated tumors in humans.[13]

8.8 SUMMARY

Papillomatosis of the aero-digestive tract, including the oral cavity, hypopharynx, esophagus, and bronchial system, is one of the most common benign laryngeal tumors. Several types of HPVs, especially types 6, 11, 16, and 18, play a role in the etiology. The lesions are histologically benign; however, their recurrence or dissemination can ultimately impair the patency of the airways. The clinical behavior is variable: the lesions most often regress, occasionally persist, or can progress to cancer. Because of the recurrences and/or widespread nature of aero-digestive papillomatosis, treatment is often difficult. The current gold standard is endoscopic excision, primarily with carbon dioxide laser. Photodynamic therapy as well as immunotherapeutic and pharmacotherapeutic approaches (5-fluorouracil, methotrexate, cis-platinum, interferons, retinoic acid, cidofovir, ribavirin) are currently being investigated.

REFERENCES

1. Aaltonen LM, Peltomaa J, Rihkanen H. (1997) Prognostic value of clinical findings in histologically verified adult-onset laryngeal papillomas. *Eur Arch Oto-Rhino-Laryngol* **254**: 219–22.
2. Abramson AL, DiLorenzo TP, Steinberg BM. (1990) Is papillomavirus detectable in the plume of laser-treated laryngeal papilloma? *Arch Otolaryngol Head Neck Surg* **116**: 604–7.
3. Abramson AL, Shikowitz MJ, Mullooly VM, *et al.* (1992) Clinical effects of photodynamic therapy on recurrent laryngeal papillomas. *Arch Otolaryngol Head Neck Surg* **118**: 25–9.
4. Abramson AL, Shikowitz MJ, Mullooly VM, *et al.* (1994) Variable light-dose effect on photodynamic therapy for laryngeal papillomas. *Arch Otolaryngol Head Neck Surg* **120**: 852–5.
5. Arndt O, Brock J, Kundt O, *et al.* (1994) Detection of human papillomavirus DNA in formalin fixed invasive squamous cell carcinoma of the larynx with polymerase chain reaction (PCR). *Laryngo-Rhino-Otol* **73**: 527–32.
6. Avidano MA, Singleton GT. (1995) Adjuvant drug strategies in the treatment of recurrent respiratory papillomatosis. *Otolaryngol Head Neck Surg* **112**: 197–202.
7. Balazic J, Masera A, Poljak M. (1997) Sudden death caused by laryngeal papillomatosis. *Acta Oto-Laryngol* **527**(Suppl.): 111–13.
8. Bell R, Hong WK, Itri LM, *et al.* (1988) The use of cis-retinoic acid in recurrent respiratory papillomatosis of the larynx: a randomized pilot study. *Am J Otolaryngol* **9**: 161–4.
9. Bergler W, Riedel F, Gotte K, *et al.* (1997) The treatment of juvenile laryngeal papillomatosis with argon plasma coagulation. *Deut Medizin Wochensch* **122**: 1033–6.
10. Bomholt A. (1988) Laryngeal papillomas with adult onset. An epidemiological study from the Copenhagen region. *Acta Oto-Laryngol* **106**: 140–4.
11. Bower CM, Waner M, Parkin D, *et al.* (1998) Flash pump dye laser treatment of laryngeal papillomas. *Ann Otol Rhinol Laryngol* **107**: 1001–5.
12. Byhardt R., Almagro U. (1988) The role of radiation therapy in the treatment of recurrent adult laryngeal papillomatosis. [Review]. *Am J Clin Oncol* **11**: 131–7.
13. Campo MS. (1991) Vaccination against papillomavirus. [Review]. *Cancer Cells* **3**: 421–6.
14. Chipps BE, Mcclurg FL, Jr, Freidman EM, *et al.* (1990) Respiratory papillomas: presentation before six months. *Pediatr Pulmonol* **9**: 125–30.
15. Clarke J, Terry RM, Lacey CJ. (1991) A study to estimate the prevalence of upper respiratory tract papillomatosis in patients with genital warts. *Int J STD AIDS* **2**: 114–5.
16. Colquhoun-Flannery, W., Carruth, J.A. (1995) Diet-modified sex hormone metabolism: is this the way forward in recurrent respiratory papillomatosis and squamous carcinoma prophylaxis? *J Laryngol Otol* **109**: 873–5.
17. de Clercq E. (1996) Therapeutic potential of Cidofovir (HPMPC, Vistide) for the treatment of DNA virus (i.e. herpes-, papova-, pox- and adenovirus) infections. *Verh K Acad Geneesk Belg* **58**: 19–47.
18. Derkay CS. (1995) Task force on recurrent respiratory papillomas. A preliminary report. *Arch Otolaryngol Head Neck Surg* **121**: 1386–91.
19. Deunas L, Alcantud V, Alvarez F, *et al.* (1997) Use of interferon-alpha in laryngeal papillomatosis: eight years of the Cuban national programme. *J Laryngol Otology* **111**: 134–40.
20. Dickens P, Srivastava E, Loke SL, *et al.* (1991) Human papillomavirus 6, 11, and 16 in laryngeal papillomas. *J Pathol* **165**: 243–6.
21. Doyle DJ, Gianoli GJ, Espinola T, *et al.* (1994) Recurrent

respiratory papillomatosis: juvenile versus adult forms. *Laryngoscope* **104**: 523–7.

22. Eicher SA, Taylor-Cooley LD, Donovan DT. (1994) Isotretinoin therapy for recurrent respiratory papillomatosis. *Arch Otolaryngol Head Neck Surg* **120**: 405–9.

23. Endres DR, Bauman NM, Burke D, *et al.* (1994) Acyclovir in the treatment of recurrent respiratory papillomatosis. A pilot study. *Ann Otol Rhinol Laryngol* **103**: 301–5.

24. Fouret P, Martin F, Flahault A, *et al.* (1995) Human papillomavirus infection in the malignant and premalignant head and neck epithelium. *Diagn Mol Pathol* **4**: 122–7.

25. Fukushima K, Ogura H, Watanabe S, *et al.* (1994) Human papillomavirus type 16 DNA detected by the polymerase chain reaction in non-cancer fissures of the head and neck. *Eur Arch Oto-Rhino-Laryngol* **251**: 109–12.

26. Guillou L, Sahli R, Chaubert P, *et al.* (1991) Squamous cell carcinoma of the lung in a nonsmoking, nonirradiated patient with juvenile laryngotracheal papillomatosis. Evidence of human papillomavirus-11 DNA in both carcinoma and papillomas. *Am J Surg Pathol* **15**: 891–8.

27. Hallden C, Majmudar B. (1986) The relationship between juvenile laryngeal papillomatosis and maternal condylomata acuminata. *J Reprod Med* **31**: 804–7.

28. Hallmo P, Naess O. (1991) Laryngeal papillomatosis with human papillomavirus DNA contracted by a laser surgeon. *Eur Arch Oto-Rhino-Laryngol* **248**: 425–7.

29. Hartley C, Hamilton J, Birzgalis AR, *et al.* (1994) Recurrent respiratory papillomatosis – the Manchester experience, 1974–1992. *J Laryngol Otol* **108**: 226–9.

30. Hasan S, Dutt SN, Kini U, *et al.* (1995) Laryngeal carcinoma ex-papilloma in a non-irradiated, non-smoking patient: a clinical record and review of the literature. *J Laryngol Otol* **109**: 762–6.

31. Healy GB, Gelber RD, Trowbridge AL, *et al.* (1988) Treatment of recurrent respiratory papillomatosis with human leukocyte interferon. Results of a multicenter randomized clinical trial. *N Engl J Med* **319**: 401–7.

32. Kashima H, Leventhal B, Clark K, *et al.* (1988) Interferon alfa-nil (Wellferon) in juvenile onset recurrent respiratory papillomatosis: results of a randomized study in twelve collaborative institutions. *Laryngoscope* **98**: 334–40.

33. Kashima H, Mounts P, Leventhal B, *et al.* (1993) Sites of predilection in recurrent respiratory papillomatosis. *Ann Otol Rhinol Laryngol* **102**: 580–3.

34. Kashima H, Wu TC, Mounts P, *et al.* (1988) Carcinoma ex-papilloma: histologic and virologic studies in whole-organ sections of the larynx. *Laryngoscope* **98**: 619–24.

35. Kashima HK, Kessis T, Mounts P, *et al.* (1991) Polymerase chain reaction identification of human papillomavirus DNA in CO_2 laser plume from recurrent respiratory papillomatosis. *Otolaryngol Head Neck Surg* **104**: 191–5.

36. Kashima HK, Shah F, Lyles A, *et al.* (1992) A comparison of risk factors in juvenile-onset and adult-onset recurrent respiratory papillomatosis. *Laryngoscope* **102**: 9–13.

37. Kavuru MS, Mehta AC, Eliachar I. (1990) Effect of photodynamic therapy and external beam radiation therapy on juvenile laryngotracheobronchial papillomatosis. *Am Rev Resp Dis* **141**: 509–10.

38. Kjer JJ, Eldon K, Dreisler A. (1988) Maternal condylomata and juvenile laryngeal papillomas in their children. *Zentralb Gynakol* **110**: 107–10.

39. Kpemissi E, Agbere AR, Sossou K. (1995) Laryngeal papillomatosis in children: therapeutic problems apropos of 39 cases at the Lome University Hospital Center. *Rev Laryngol Otol Rhinol* **116**: 335–8.

40. Leventhal BG, Kashima HK, Mounts P, *et al.* (1991) Long-term response of recurrent respiratory papillomatosis to treatment with lymphoblastoid interferon alfa-N1. Papilloma Study Group. *N Engl J Med* **325**: 613–7.

41. Lin KY, Westra WH, Kashima HK, *et al.* (1997) Coinfection of HPV-11 and HPV-16 in a case of laryngeal squamous papillomas with severe dysplasia. *Laryngoscope* **107**: 942–7.

42. Lindeberg H, Elbrond O. (1990a) Laryngeal papillomas: the epidemiology in a Danish subpopulation 1965–1984. *Clin Otolaryngol* **15**: 125–31.

43. Lindeberg H, Elbrond O. (1991) Malignant tumours in patients with a history of multiple laryngeal papillomas: the significance of irradiation. *Clin Otolaryngol* **16**: 149–51.

44. Lindeberg H, Johansen L. (1990) The presence of human papillomavirus (HPV) in solitary adult laryngeal papillomas demonstrated by in-situ DNA hybridization with sulphonated probes. *Clin Otolaryngol* **15**: 367–71.

45. Lopez Aguado D, Perez Pinero B, Betancor L, *et al.* (1991) Acyclovir in the treatment of laryngeal papillomatosis. *Int J Pediatr Otorhinolaryngol* **21**: 269–74.

46. Lusk RP, McCabe BF, Mixon JH. (1987) Three-year experience of treating recurrent respiratory papilloma with interferon. *Ann Otol Rhinol Laryngol* **96**: 158–62.

47. Mattot M, Ninane E, Hamoir M, *et al.* (1990) Combined CO_2-laser and alpha recombinant interferon treatment in five children with juvenile laryngeal papillomatosis. *Acta Clin Belg* **45**: 158–63.

48. McGlennen RC, Adams GL, Lewis CM, *et al.* (1993) Pilot trial of ribavirin for the treatment of laryngeal papillomatosis. *Head Neck* **15**: 504–12.

49. Morrison GA, Evans JN. (1993) Juvenile respiratory papillomatosis: acyclovir reassessed. *Int J Pediatr Otorhinolaryngol* **26**: 193–7.

50. Morrison GA, Kotecha B, Evans JN. (1993) Ribavirin treatment for juvenile respiratory papillomatosis. *J Laryngol Otol* **107**: 423–6.

51. Nunez DA, Astley SM, Lewis FA, *et al.* (1994) Human papilloma viruses: a study of their prevalence in the normal larynx. *J Laryngol Otol* **108**: 319–20.

52. Obalek S, Misiewicz J, Jablonska S, *et al.* (1993) Childhood condyloma acuminatum: association with genital and cutaneous human papillomaviruses. *Pediatr Dermatol* **10**: 101–6.

53. Padayachee A, Prescott CA. (1993) Relationship between the clinical course and HPV typing of recurrent laryngeal papillomatosis. The Red Cross War Memorial Children's Hospital experience 1982–1988. *Int J Pediatr Otorhinolaryngol* **26**: 141–7.

54. Peng TC, Searle CP, Shah KV, *et al.* (1990) Prevalence of human papillomavirus infections in term pregnancy. *Am J Perinatol* **7**: 189–92.

55. Petersen BL, Buchwald C, Gerstoft J, *et al.* (1998) An aggressive and invasive growth of juvenile papillomas

involving the total respiratory tract. *J Laryngol Otol* **112**: 1101–4.

56. Pou AM, Rimell FL, Jordan JA, *et al.* (1995) Adult respiratory papillomatosis: human papillomavirus type and viral coinfections as predictors of prognosis. *Ann Otol Rhinol Laryngol* **104**: 758–62.

57. Quiney RE, Wells M, Lewis FA, *et al.* (1989) Laryngeal papillomatosis: correlation between severity of disease and presence of HPV 6 and 11 detected by in situ DNA hybridisation. *J Clin Pathol* **42**: 694–8.

58. Rady PL, Schnadig VJ, Weiss RL, *et al.* (1998) Malignant transformation of recurrent respiratory papillomatosis associated with integrated human papillomavirus type 11 DNA and mutation of p53. *Laryngoscope* **108**: 735–40.

59. Rehberg, E., Kleinsasser, O. (1999) Malignant transformation in non-irradiated juvenile laryngeal papillomatosis. *Eur Arch Oto-Rhino-Laryngol* **256**: 450–4.

60. Reppucci AD, DiLorenzo TP, Abramson AL, *et al.* (1991) In vitro modulation of human laryngeal papilloma cell differentiation by retinoic acid. *Otolaryngol Head Neck Surg* **105**: 528–32.

61. Salam MA, Rockett J, Morris A. (1995) General primer-mediated polymerase chain reaction for simultaneous detection and typing of human papillomavirus DNA in laryngeal squamous cell carcinomas. *Clin Otolaryngol* **20**: 84–8.

62. Schnadig VJ, Clark WD, Clegg TJ, *et al.* (1986) Invasive papillomatosis and squamous carcinoma complicating juvenile laryngeal papillomatosis. *Arch Otolaryngol Head Neck Surg* **112**: 966–71.

63. Shah K, Kashima H, Polk BF, *et al.* (1986) Rarity of cesarean delivery in cases of juvenile-onset respiratory papillomatosis. *Obstet Gynecol* **68**: 795–9.

64. Shapiro AM, Rimell FL, Shoemaker D, *et al.* (1996) Tracheotomy in children with juvenile-onset recurrent respiratory papillomatosis: the Children's Hospital of Pittsburgh experience. *Ann Otol Rhinol Laryngol* **105**: 1–5.

65. Shikowitz MJ, Abramson AL, Freeman K, *et al.* (1998) Efficacy of DHE photodynamic therapy for respiratory papillomatosis: immediate and long–term results. *Laryngoscope* **108**: 962–7.

66. Smith HG, Healy GB, Vaughan CW, *et al.* (1980) Topical chemotherapy of recurrent respiratory papillomatosis. A preliminary report. *Ann Otol Rhinol Laryngol* **89**: 472–8.

67. Snoeck R, Wellens W, Desloovere C, *et al.* (1998) Treatment of severe laryngeal papillomatosis with intralesional injections of cidofovir [(S)-1-(3-hydroxy-2-phosphonylmethoxypropyl)cytosine]. *J Med Virol* **54**: 219–25.

68. St Louis ME, Icenogle JP, Manzila T, *et al.* (1993) Genital types of papillomavirus in children of women with HIV-1 infection in Kinshasa, Zaire. *Int J Cancer* **54**: 181–4.

69. Strong MS, Vaughan CW, Healy GB, *et al.* (1976) Recurrent respiratory papillomatosis. *Ann Otol Rhinol Laryngol* **85**: 508–16.

70. Walther EK, Herberhold C. (1993) Treatment of laryngotracheal papillomatosis with combined use of laser surgery and intralesional administration of alpha-interferon (Roferon). *Laryngo-Rhino-Otologie* **72**: 485–91.

71. Wilde E, Duggan MA, Field SK. (1994) Bronchogenic squamous cell carcinoma complicating localized recurrent respiratory papillomatosis. *Chest* **105**: 1887–8.

72. Williams SD, Jamieson DH, Prescott CA. (1994) Clinical and radiological features in three cases of pulmonary involvement from recurrent respiratory papillomatosis. *Int J Pediatr Otorhinolaryngol* **30**: 71–7.

73. Wood CL. (1991) Laryngeal papillomas in infants and children. Relationship to maternal venereal warts. *J Nurse Midwifery* **36**: 297–302.

9

Epidermodysplasia verruciformis

Slawomir Majewski and Stefania Jablonska

9.1 INTRODUCTION

Epidermodysplasia verruciformis (EV) is a human papillomavirus (HPV)-associated, life-long, genetically determined disease, originally described as a genodermatosis.[65] The lesions start to appear in early childhood and multiple carcinomas develop later in life in about half of the patients, mostly in the fourth to fifth decades.[78,79] Thus, EV is in essence a genetic cancer of viral origin, and could also be regarded as a model of cutaneous HPV oncogenesis.[53,69]

Although EV is a genetically transmitted disease, it differs from other genodermatoses by association with specific HPVs and the development of cancers from HPV-harboring lesions. It differs from other HPV infections of the skin by life-long persistence of viruses, which are not infectious for immunocompetent individuals.

A characteristic feature of EV is immunotolerance toward the EV-specific HPV types which persist during the whole lifespan. It could be speculated that immune tolerance results from a possible vertical transmission of EV HPV *in utero*, as documented by the case of a EV patient who has given birth to healthy child. DNA of EV HPVs was found in the newborn as well as in the amniotic fluid and placenta, and was demonstrated to be of the same type as that found in the mother.[34] Recently, it has been shown that maternal hematopoietic cells can pass through the placenta and, conversely, the fetal DNA can pass into the circulation of the mother. The transfer through the placenta starts as early as 5–6 weeks of gestation,[103] and could stimulate the development of tolerance due to exposure of the developing fetal thymus to antigens present in maternal circulation.[75] Alternatively, the mother's cells may persist in the child's circulation and, by HLA compatibility, may also induce or aggravate immune tolerance. Recently, it was also shown that the *in utero* HPV infection primarily involves the trophoblast, as found in spontaneously aborted products of conception.[48] As a rapidly proliferating part of the placenta, the trophoblast presents a preferential target for HPV.

EV is associated with disease-specific HPVs, EV HPVs, that are harmless for the general population due to host restriction of EV HPV. Thus, a genetically transmitted, specific immune defect appears to be a crucial factor for development of the disease. Cutaneous responses to various locally applied sensitizers are, as a rule, absent, which is suggestive of defective local cellular immunity dependent on antigen-presenting cells and/or EV HPV-harboring keratinocytes.[25] However, in several patients, the immunosuppression is more severe and not limited to the patient's own EV HPVs.[55] This could be in part due to the persistence and extent of the viral load.

We found that the decrease of cell-mediated immunity (CMI) is most pronounced in patients with EV HPVs and HPV 3 or related HPVs responsible for plane warts in the general population.[71] In immunosuppressed populations, EV HPVs were co-detected in lesions displaying clinical and histologic features of plane warts,[77] with no EV phenotype, probably as a consequence of preserved host cell restriction of the EV HPV genome. Thus, viral proteins of some HPVs appear to enable persistence of episomal EV HPV DNA in a latent form. Immunosuppression that facilitates HPV infection accounts for the lack of regression of lesions, which may result in accumulation of mutational errors and lead to malignant conversion. Interestingly, the only successful transepidermal inoculation of

EV HPVs was performed with the use of antigens obtained from patients having mixed EV HPVs and HPV 3 infection.[53,54] Also, a more recent study in immunosuppressed patients stresses a frequent co-detection of HPV 3-related HPVs in patients infected with EV HPVs.[93] Moreover, changes may appear in the immunosuppressed population having clinical and histologic characteristics of EV and harboring EV HPV DNA.[43,66,81] Of special interest is the development of EV lesions in a heavily immunosuppressed patient with Hodgkin's disease after X-ray irradiation. This is highly suggestive of the role of cofactors in virally induced oncogenesis. The significance of immunosuppression in EV is also evidenced by reported cases of symptomatic disease in patients co-infected with HIV and EV-type HPVs.[5,7,86]

Because the risk of developing cancers in immunosuppressed populations depends on the duration and severity of immunosuppression and parallels the presence and extent of warts,[14,36,74,85] an intriguing question is whether EV HPVs are involved in cutaneous oncogenesis in immunocompromised individuals. The introduction of a most sensitive technique of nested polymerase chain reaction (PCR) with the use of degenerate primers allowed the detection of EV HPVs or EV HPV-related DNA sequences in a high proportion of tumors in immunosuppressed populations.[8,28,93,94,101,102,111] Most importantly, similar diverse EV-related or EV HPV DNAs were found in tumors of immunocompetent populations.[3,8,29,94,111]

Of special interest is a possible ubiquitous presence of EV HPVs in a latent form in normal individuals, both in hair follicles[15,16] and in skin,[3] with detectability of EV HPVs or EV-related HPV DNA sequences in cutaneous tumors.[30,47,82,94] Most of the newly detected EV HPVs or EV-related HPVs are not yet cloned, and their role in cancers in the general population must still be confirmed. A high frequency of EV HPVs in cutaneous cancers is suggestive of their participation in cutaneous oncogenesis. However, the presence of DNA sequences of divergent EV HPVs, but not of the most oncogenic HPV 5, and no evidence for E6 and E7 gene expression do not support the primary role of EV HPV in non-melanoma skin cancer in non-EV patients.

9.2 EPIDERMODYSPLASIA VERRUCIFORMIS HPVs

9.2.1 The phylogenetic tree

The phylogenetic tree for EV HPVs was constructed on the basis of nucleotide homology.[9,24,27] EV HPVs were found to be in a main branch, with two subgroups consisting of the following HPVs (Figure 9.1.):

first subgroup: HPVs 5, 8, 12, 19, 20, (20b = 46), 21, 24, 25, 36, and 47;
second subgroup: HPVs 9, 15, 17, 22, 23, 37, 38, and 49; more distantly related: HPVs 48 and 50.

The location of HPV 14 on the sub-branches of the tree is unknown. This classification will certainly be modified after new HPV types are characterized and cloned.

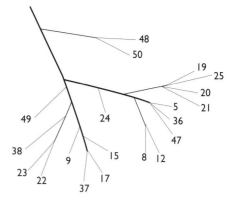

Figure 9.1
The branch of the phylogenetic tree for EV HPVs according to Chan et al.[24]

It is to be stressed that, in contrast to benign EV lesions in which a large spectrum of EV HPVs is found, HPV 5 and HPV 8 predominate in EV skin cancers; HPVs 14, 17, 20, and 47[78] are detected much less frequently.

Because HPV 5 and HPV 8 show a strong genetic heterogeneity and the presence of stable variants,[31,61] it is conceivable that the diversity of HPVs associated with EV is still greater.

9.2.2 Molecular biology of EV HPVs and their role in cutaneous carcinogenesis

EV HPVs exhibit some important differences in their organization of DNA and in the expression of some genes as compared to other HPVs, including high-risk genital types.[1,38] The main differences are:

- The non-coding regulatory region (NCR) of EV HPVs is only half as large as the NCR of all other HPVs,[37,38] suggesting a distinct nature of mechanisms regulating viral gene expression and response to regulatory transcription factors.
- There is no gene coding for E5 protein.
- E6 and E7 oncoproteins of oncogenic EV HPVs are very frequently expressed in EV tumors despite a very rare integration of viral DNA into the host DNA,[31,110] except for metastatic tumors.[108]
- E6 and L1 of EV HPVs show unusual genomic heterogeneity, which might reflect immunological selective mechanisms related to the formation of antibodies against these proteins[61]
- E6 oncoprotein of EV HPVs, in contrast to genital HPVs, does not degrade p53,[50,98] and E7 oncoprotein has a very low, if any, transforming activity.[1,50]

Thus, the mechanisms of cell transformation by oncogenic EV HPVs are much less known and seem to differ considerably from those of genital high-risk HPV 16 and HPV 18.[1] Our recent studies suggest that EV HPV-associated carcinogenesis also differs from cutaneous oncogenesis in the general population. Both in skin cancers in the general population and in EV tumors mutations of p53 were found in comparable frequencies (about 50%) (submitted). However, DNA sequencing revealed $C \rightarrow G$ and $C \rightarrow A$ mutations different from ultraviolet (UV)-induced mutations $C \rightarrow T$

and CC→TT[18,19] in non-EV patients. Immunohistochemical staining suggested that, in the majority of EV cancers, there was accumulation of p53, accompanied by a marked down-regulation of bcl-2 protein. It is conceivable that these changes in p53 and bcl-2 could enhance apoptosis in EV tumors, which is a characteristic feature of these neoplasms.[53,64]

9.3 IMMUNOLOGIC ASPECTS OF EPIDERMODYSPLASIA VERRUCIFORMIS

9.3.1 Immunogenetics

The immune response to various pathogens, including HPVs, is genetically determined and depends on major histocompatibility complex (MHC) class I and class II molecules involved in the process of antigen presentation and in the development of specific effector T cytotoxic cells or anti-HPV antibodies.[17] Therefore, it is believed that particular MHC alleles involved in antigen presentation could determine the host reactions of immunity or immunotolerance, leading to regression or progression of HPV-associated tumors. In the rabbit Shope papilloma–carcinoma complex, which is considered an animal model of EV, malignant progression or regression of rabbit papillomas was shown to be closely linked to MHC class II genes.[20,45] In these studies, analysis of the polymorphism of class II MHC in the rabbits revealed strong linkage between papillomavirus regression and a DR EcoRI fragment, whereas malignant conversion of the lesions was found to be associated with a DQ PvuII fragment. The preliminary studies in a large series of 57 EV patients also revealed positive and negative associations of specific MHC class II (DR-DQ) haplotypes.[35] These haplotypes could represent susceptibility alleles or markers in linkage disequilibrium with gene(s) predisposing to the disease. However, no specific EV gene within MHC class I, II, and III has yet been identified. Recently, a susceptibility locus for EV (EV1) was mapped to the 17qter region, in close proximity to Psors 2 major susceptibility locus for psoriasis.[87]

9.3.2 Immunotolerance in EV patients

EV patients show cutaneous unresponsiveness to EV HPVs and to epicutaneously applied antigens, eg., dinitrochlorobenzene (DNCB).[41] A defect of local CMI is probably responsible for the inability of natural cytotoxic cells to lyse EV HPV-harboring keratinocytes[71] and for the unresponsiveness of EV patients' lymphocytes to autologous keratinocytes infected by the EV HPVs.[25] The mechanisms of this specific and non-specific immunotolerance are still unknown, but recent studies suggest that UV irradiation may play an important role.

The role of ultraviolet irradiation in the development of immune defects in EV

Ultraviolet irradiation (especially UVB) is known as an environmental factor inducing both local and systemic immuno-suppression. UVB was found to impair the induction of contact hypersensitivity,[109] and the extent of this defect was suggested to present a risk factor for skin cancer.[76,100,109] The inhibitory effect of UVB on the development of immune reactions could be related to a local generation in the epidermis of cis-urocanic acid (c-UCA) (for review, see reference 76). It was shown that application of c-UCA on the skin suppressed CMI reactions against herpes simplex virus and various contact sensitizers.[46,91] We found that the stratum corneum of the epidermis from sun-exposed areas in EV patients contained markedly increased concentrations of c-UCA.[55] Interestingly, increased levels of c-UCA were also found in healthy members of the families of EV patients. The immunosuppressive effects of c-UCA could be related to its capability of disturbing antigen presentation by Langerhans' cells. Although the number and distribution of Langerhans' cells in the epidermis of EV patients were found to be unchanged,[25,44] it is possible that some locally generated UVB-inducible cytokines could alter the function of antigen-presenting cells in EV.

The role of cytokines and adhesion molecules

Ultraviolet B is a factor capable of inducing not only proinflammatory cytokines in the skin but also various cytokines with immunosuppressive properties, e.g., tumor necrosis factor-α (TNFα), transforming growth factor-β (TGFβ), interleukin-10 (IL-10), α-melanocyte-stimulating hormone (αMSH), and others. Two of them, TNFα and TGFβ, were found to be overexpressed in both benign and malignant EV lesions.[68] An increased expression of TNFα could contribute to the induction of local immunosuppression or immunotolerance toward EV HPV- infected cells because TNFα was shown to prevent Langerhans cells from migrating to the regional lymph node.[76,99] Moreover, TNFα seems to be a mediator of c-UCA-induced immunosuppression after UVB exposure.

TGFβ has a variety of immunosuppressive effects, including inhibition of T-cell proliferation, decrease of IL-1-dependent antigen presentation, and inhibition of natural killer (NK) and lymphokine-activated killer (LAK) cell cytotoxicity.[89]

IL-10 was not studied in EV, although this cytokine was found to be expressed in some squamous cell and basal cell carcinomas.[62] The production of IL-10 in keratinocytes is stimulated by UVB.[88] The immunosuppressive effects on T-helper 1 cells (Th1) are due to inhibition of B7/BB1-dependent Th1 cell proliferation and inhibition of production of interferon-gamma (IFNγ) and IL-12[92,96] Thus, IL-10 could render T-cells anergic to HPV antigens or to putative tumor-associated antigens.

Another important immunosuppressive factor is αMSH, initially recognized as a main cytokine-stimulating melanogenesis.[107] Although αMSH was not studied in EV, it is striking that the exposed skin lesions of these patients are frequently hyperpigmented[51] and production of this cytokine is induced by UVB.[23] The local immunosuppressive action of αMSH is related to its capability to antagonize the effects of IL-1a, IL-1b, IL-6 and IFNγ as well as to induce the production of Th2-derived IL-10.[12,22,49] Most importantly, αMSH was found not only to induce local suppression of contact hypersensitivity but also to induce hapten-specific immunotolerance.[42]

Cytokines and adhesion molecules could also be of significance for the relatively slow progression of EV tumors, which rarely form metastases. Overexpression of TGFβ in the skin lesions of EV patients may play an important role. A strong correlation was reported between the loss of TGFβ and malignant progression of mouse papillomas,[39] and it was shown that genetic depletion of this cytokine stimulates progression to squamous cell carcinomas.[40] The anti-tumor and anti-invasive properties of TGFβ could be linked to its ability to decrease cell proliferation[89] and to inhibit angiogenesis induced by angiogenic factors, e.g., β-fibroblast growth factor (βFGF).[80]

9.4 CLINICAL AND HISTOLOGIC FINDINGS

9.4.1 Polymorphic cutaneous lesions associated with EV HPVs

The cutaneous lesions in EV are highly polymorphic, although the most typical findings are red macules and plaques, plane wart-like and pityriasis versicolor-like lesions.

Red macules and *plaques* have irregular borders and somewhat scaly surfaces (Figure 9.2), are localized mainly on the thorax and neck, but not infrequently also involve the pubic area, arms, and thighs. Larger and more irregular *brownish plaques*, often confluent and widespread (Figure 9.3), are seen in some patients.

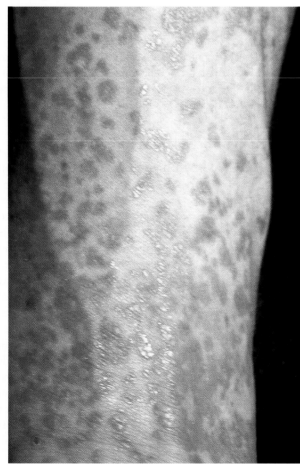

Figure 9.2
Red plaques, very flat or somewhat elevated, with irregular borders, some confluent, found to be associated with EV HPV 20 and HPV 5.

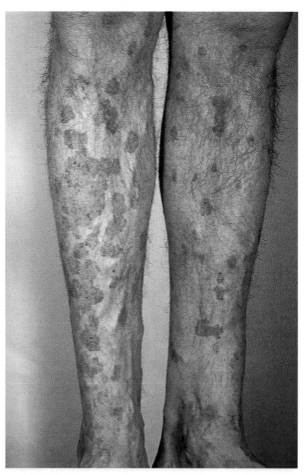

Figure 9.3
Brownish plaques on the legs, larger and more irregular than red plaques, associated with HPV 8.

Plane wart-like lesions may have all the features of plane warts in the general population, or may be somewhat smaller or larger, and are sometimes reddish. Not infrequently, scratching produces a Koebner phenomenon as in plane warts in the general population.

Pityriasis versicolor-like lesions are polymorphous, reddish, pigmented and depigmented lesions which resemble pityriasis versicolor (Figure 9.4). Due to the striking similarity, these cases are sometimes recognized as pityriasis versicolor with coexisting plane warts. We have also seen very *small achromic papules* involving almost all the trunk and extremities.

Papillomas and seborrheic keratosis-like lesions have also been described. Some of these proliferative lesions are flat and pigmented, resembling lentigo, whereas others are highly hyperkeratotic. Lesions of this type were also described in black individuals.[58,60]

Histology of EV lesions associated with EV HPVs

Regardless of clinical characteristics, all EV benign lesions have a similar histologic pattern. Large clarified keratinocytes start to appear suprabasally, are more abundant, and arranged in nests in upper layers, and may replace almost the entire epidermis.

The characteristic cytopathic effect consists of clarification of the cytoplasm and nucleoplasm. Nuclei become very small and pyknotic within fully koilocytic cells. Pepper-like, small, basophilic granules appear in the uppermost layers whereas the stratum corneum is completely disorganized

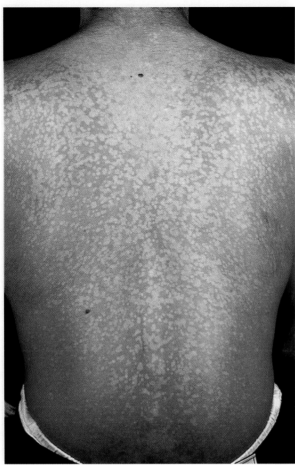

Figure 9.4
Pityriasis versicolor-like lesions on the trunk. Such changes cannot be clinically distinguished from pityriasis versicolor. In this patient, infection was associated with HPV 5, 9, and 24.

(Figure 9.5). The cytopathic effect is most pronounced in active lesions. Single dysplastic cells may be found in benign lesions associated with EV HPV.

Electron microscopy
The cytopathic effect is manifested by a complete disappearance of mitochondria and other cytoplasmic organelles. The granular appearance of cytoplasm is due to the remaining ribosomes. The cytoplasm also contains large keratohyaline granules not associated with rarified tonofilaments. The

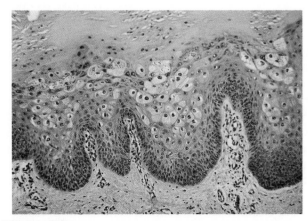

Figure 9.5
Typical cytopathic effect of EV. Nests of clarified or koilocytic cells start to appear suprabasally. Keratohyaline granules appear within clarified cells in the upper parts of the epidermis; the stratum corneum is disorganized with focal parakeratosis (H + E, × 200).

nuclei are clarified with marginated chromatin, and crystalline viral particles are present in the nucleoplasm and in the prominent nucleoli.

9.4.2 Mixed infection with HPV3 and EV HPVs

The lesions are usually typical plane warts. The difference is that the cutaneous changes are very widespread, involving the extremities, face, and trunk, and are not infrequently larger and more irregular than usual plane warts. The mixed EV HPV and HPV 3/10 infection is much more common than previously believed. Repeated examinations during a long follow-up period have shown very frequent multiple infections with three to four or more EV HPV types, and co-infection with HPV 3 or the related HPVs 10 and 28. After 10–20 or even 30 years, numerous red plaques developed in all our five patients with disseminated or generalized plane wart-like lesions associated with HPV 3; virological study disclosed a mixture of EV HPVs. All these patients had a severe defect of cell-mediated immunity,[71] and EV HPV infection could be due to activation of potentially oncogenic viruses, characteristic of immunosuppression.

Histology of HPV 3-induced lesions in EV
The histology is characteristic of HPV 3-induced warts in the general population, i.e., vacuolization of cells in the upper layers with small, strongly stained nuclei and well-defined borders ('bird's eyes'). The stratum corneum has a loose, basket weave-like appearance.

Electron microscopy
The cytoplasmic organelles and tonofilaments are pushed to the periphery, forming well-marked borders of the vacuolized cells. Despite the presence of viral particles, the chromatin is not destroyed as in EV HPV-induced warts.

9.4.3 Malignant tumors in EV

Malignant conversion occurs preferentially in sun-exposed areas, mainly on the forehead, and starts from benign lesions that become larger, deeper, scaly, hyperkeratotic, erosive or ulcerative. The progression from pre-malignant changes to tumors is very slow, and the tumors remain only locally destructive, usually with little metastatic potential (Figure 9.6). The first pre-malignant lesions of the actinic keratoses type appear preferentially in the temporal region; they start to develop in the third and fourth decades, and malignant transformation occurs progressively in numerous lesions within a few years (Figure 9.7). Not infrequently, the changes are so abundant that almost all the forehead is involved. Malignant tumors may also occur on the dorsa of the hands and in the inguinal, retroauricular and other folds, i.e., in the chronically traumatized areas. In older patients, tumors can develop in different skin areas; however, the most frequent inducing factor is chronic sun exposure. Malignant transformation and tumor growth are usually slow, but cancers localized on the lips and peri-orbicularly may become invasive.

Tumors are reported in about 50% of EV patients.[78] However, we have seen pre-malignant and early malignant changes in all EV patients followed for 20 to 30 years. It should be stressed that the oncogenic potential of EV

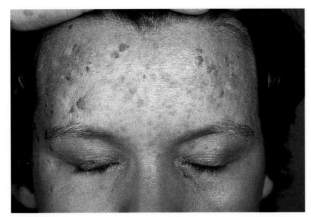

Figure 9.6
Very early malignancies on the forehead and palpebra. Some lesions are of seborrheic keratosis type. There is no involvement of the eyeball. This patient was found to be infected with HPV 8 and HPV 3.

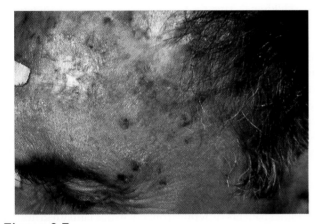

Figure 9.7
Multiple tumors on the forehead, partly coalescent, found to be associated with HPV 5.

HPVs differs considerably, and the development of tumors depends upon the extent of infection with oncogenic HPVs and on the action of cofactors of oncogenesis, mainly chronic sun exposure.

Metastases usually occur only in tumors irradiated with gamma-rays or upon applying some other cocarcinogens.[26,55] The most characteristic feature of EV-associated tumors is non-invasive or microinvasive growth, even with a very long persistence of tumors.

Histology of EV tumors

The onset of malignant conversion is characterized by disappearance of the cytopathic effect and downward proliferation of the epidermis. Dyskeratotic cells and Bowen's atypia are very much like in actinic keratoses in the general population, but are usually much more pronounced (Figures 9.8a, b). The process of oncogenesis frequently starts within and around hair follicles. It is conceivable that EV HPVs are present in a latent form in the keratinocyte stem cells, believed to be in hair follicles.[90]

Microinvasive and invasive squamous cell carcinomas in EV retain features of Bowen's atypia, with numerous dyskeratotic, pleomorphic and multinucleated cells (Figure 9.9). Not infrequently, squamous cell carcinomas show basaloid differentiation (Figure 9.10), reported also in HPV-associated anal cancers,[95] and are recognized as basal cell cancers. It is usually possible, however, to find dyskeratotic cells and Bowen's atypia in serial sections of these tumors. It should be stressed that typical basal cell cancers may also occur in EV patients.

Electron microscopy

Apoptosis is seen in carcinomas displaying histologic features of Bowen's atypia. Numerous apoptotic bodies containing disorganized chromatin intermingled with tonofilaments and remnants of cytoplasmic organelles are found engulfed by the neighboring keratinocytes and undergoing progressive lysis.[52,64] Apoptosis appears to be an important phenomenon in EV tumors, possibly responsible for a low invasive and metastatic potential of these carcinomas. The other contributing factor could be a high amount of TGFβ found in EV lesions,[68] which in addition to antitumor effects, enhances repair processes. Therefore, in EV patients, the wounds, after tumor excision, show much faster healing than in the general population.

9.4.4 The development and course of EV: follow-up of three generations

We had a quite unique possibility to follow-up for many years some familial and sporadic EV cases and to study three generations of these families; this made possible the detection of the first cutaneous changes.

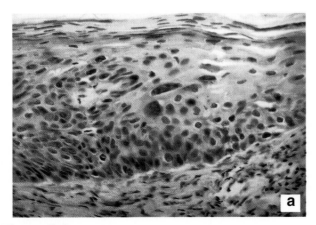
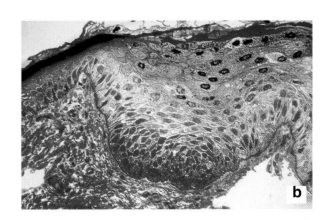

Figure 9.8
(a) Histology of an early actinic keratosis-like lesion. Note the hyperkeratosis and abundant parakeratosis, partly with large, irregular nuclei. Numerous atypical cells with features of dyskeratosis are seen in the stratum malpighii. (H + E, × 320). (b) *In situ* hybridization showing EV HPV 5 DNA in the upper epidermis, abundant in parakeratotic cells (H+ E, × 320).

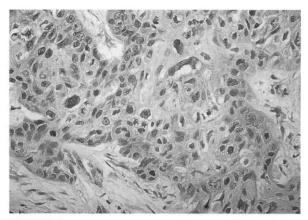

Figure 9.9
Microinvasive squamous cell carcinoma with pronounced Bowen's atypia (H + E, × 200).

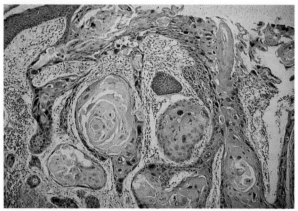

Figure 9.10
Histology of the tumor shown in Figure 9.7. There is malignant proliferation displaying features of Bowen's atypia with basaloid differentiation (H + E, × 200).

The onset of the disease is at the age of 5–8 years. Usually, the first lesions are plane warts, localized on the dorsa of the hands and dorsal sides of the fingers. The appearance of the warts in other locations, especially on the forearms, face,

and trunk, is suggestive of the development of EV. However, we have seen warts in the children and/or grandchildren of EV patients which disappeared either spontaneously or did not recur after excision (Figure 9.11).

Two sisters in one family suffered from EV. One sister, two of whose daughters also developed EV, originally had a high prevalence of HPV 3 in addition to specific EV HPV infection. Disseminated plane wart-like lesions persisted from early childhood, and red plaques appeared in the fourth decade, mainly on the face, neck, and trunk. In the fifth decade, pre-malignant and malignant lesions developed in the retroauricular location, and later on the neck and arms. She died from lymphoblastic lymphoma, which could be a consequence of a severe cellular immune defect, but was not related to EV, i.e., not associated with EV HPVs. One daughter had widespread plane warts, found to be induced exclusively by HPV 3. In this daughter, the lesions, present since early childhood, regressed spontaneously after the birth of two children.[56] After the first delivery, we noticed flattening of the warts and, 2 years later, after delivery of the second child, she became free of lesions. It is the only case of regression of EV, with no relapse. However, in this woman there was no co-infection with specific EV HPVs. In another daughter, infected with both HPV 8 and HPV 3, the lesions were present from the age of 6 years, and red plaques appeared on the trunk somewhat later. In the second decade, seborrheic keratoses-like papillomas associated with HPV 3 developed, mainly on the forehead and on the palpebrae. At about 38–40 years of age, pre-malignant tumors and carcinomas *in situ* associated with oncogenic HPV 8 started to appear, mainly on the forehead and the neck.

Other patients suffering from EV in this family had healthy children and two of them also had healthy grandchildren.

9.5 TREATMENT

There is no drug with specific anti-HPV DNA efficacy and no therapy that produces sustained clearances.

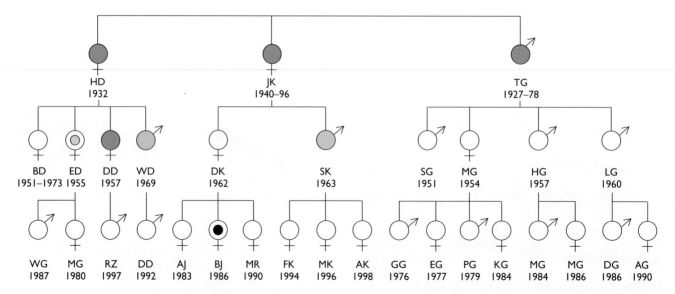

Figure 9.11
A family tree of EV in three generations. Key: ●, EV cases, ● Cases with no signs of EV. Cutaneous warts were transiently present in childhood, ◉, 14-year-old girl (third generation), in whom plane warts started to appear at the age of 6 years and are steadily present in spite of treatment. The warts were primarily associated with HPV3, but subsequently HPV5 was also disclosed. No signs of EV up to now, ◎, Unusual EV case with typical widespread clinical manifestations, in which the lesions regressed after 2 deliveries.

9.5.1 Benign lesions

The lesions can be treated locally with 0.05–0.1% retinoic acid combined with 5% 5-fluorouracil ointment. We have seen amelioration of the pronounced verruca-like lesions on the dorsa of the hands after several months of this topical treatment. However, because it may produce inflammation, the application should be cautious and interrupted as necessary. A new treatment modality is imiquimod cream – an immunomodulating agent for local application. Although it does not act directly on HPV DNA, it stimulates immune responses to HPV-infected cells by inducing the production of pro-inflammatory cytokines (TNFα, IFNs, IL-1, etc.).[104] This drug is highly effective for genital warts[11] and was also found to be beneficial for basal cell cancers.[10]

9.5.2 Pre-malignant and malignant lesions

Either 5-fluorouracil ointment or imiquimod cream can be used for pre-malignant lesions. Tumors should be removed as soon as they are noticed. The excision does not need to be performed with large margins of the seemingly healthy skin because of a very low invasive potential of the tumors. Conservative surgery is usually sufficient, even for tumors in periorbital and perioral locations. Radiation therapy is contraindicated, although in *in vitro* studies X-ray irradiation of lymphocytes from EV patients has not induced altered mean chromosome aberration frequencies and DNA repair response was found to be normal.[32] However, the deleterious effect of radiation therapy in EV[26] might be due to co-carcinogenic effects on EV HPV-harboring keratinocytes.

9.5.3 Skin grafts

Observing our patients for over 20–30 years, we have noticed that it is not possible to remove all steadily appearing pre-malignant and malignant changes, which often become confluent on the forehead. Excision of the entire skin of the forehead and its replacement by the grafts taken from unexposed skin of the internal aspects of the arms or thighs proved to be a very successful preventive procedure.[70] In the grafted skin, there were no malignancies within up to 22 years of follow-up, and single, benign, red plaques started to appear after 4–6 years, while in the surrounding skin multiple malignant and pre-malignant tumors developed in this period (Figure 9.12). Thus, HPV-associated malignant conversion is an extremely chronic multistage process occurring on the skin exposed for a very long time to adverse extrinsic factors.

9.5.4 Experimental therapy with retinoids or interferons

Retinoids were found to be of benefit in some patients,[13] but not satisfactory in other cases associated with EV HPVs.[57] However, in patients with mixed infection or infected exclusively with HPV 3, there was a marked reduction of the number of warts and/or of the viral load.

IFNα, due to its antiproliferative effect, has been applied in several cases of EV.[2,6,106] We have used IFNα2 or IFNβ in dosages of 5–9 million units, three times a week for several months, with minimal and only transient effects. Some

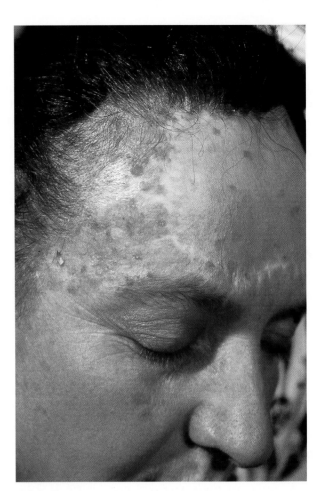

Figure 9.12
Grafted skin taken from the internal aspect of the arm and transplanted into the forehead after removal of multiple carcinomas. Single red plaques are appearing within the grafted skin and multiple pre-malignant and malignant lesions are present around the graft 4 years after transplantation.

lesions disappeared during treatment and reappeared after its cessation. Androphy *et al.*[2] reported a decrease in viral load in cases of mixed infection with EV HPVs and HPV 3 during IFNα therapy, with relapse several weeks after the therapy was discontinued. No complete clearance has been achieved either in our study or in the studies of others. Thus, IFNs alone are not effective for benign EV lesions. However, there was a single report on the beneficial effect of intralesional IFNα in Bowen's carcinoma of EV patients.[13] We used IFNα and IFNβ intralesionally in dosages of 3 million units three times weekly for 3 months in early malignant lesions of EV patients, with transient effects in some individuals.

9.5.5 Combinations of retinoids and IFNα

The combination of retinoids and IFNα was found to have both antiproliferative and anti-angiogenic synergistic effects on HPV-harboring cell lines.[67,72] IFNs combined with 1,25-dihydroxyvitamin D3 (VD3) derivatives were shown to have synergistic antiproliferative and anti-angiogenic effects in *in vitro* studies.[72,73] Application of this regimen in multiple early malignancies significantly decreased the number and extent of the changes.[97] However, it is not yet known whether such therapy will be effective in EV patients.

9.5.6 Prevention

It is most important to prevent malignant conversion. Because the role of chronic UV exposure is well established, the patient should be advised to use sunscreens having both UVA and UVB protection and a sun protection factor (SPF) of at least 50. Sunscreen use should be initiated in early childhood, before the onset of the benign lesions. Sun avoidance and protective clothing should also be recommended. Skin pigmentation in black Africans was found to be a protective factor in EV patients, as this population was found to have very rare cutaneous malignancies despite generalized infection with potentially oncogenic HPVs.[59,60]

9.5.7 Experimental vaccination

Vaccination using L1 or L1–L2 proteins of EV HPV5 self-assembled *in vitro* into virus-like particles[33,34,63] potentially could be useful for the prevention of the spreading of EV HPV5 infection. Such experimental vaccination in EV has now started in some of our patients and family members.

REFERENCES

1. Androphy EJ. (1994) Molecular biology of human papillomavirus infection and oncogenesis. *J Invest Dermatol* **103**: 248–56.
2. Androphy EJ, Dvoretzky I, Malnish A.E. (1984) Response of warts in epidermodysplasia verruciformis to treatment with systemic oral and intralesional alpha interferon. *J Am Acad Dermatol* **11**: 197–202.
3. Astori G, Lavergne D, Benton C, *et al.* (1998) Human papillomaviruses are commonly found in normal skin of immunocompetent hosts. *J Invest Dermatol* **110**: 752–5.
4. Banks RE, Patel PM, Selby PJ. (1995) Interleukin-12: a new clinical player in cytokine therapy. *Br J Cancer* **71**: 655–9.
5. Barzegar C, Paul C, Saiag P, *et al.* (1998) Epidermodysplasia verruciformis-like eruption complicating human immunodeficiency virus infection. *Br J Dermat* **139**: 122–7.
6. Beaulien PH, Blanchet-Bardon C, Breitburd F, *et al.* (1993) Epidermodysplasia verruciforme et carcinome syringoide eccrine. *Ann Dermatol Venereol* **120**: 833–5.
7. Berger TG, Sawchuk WS, Leonardi C, *et al.* (1991) Epidermodysplasia verruciformis-associated with human immunodeficiency virus disease. *Br J Dermatol* **124**: 79–83.
8. Berkhout RJ, Tieben LM, Smiths H, *et al.* (1995) Nested PCR approach for detection and typing of epidermodysplasia verruciformis-associated human papillomavirus types in cutaneous cancers from renal transplant recipients. *J Clin Microbiol* **33**: 690–5.
9. Bernard HU, Chan SY, Delius H. (1994) Evaluation of papillomaviruses. In *Current topics in microbiology and immunology*, Vol. 186, ed. H zur Hausen. Berlin, Heidelberg, Springer-Verlag, 33–54.
10. Beutner KR, Geisse JK, Helman D, et al. (1999) Therapeutic response of basal cell carcinoma to the immune response modifier imiquimod 5% cream. *J Am Acad Dermatol* **41**: 1002–7.
11. Beutner KR, Spruance SL, Hougham A.J, *et al.* (1998) Treatment of genital warts with an immune response modifier (imiquimod). *J Am Acad Dermatol* **38**: 230–9.
12. Bhardwaj RS, Arange Y, Becher E, *et al.* (1994) Alpha melanocyte stimulating hormone differentially regulates IL-10 by human peripheral blood mononuclear cells. *J Invest Dermatol* **102**: 586–90.
13. Blanchet-Bardon C, Lutzner MA. (1985) Interferon and retinoids in the therapy of HPV-induced lesions. *Clin Dermatol* **3**: 195–9.
14. Bouwes Bavinck J., Berkhout RJM, Tieben LM, *et al.* (1995) DNA of EV-associated human papillomavirus in skin cancers from non-immunosuppressed patients. *Abstract Book, International Conference Papillomavirus,* Quebec, p. 93.
15. Boxman I, Berkhout R, Mulder L, *et al.* (1997) Detection of human papillomavirus DNA in plucked hairs from renal transplant recipients and healthy volunteers. *J Invest Dermatol* **108**: 712–15.
16. Boxman ILA, Mulder LHC, Russell A., *et al.* (1999) Human papillomavirus type 5 is commonly present in immunosuppressed and immunocomponent individuals. *Br J Dermatol* **141**: 246–9.
17. Braciale TJ, Braciale VL. (1991) Antigen presentation: structural themes and functional variations. *Immunol Today* **12**: 124–9.
18. Brash DE, Rudolph JA, Simon JA, *et al.* (1991) A role of sunlight in skin cancer: UV-induced p53 mutations in squamous cell carcinoma. *Proc Nat Acad Sci USA* **88**: 10124–8.
19. Brash DE, Ziegler A, Jonason AS, Simon JA, *et al.* (1996) Sunlight and sunburn in human skin cancer: p53, apoptosis, and tumor promotion. *J Invest Dermatol Symp Proc* **1**: 136–42.
20. Breitburd F, Ramoz N, Salmon J, Orth G. (1996) HLA control in the progression of human papillomavirus infections. *Semin Cancer Biol* **7**: 359–71.
21. Campbell C, Quinn AG, Angus B, Rees JL. (1993) The relation between p53 mutation and p53 immunostaining in nonmelanoma skin cancer. *Br J Dermatol* **129**: 235–41.
22. Cannon JG, Tatro JB, Reichlin S, *et al.* (1986) α-Melanocyte-stimulating hormone inhibits immunostimulatory and inflammatory action of interleukin 1. *J Immunol* **137**: 2232–8.
23. Chakraborty A, Slominski A, Ermark G. (1995) Ultraviolet B and melanocyte-stimulating hormone (MSH) stimulate mRNA production for αMSH receptors and propiomelanocortin-derived peptides in mouse melanoma cells and transformed keratinocytes. *J Invest Dermatol* **105**: 655–9.
24. Chan SY, Bernard HU, Ong CK, *et al.* (1994) Phylogenetic analysis of 48 papillomavirus types and 28 subtypes and variants: a showcase for the molecular evaluation of DNA viruses. *J Virol* **66**: 5714–25.
25. Cooper KD, Androphy EJ, Lowy DR, *et al.* (1990) Antigen presentation and T cell activation in epidermodysplasia verruciformis. *J Invest Dermatol* **94**: 769–76.

26. Cortes-Franco R, Tyring SK, Vega E, *et al.* (1997) Divergent clinical course of epidermodysplasia verruciformis in siblings. *Int J Dermatol* **36**: 435–52.

27. de Villiers, EM. (1994) Human pathogenic papillomavirus types: an update. In *Current topics in microbiology and immunology*, Vol. 186, ed. H zur Hausen. Berlin, Heidelberg, Springer-Verlag, 1–12.

28. de Villiers EM. (1997) Papillomavirus and HPV typing. *Clin Dermatol* **15**: 199–206.

29. de Villiers EM. (1998) Human papillomavirus infections in skin cancers. *Biomed Pharmacother* **52**: 26–33.

30. de Villiers, EM, Lavergne D, McLaren K, Benton EC. (1997) Prevailing papillomavirus types in non-melanoma carcinomas of the skin in renal allograft recipients. *Int J Cancer* **73**: 356–61.

31. Deau MC, Favre M, Orth G. (1991) Genetic heterogeneity among papillomaviruses (HPV) associated with epidermodysplasia verruciformis: evidence for multiple allelic forms of HPV 5 and HPV 8 E6 genes. *Virology* **184**: 492–503.

32. El-Zein R, Shaw P, Tyring SK, *et al.* (1995) Chromosomal radiosensitivity of lymphocytes from skin cancer-prone patients. *Mut Res* **335**: 143–9.

33. Favre M, Majewski S, Noszczyk B, *et al.* (2000) Antibodies to human papillomavirus type 5 are generated in epidermal repair processes. *J Invest Dermatol* **114**: 403–7.

34. Favre M, Orth G, Majewski S, *et al.* (1998) Psoriasis: a possible reservoir for human papillomavirus type 5, the virus associated with skin carcinomas of epidermodysplasia verruciformis. *J Invest Dermatol* **110**: 311–17.

35. Favre M, Ramoz N, Jablonska S, *et al.* (1995) Search for a gene predisposing to epidermodysplasia verruciformis within the major histocompatibility complex. In *14ᵗʰ International Papillomavirus Conference*, Abstract Book, Quebec, 198.

36. Fernándiz C, Fuente MJ, Ribera M, *et al.* (1995) Epidermal dysplasia and neoplasia in kidney transplant recipients. *J Am Acad Dermatol* **33**: 590–6.

37. Fuchs PG, Pfister H. (1996) Papillomaviruses in epidermodysplasia verruciformis. In *Papillomavirus reviews: current research on papillomaviruses*, ed. C Lacey. Leeds, Leeds University Press, 253–62.

38. Fuchs PG, Pfister H. (1997) Molecular biology of HPV and mechanisms of keratinocyte transformation. In *Human papillomavirus infections in dermatovenereology,* eds G Gross, G von Krogh. Boca Raton, CRC Press, 15–46.

39. Glick AB, Kulkarni AB, Tennenbaum T, *et al.* (1993) Loss of expression of transforming growth factor beta in skin and skin tumors is associated with hyperproliferation and a high risk for malignant conversion. *Proc Nat Acad Sci USA* **90**: 6076–80.

40. Glick AB, Lee MM, Darwiche N, *et al.* (1994) Targeted depletion of the TGF-β1 gene causes rapid progression to squamous cell carcinoma. *Genes Dev* **8**: 2429–40.

41. Glinski W, Obalek S, Jablonska S, *et al.* (1981) T cell defect in patients with epidermodysplasia verruciformis due to human papillomavirus type 3 and 5. *Dermatologica* **162**: 141–7.

42. Grabbe S, Bhardwaj RS, Mahnke K, *et al.* (1996) Alpha-melanocyte-stimulating hormone induces hapten-specific tolerance in mice. *J Immunol* **156**: 473–8.

43. Gross G, Ellinger K, Roussaki A, *et al.* (1988) Epidermodysplasia verruciformis in a patient with Hodgkins disease: characterization of a new papillomavirus type and interferon treatment. *J Invest Dermatol* **91**: 43–8.

44. Haftek M, Jablonska S, Szymanczyk J, *et al.* (1987) Langerhans cells in epidermodysplasia verruciformis. *Dermatologica* **174**:173–9.

45. Han R, Breitburd F, Marche PN, *et al.* (1994) Analysis of the nucleotide sequence variation of the antigen-binding domain of DRα and DQα molecules as related to the evolution of papillomavirus-induced warts in rabbits. *J Invest Dermatol* **103**: 376–80.

46. Harriot-Smith TG, Halliday WJ. (1988) Suppression of contact hypersensitivity by short-term ultraviolet irradiation. The role of urocanic acid. *Clin Exp Immunol* **72**: 432–3.

47. Harwood CA, Spink PJ, Surentheran T, Leigh IM. (1998) Detection of human papillomavirus DNA in PUVA-associated non-melanoma skin cancers. *J Invest Dermatol* **111**: 123–7.

48. Hermonat PL, Kechelava S, Lowery CL, Korourian K. (1998) Trophoblasts are the preferential target for human papilloma virus infection in spontaneously aborted products of conception. *Hum Pathol* **29**: 170–4.

49. Hiltz ME, Catania EA, Lipton JM. (1992) α-MSH peptides inhibit acute inflammation induced in mice by rIL-1beta, rIL-6, rTNFa and endogeneous pyrogen but not that caused by LTB4, PAF and rIL. *Cytokine* **4**: 320–8.

50. Iftner T, Sagner G, Pfister H, *et al.* (1990) The E7 protein of human papillomavirus 8 is a nonphosphorylated protein of 17 kDa and can be generated by two different mechanisms. *Virology* **179**: 428–36.

51. Jablonska S. (1991) Epidermodysplasia verruciformis. In *Cancer of the skin*, eds RJ Friedman, *et al.* Philadelphia, W.B. Saunders Co, 101–13.

52. Jablonska S, Biczysko W, Jakubowicz K, *et al.* (1970) The ultrastructure of transitional states of Bowen's disease and invasive Bowen's carcinoma in epidermodysplasia verruciformis. *Dermatologica* **140**: 186–94.

53. Jablonska S, Dabrowski J, Jakubowicz K. (1972) Epidermodysplasia verruciformis as a model in studies on the role of papillomavirus in oncogenesis. *Cancer Res* **32**: 585–9.

54. Jablonska S, Fabianska L, Formas I. (1966) On the viral etiology of epidermodysplasia verruciformis. *Dermatologica* **132**: 369–85.

55. Jablonska S, Majewski S. (1994) Epidermodysplasia verruciformis: immunological and clinical aspects. In *Current topics microbiology and immunology*, Vol. 186, ed. H zur Hausen. Berlin, Heidelberg, Springer-Verlag, 157–75.

56. Jablonska S, Obalek S, Orth G, *et al.* (1982) Regression of the lesions of epidermodysplasia verruciformis. *Br J Dermatol* **107**: 109–16.

57. Jablonska S, Obalek S, Wolska H, *et al.* (1981) Ro-10-9359 in epidermodysplasia verruciformis. Preliminary report. In *Retinoids*, eds CE Orfanos, *et al.* Berlin, Springer-Verlag, 401–5.

58. Jacyk WK, de Villiers EM. (1993) Epidermodysplasia verruciformis in Africans. *Int J Dermatol* **32**: 806–10.

59. Jacyk WK, Dreyer L, de Villiers EM. (1993) Seborrheic

keratoses of black patients with epidermodysplasia verruciformis contain human papillomavirus DNA. *Am J Dermatopathol* **15**: 1–6.

60. Jacyk WK, Subbuswamy SG. (1979) Epidermodysplasia verruciformis in Nigerians. *Dermatologica* **159**: 256–65.

61. Kawase M, Orth G, Jablonska S, *et al.* (1996) Variability and phylogeny of the L1 capsid protein gene in human papillomavirus type 5: contribution of clusters of non-synonymous mutations and a 30-nucleotide duplication. *Virology* **221**: 189–98.

62. Kim J, Modlin RL, Moy RL, *et al.* (1995) IL-10 production in cutaneous basal and squamous cell carcinomas. *J Immunol* **155**: 2240–7.

63. Kirnbauer R, Taub J, Greenstone H. (1993) Efficient self-assembly of human papillomavirus type 16 L1 and L1-L2 into virus-like particles. *J Virol* **67**: 6929–36.

64. Kuligowski M, Dabrowski JH, Jablonska S. (1989) Apoptosis in Bowen's disease. An ultrastructural study. *Am J Dermatopathol* **11**: 13–21.

65. Lewandowsky F, Lutz W. (1922) Ein Fall einer bisher nicht beschriebenen Hauterkrankung (Epidermodysplasia verruciformis). *Arch Dermatol Syph (Berlin),* **141**: 193–203.

66. Lutzner MA, Orth G, Dutronquay V, *et al.* (1983) Detection of human papillomavirus type 5 DNA in skin cancers of an immunosuppressed renal allograft recipient. *Lancet* **ii**: 422–4.

67. Majewski S, Breitburd F, Skopinska M, *et al.* (1994) A mouse model for studying epidermodysplasia verruciformis-associated carcinogenesis. *Int J Cancer* **56**: 727–30.

68. Majewski S, Hunzelmann N, Nischt R, *et al.* (1991) TGFβ-1 and TNF expression in the epidermis of patients with epidermodysplasia verruciformis. *J Invest Dermatol* **97**: 862–7.

69. Majewski S, Jablonska S. (1995) Epidermodysplasia verruciformis as a model of human papillomavirus-induced genetic cancer of the skin. *Arch Dermatol* **131**:1312–18.

70. Majewski S, Jablonska S. (1997) Skin autografts in epidermodysplasia verruciformis: human papillomavirus-associated cutaneous changes need over 20 years for malignant conversion. *Cancer Res* **57**: 4214–16.

71. Majewski S, Malejczyk J, Jablonska S, *et al.* (1990) Natural cell-mediated cytotoxicity against various target cells in patients with epidermodysplasia verruciformis. *J Am Acad Dermatol* **22**: 423–7.

72. Majewski S, Marczak M, Szmurlo A, *et al.* (1995) Retinoids combined with interferon alpha or 1,25-dihydroxyvitamin D3 synergistically inhibit angiogenesis induced by non-HPV harboring tumor cell lines. *Cancer Lett* **89**: 117–24.

73. Majewski S, Szmurlo A, Marczak M. (1993) Inhibition of tumor cell-induced angiogenesis by retinoids, 1,25-dihydroxyvitamin D3 and their combination. *Cancer Lett* **75**: 35–9.

74. McGregor JM, Morris R, Smith Ch, *et al.* (1995) Skin cancer morbidity amongst renal allograft recipients. A 25 year retrospective follow-up study. *Br J Dermatol* **133** (Suppl. 45): 40.

75. Nelson JL, Campbell MJ, Goldblatt PO, *et al.* (1998) Microchimerism and HLA-compatible relationships of pregnancy in scleroderma. *Lancet* **351**: 559–62.

76. Nishigori C, Yarosh DB, Donawho C, *et al.* (1996) The immune system in ultraviolet carcinogenesis. *J Invest Dermatol Symp Proc* **1**: 143–6.

77. Obalek S, Favre M, Szymanczyk J, *et al.* (1992) Human papillomavirus (HPV) types specific of epidermodysplasia verruciformis detected in warts induced by HPV 3 or HPV 3-related types in immunosuppressed patients. *J Invest Dermatol* **98**: 936–41.

78. Orth G. (1986) Epidermodysplasia verruciformis: a model for understanding the oncogenicity of human papillomaviruses. Ciba Foundation Symposium 120, *Papillomaviruses.* Chichester, Wiley. 157–74.

79. Orth G, Jablonska S, Favre M, *et al.* (1978) Characterization of two types of human papillomaviruses in lesions of epidermodysplasia verruciformis. *Proc Nat Acad Sci USA* **75**: 1537–41.

80. Pepper MS, Belin D, Montesano R, *et al.* (1990) Transforming growth factor-beta 1 modulates basic fibroblast growth factor-induced proteolytic and angiogenic properties of endothelial cell in vitro. *J Cell Biol* **111**: 743–55.

81. Pfister H, Iftner T, Fuchs PG. (1985) Papillomaviruses from epidermodysplasia verruciformis patients and renal allograft recipients. *UCLA Symp Mol Cell Biol New Ser* **32**: 85–100.

82. Pfister H, ter Schegget J. (1997) Role of HPV in cutaneous premalignant and malignant tumors. *Clin Dermatol* **15**: 335–48.

83. Pizarro A, Gamallo C, Castresana JS, *et al.* (1995) p53 expression in viral warts from patients with epidermodysplasia verruciformis. *Br J Dermatol* **132**: 513–19.

84. Proby C, Storey A, McGregor J, Leigh I. (1996) Does human papillomavirus infection play a role in non-melanoma skin cancer? *Papillomavirus Rep* **7**: 53–60.

85. Proby CM, Shamanin IV, Rausch C, *et al.* (1995) Novel human papillomaviruses identified in skin cancers and keratinocyte cell lines from renal transplant recipients. *Br J Dermatol* **132**: 644.

86. Prose N, von Knebel-Doeberitz C, Miller S, *et al.* (1990) Widespread flat warts associated with human papillomavirus type 5: a cutaneous manifestation of human immunodeficiency virus infection. *J Am Acad Dermatol* **23**: 978–81.

87. Ramoz N, Rueda LA, Bouadjar B, *et al.* (1999) A susceptibility locus for epidermodysplasia verruciformis, an abnormal predisposition to infection with the oncogenic human papillomavirus type 5, maps to chromosome 17qter in a region containing a psoriasis locus. *J Invest Dermatol* **112**: 259–63.

88. Rivas JH, Ullrich SE. (1992) Systemic suppression of delayed-type hypersensitivity by supernatants from UV-irradiated keratinocytes: an essential role for keratinocyte-derived IL-10. *J Immunol* **149**: 3865–71.

89. Roberts AB, Sporn MB. (1990) The transforming growth factor-beta. In *Handbook of experimental pharmacology*, Vol. 95, eds MB Sporn, AB Roberts. Berlin, Springer, 419–72.

90. Rochat A, Kobayashi K, Bernardon Y, *et al.* (1994) Location of stem cells of human hair follicles by clonal analysis. *Cell* **76**: 1063–73.

91. Ross JA, Howie SEM, Norval M, *et al.* (1986) Ultraviolet-irradiated urocanic acid suppresses delayed-type hypersensitivity to herpes simplex virus in mice. J *Invest Dermatol* **87**: 630–3.

92. Schwarz A, Grabbe S, Rieman H, *et al.* (1994) In vivo effects of interleukin-10 on contact hypersensitivity and delayed-type hypersensitivity reactions. *J Invest Dermatol* **103**: 211–16.

93. Shamanin V, Glover M, Rausch CH, *et al.* (1994) Specific types of human papillomavirus found in benign proliferations and carcinomas of the skin in immunosuppressed patients. *Cancer Res* **54**: 4610–13.

94. Shamanin EV, zur Hausen H, Lavergne D, *et al.* (1996) Human papillomavirus infections in nonmelanoma skin cancers from renal transplant recipients and non-immunosuppressed patients. *J Nat Cancer Inst* **88**: 802–11.

95. Shoyer KR, Brookes CG, Markham NE, *et al.* (1995) Detection of human papillomavirus in anorectal squamous cell carcinoma: correlation with basaloid pattern of differentiation. *Am J Clin Pathol* **104**: 299–305.

96. Sieling PA, Abrams JS, Yamamura M, *et al.* (1993) Immunosuppressive roles for IL-10 in human infection. *J Immunol* **150**: 5501–6.

97. Skopinska M, Majewski S, Bollag W, et al. (1996) Calcitrol and isotretinoin: combination therapy for precancerous and cancerous skin lesions. *J Dermatol Treat* **9**: 418–22.

98. Steger G, Pfister H. (1992) In vitro expressed HPV8 E6 protein does not bind p53. *Arch Virol* **125**: 355.

99. Streilein JW. (1993) Sunlight and skin-associated lymphoid tissues (SALT): if UVB is the trigger and TNFα is its mediator, what is the message? *J Invest Dermatol* **100**: 47s–52s.

100. Tie C, Golumb C, Taylor JR, *et al.* (1995) Suppressive and enhancing effects of ultraviolet B radiation on expression of contact hypersensitivity in man *J Invest Dermatol* **104**: 18–22.

101. Tieben-de Jong IM, Berkhout RJM, Smiths HL, *et al.* (1994) Detection of epidermodysplasia verruciformis-like human papillomavirus types in malignant and pre-malignant lesions of renal transplant recipients. *Br J Dermatol* **131**: 226–30.

102. Tieben-de Jong LM, Berkhout RJM, Smits HI, *et al.* (1995) High frequency of detection of epidermodysplasia verruciformis-associated human papillomavirus DNA in biopsies from malignant and premalignant skin lesions from renal transplant recipients. *J Invest Dermatol* **105**: 367–71.

103. Tyndall A, Grathwohl A. (1998) Microchimerism: friend or foe? *Nat Med* **4**: 386–8.

104. Tyring SK, Arany I, Stanley MA, *et al.* (1998) A randomized, controlled, molecular study of condylomata acuminata clearance during treatment with imiquimod. *J Infect Dis* **178**: 551–5.

105. Van der Leest RJ, Dacjow KR, Ostrow RS, *et al.* (1987) Human papillomavirus heterogeneity in 36 renal transplant recipients. *Arch Dermatol* **123**: 354–7.

106. Weber BP, Fierlbeck G, Kempf. (1994.) Multiple metachronous skin squamous cell carcinomas and epidermodysplasia verruciformis in the head region: a human papilloma virus-associated disease. *Eur Arch Otorhinolaryngol* **252**: 342–6.

107. Wintzen M, Gilchrest BA. (1996) Propiomelanocortin, its derived peptides, and the skin. *J Invest Dermatol* **106**: 3–10.

108. Yabe Y, Sakai A, Hitsumoto T, *et al.* (1999) Human papillomavirus-5b DNA integrated in a metastatic tumor: cloning, nucleotide sequence and genomic organization. *Int J Cancer* **80**: 334–5.

109. Yoshikawa T, Streilein JW. (1990) Genetic basis of the effects of ultraviolet light B on cutaneous immunity. Evidence that polymorphism at the TNFα and Lps loci governs susceptibility. *Immunogenetics* **32**: 398–405.

110. Yutsudo M, Tanigaki T, Kanda R, *et al.* (1994) Involvement of human papillomavirus type 20 in epidermodysplasia verruciformis skin carcinogenesis. J *Clin Microbiol* **32**: 1076–8.

111. zur Hausen H. (1996) Roots and perspectives of contemporary papillomavirus research. *J Cancer Res Clin Oncol* **122**: 3–13.

10

Human papillomavirus and immunosuppression

Catherine A. Harwood and Charlotte M. Proby

10.1 INTRODUCTION

The immune system plays an important part in the control of human papillomavirus (HPV) infection, and cell-mediated immunity (CMI) in particular is regarded as the principal mechanism involved in the host's defenses against HPV. For an immunocompetent individual, viral warts are usually little more than a minor inconvenience as spontaneous resolution tends to occur. However, for those with abnormalities of CMI, cutaneous and mucosal HPV infection may be extensive, persistent, refractory to treatment, and associated with malignancy.[83]

Epidermodysplasia verruciformis (EV), discussed in Chapter 9, is perhaps the most distinctive condition associated with an immunological deficit in defense against HPV infection. This rare disorder is characterized by a genetic predisposition to infection with specific types of HPV (EV HPV types), and two susceptibility loci have been linked to chromosomes 17qter[127] and 2p21–p24.[128] Cutaneous manifestations include red-brown plaques and pityriasis versicolor-like lesions in addition to extensive common and plane warts.[93] Cutaneous squamous cell carcinomas develop on ultraviolet (UV)-exposed sites in up to 60% of patients, and specific EV HPV types, including HPV 14, 17, 20 and 47 but predominantly HPV 5 and 8 are found in over 90% of tumors.[93,109] In several other primary immunodeficiency states, persistent HPV infection may also present as widespread viral warts or may resemble EV. Secondary immunodeficiency states are more common, and human immunodeficiency virus (HIV) infection and organ transplantation are emerging as important causes of extensive

HPV infection. In recent years, considerable attention has focused on the possible contribution of HPV to the pathogenesis of non-melanoma skin cancer associated with immunosuppression, and in this chapter particular emphasis is placed on discussion of the evidence for this.

10.2 PRIMARY IMMUNODEFICIENCY

Many diseases associated with defined primary abnormalities of the immune system predispose to HPV infection. The range of defects observed in these disorders emphasizes the complexity of the immune repertoire in the control of HPV infection. These conditions are relatively uncommon and there have been few reports of the HPV types found in such lesions. In otherwise apparently healthy individuals, extensive and persistent HPV infection may also result from subtle primary defects in the immune response to HPV which have yet to be characterized.

10.2.1 Defined primary immunodeficiency states

Cutaneous warts may appear in early childhood and may even be the first indication of an immunological abnormality in certain defined primary immunodeficiency disorders. Infection is often extensive and resistant to treatment and, in addition to common warts and plane warts, EV-like presentations have also been reported.

Multiple viral warts have been described in ataxia telangiectasia,[8] Wiskott–Aldrich syndrome,[157,184] X-linked combined immunodeficiency disease,[23] and severe combined immunodeficiency.[99] Palmoplantar and genital warts occur in common variable immunodeficiency,[8,130] and EV-like features associated with HPV 5-related infection have also been described.[55] Fanconi's anemia and dyskeratosis congenita have both been associated with extensive HPV infection including features reminiscent of EV.[26,118] In one report, malignant thymoma associated with immunodeficiency was preceded by multiple common warts and EV-like lesions from which HPV 4 and 9 were co-detected.[74] Selective IgA deficiency may present with extensive palmoplantar warts,[8] and IgA levels are also low and associated with impaired CMI in Bittner's syndrome, in which florid common warts have been reported in association with multiple seborrheic keratoses and cutaneous carcinoma in situ.[159]

10.2.2 Other primary abnormalities of cell-mediated immunity

A proportion of individuals with extensive and persistent HPV infection may appear otherwise entirely healthy, and it is unclear whether the persistent infection itself might induce local impairment of CMI and persistence of the virus.[42] Consistent with this hypothesis, two studies have reported reductions in CMI in patients with warts when compared with controls.[21,101] This was dependent on the duration and type of infection, with T-cell function most depressed in those with flat warts.[107] There is also evidence that total T-cell numbers increase after successful treatment of genital warts.[100] An alternative explanation for persistent HPV infection in apparently normal individuals is the possibility of subtle primary abnormalities in the CMI cascade, perhaps specific for HPV infection.[10] As our understanding of the complexity of the pathways of the immune response to HPV improves, such abnormalities are increasingly likely to be recognized.

10.3 SECONDARY IMMUNODEFICIENCY

Secondary immunodeficiency states are generally more common than primary disorders. These may result from either the disease process itself, as in HIV infection, hematological malignancies, and systemic lupus erythematosus, or from iatrogenic immunosuppression, for example psoralen and UVA (PUVA) therapy and, most notably, following organ transplantation. Persistent benign HPV infection is frequent, and HPV-related malignancies are also more prevalent.[83] In contrast to primary immunodeficiency states, rather more is known of the spectrum of HPV types harbored by these patients.

10.3.1 HIV infection

The gradual loss of immune control in HIV-positive individuals produces increasing susceptibility to viral infections, and HPV is one of the more common viral causes of mucocutaneous lesions.[30,112] Improved medical therapy for HIV infection means that illnesses with potentially long latency periods, as characterized by many HPV-associated diseases, are assuming increasing importance as causes of morbidity and mortality in these individuals.

Interaction between HIV and HPV

The precise nature of the changes in immunity to HPV that accompany more generalized HIV-induced immune deficiency has not been determined. Similarly, the mechanisms by which HIV and HPV interact at the molecular and cellular level are unclear. The primary target cells for HPV are epithelial cells and for HIV are lymphoid as well as related cells bearing CD4 receptors, so dual cellular infection is unlikely. However, interaction between these viruses is still possible. It is known, for example, that HIV *tat* can drive the replication of HPV 16 and 18,[166,170] and that there are alterations of cell-cycle regulatory genes within HIV-positive viral warts compared with HIV-negative lesions.[2] In addition, HPV replication occurs in epithelia containing trafficking T-cells and resident dendritic cells. It is therefore likely that the increased prevalence of HPV disease in the context of HIV infection is mediated not only by epidermal, dermal, and regional lymph node impairment of T-cell and antigen-presenting cell function, but also by local effects of HIV *tat* in up-regulating HPV replication.[62]

Cutaneous HPV infection in HIV
Cutaneous warts

The incidence of cutaneous warts in both adult and pediatric HIV infection is estimated to be between 5% and 27%.[117] Warts affecting the hands, face, and feet were observed in over 18% of adult patients compared with 1% of non-infected controls in one prospective study;[168] and, in another series, 8/39 (21%) HIV-positive individuals had plantar warts compared to 7/341 (2%) of HIV-negative controls.[79] Warts are often multiple, large, rapidly growing, refractory to treatment, and may result in considerable morbidity.[77] EV-like presentations have been reported, and in three patients HPV 5 and/or HPV 8 were detected.[11,124] Our group has analysed cutaneous warts from two HIV-positive patients using the methods described in section 10.4.[65] We have also detected EV HPV types, particularly HPV 5, often in mixed infections with cutaneous HPV types (unpublished observations); HPV 5 and 20 were found in an EV-like plaque and HPV 5, 14 and 27 in a plantar wart from the same individual. In another patient, HPV 2 and 5 were identified in a common wart on the finger and HPV 36 in a plantar wart. However, it remains to be established whether the spectrum of HPV types present in warts from HIV-positive individuals is similar to that of the general population, or whether EV HPV types are over-represented, as these preliminary data would seem to suggest.

Cutaneous malignancy

Epidermal dysplasia and cytological atypia progressing to *in situ* carcinoma may occur within the warts of HIV-positive individuals.[98] Furthermore, several retrospective and prospective studies[83,150] have suggested that HIV-positive patients are at increased risk for developing non-melanoma skin cancer, although this remains to be confirmed.[54] Basal cell carcinomas are the commonest skin malignancy, occurring earlier in the course of HIV infection than squamous cell carcinomas.[94] Although UV appears to be the most important etiological factor, a possible co-carcinogenic role for HPV has been proposed.[83] The role of HPV in the pathogenesis of HIV-associated non-melanoma skin cancer has not been as comprehensively studied as in transplant recipients (see section 10.4.2), but there have been case reports describing the detection of HPV DNA in these malignancies.[115] More recently, Maurer et al.[94] analysed a series of non-melanoma skin cancers from HIV-positive patients and observed HPV 18 and 38 in 2 of 12 (17%) squamous cell carcinomas using a dot-blot method and consensus primers. However, a higher prevalence of HPV might have been observed if a more comprehensive degenerate primer-based detection method had been used (see below).

Anogenital HPV infection in HIV

There is an increased incidence of anogenital warts and squamous intraepithelial neoplasia in HIV infection. Surprisingly, evidence of an elevated rate of invasive cervical and anal cancer has not been unequivocally demonstrated.[62,112] Nonetheless, with extended life expectancy associated with combination anti-retroviral therapy, a significant increase may yet be observed.[112,114]

Anogenital warts

Anogenital warts are a common problem in HIV infection. Two studies found the incidence of genital warts was 9.2% and 0.8%[41] and the prevalence 5.6% and 0.8%[29] in HIV-positive and HIV-negative women, respectively. Several studies have suggested that they may be a marker of early impaired immunity in both adult and pediatric populations.[46,78,82,136] Recurrence is also common; in one study, HIV-positive women were 16 times more likely to develop recurrent genital warts than HIV-negative women, and this correlated with CD4 count.[43] Such clinically benign genital warts are also more often associated with intraepithelial neoplasia and the presence of high-risk oncogenic HPV types.[6,25]

Cervical intraepithelial neoplasia

Many case-control studies using cervical cytology have shown an excess prevalence of cervical pre-cancer in HIV-positive women.[71] One population-based study from Edinburgh analysed HIV-positive intravenous drug users, HIV-negative intravenous drug users, and controls and showed prevalences of moderate/severe dyskaryosis of 24%, 10%, and 6% respectively.[76] More recent studies have incorporated colposcopy and biopsy. In one series, low-grade cervical intraepithelial neoplasia (CIN) was observed in 13% and 4%, and CIN 2/3 in 7% and 1% of HIV-positive and HIV-negative women, respectively.[179] Regression analysis confirmed the association of CIN with HPV and also showed CD4 <200 μL^{-1} and age more than 34 years to be independent risk factors. Longitudinal studies have shown that 20% of HIV-positive women had persistent infection with high-risk oncogenic HPV, compared to 3% of HIV-negative women,[162] and that persistence was most frequent with CD4 <200 μL^{-1}.[149,162] In one large study, progression from normal cytology to biopsy-proven intraepithelial neoplasia occurred in 20% of HIV-positive women within 3 years compared with 5% of HIV-negative women.[37] In addition to persistent HPV infection, co-detection of more than one HPV type is also well recognized in HIV-positive women.[22,24,161] Extensive multifocal anogenital HPV disease is more common[91] and a poorer response to treatment of CIN is also observed, with recurrence being reported in 39% and 9% of HIV-positive and HIV-negative women, respectively.[90]

Cervical cancer

Women with HIV presenting with cervical cancer have more advanced disease, and have higher recurrence rates and mortality than HIV-negative women.[90] Because of these findings, cervical cancer acquired immune deficiency syndrome was deemed an AIDS-defining condition in the USA and Europe in 1993.[28] Subsequently, a number of studies in both the developed[138] and developing world[54] have failed to detect an increase in the incidence of cervical cancer in HIV-positive women. There are a number of potential explanations for this, including earlier detection and treatment in HIV-positive women or, conversely, failure of diagnosis in women with limited access to health care, or death from other HIV-associated complications before progression to invasive malignancy occurs.[112]

Vulval intraepithelial neoplasia and anal intraepithelial neoplasia

An increased frequency of vulval intraepithelial neoplasia (VIN) of either warty or basaloid histological type, associated with high-risk HPV infection, has been described in HIV-positive women.[119] Similarly, many studies have found an increased prevalence of anal intraepithelial neoplasia (AIN) associated with high-risk oncogenic HPV.[71,112,114] In one study,[47] there was cytological evidence of anal dysplasia with features of HPV infection in 24 of 61 (39%) homosexual men, and of HPV infection without dysplasia in a further 26 (43%). Dysplasia was significantly associated with HIV positivity and a history of anal warts and frequent receptive anal intercourse. In a series of 97 male homosexuals with AIDS,[113] anal cytology demonstrated atypical changes in 39% and AIN in 15%, and these abnormalities were significantly associated with HPV infection. HPV DNA was detected in 54% and HPV 16 and 18 were the most commonly detected types, found alone or in combination with other mucosal HPV types in 29% of cases. HPV DNA has also been detected in anal swabs from 30 (29%) of 102 HIV-positive women compared with 2 (2%) of 96 seronegative controls, and the prevalence of anal cytological abnormalities was significantly increased in the seropositive group.[67] An even higher prevalence of anal HPV infection was detected in another group of HIV-positive women.[178] As with CIN in HIV-positive women, the rates of anal disease in both HIV-positive men and women are inversely related to CD4 counts.[112] However, it remains unclear whether these pre-malignancies are associated with an increased risk of invasive disease and, to date, as with the cervix, studies have failed to observe an increase of anal cancer in HIV-infected populations.[54,138]

Oral HPV infection in HIV
Intraoral warts

An increased prevalence of oral warts in HIV infection is well established.[148] In one study, HPV-7 was demonstrated in warts from 7 of 17 (41%) HIV-positive individuals,[57] and the same group subsequently reported the presence of HPV 7 in both oral and facial warts from HIV-positive patients.[32] In an evaluation of 57 oral biopsies from patients with HIV infection,[172] HPV 7 (19%) and HPV 32 (28%) were the predominant types in benign lesions, and HPV 2a, 6b, 13, 16, 18, 55, 59, and 69 were also detected. Two new HPV types (HPV 72 and HPV 73) were identified in atypical oral warts. Focal epithelial hyperplasia (Heck's disease) harboring HPV 32 has also been described in association with HIV.[171]

Oral malignancy

Intraoral HPV infection may be associated with mild to severe epithelial atypia[129] and may have pre-malignant potential. In one study,[45] of HIV-associated intraoral squamous cell carcinoma three of four cases were found to be associated with HPV (types 6, 11, 16, 18, 31, 33, and 35).

Conjunctival HPV infection in HIV

Ateenyi-Agaba noted that the incidence of conjunctival carcinoma was constant in Uganda from 1970 to 1988 but had increased six fold by 1992. Cases were shown to have a prevalence of HIV of 75% and controls of 19%, and it was postulated that the increase in conjunctival malignancy was due to HIV, with UV light and HPV infection involved in the etiology.[5] In support of this hypothesis, further studies in Uganda and Malawi showed 35% of conjunctival carcinomas to be HPV 16 positive.[173]

10.3.2 Hematological malignancies

An increased prevalence of warts is well recognized in hematological disorders predominantly associated with impairment of CMI. In a study of 397 patients, warts were detected in 25.7% of those with Hodgkin's disease and in 17.6% with chronic lymphatic leukaemia (CLL), compared with 2.3% of controls.[102] In contrast, none of the patients with multiple myeloma, which largely affects humoral immunity, was found to have warts. Following bone marrow transplantation, an increase in oral and cutaneous warts has also been reported.[7,183] In 56 immunosuppressed patients including a number with Hodgkin's disease and CLL, common warts induced by HPV 2 and 4 and plane warts associated with HPV 3, 10, and 28 predominated.[106] EV-like clinical features in Hodgkin's disease have also been described, and in one case the EV type HPV 46 was identified.[58]

10.3.3 Systemic lupus erythematosus

Patients with systemic lupus erythematosus (SLE) have an increased susceptibility to HPV infection; in one series, 25 of 56 (45%) patients had warts compared with 19 of 160 (12%) controls, independent of immunosuppressive drug therapy.[75] A similar prevalence of warts was also observed in discoid lupus erythematosus.[181] An EV-like presentation has also been reported in another patient in whom HPV 20 was detected in pityriasis versicolor-like lesions.[164] HPV-associated malignancy may also be over-represented; multiple flat warts on the arms containing HPV 6 and 11, together with Bowenoid papulosis of the genitalia and squamous cell carcinoma of the tongue harboring HPV 16, were described in one individual, although this patient had received treatment with systemic steroids.[87] HPV 2 has been found in both basal cell carcinomas and plane warts from a patient with SLE.[105] An increased prevalence of lower genital tract intraepithelial neoplasia has been reported in women with SLE, although such patients have usually been receiving immunosuppressive therapy.[119,147]

10.3.4 Other diseases associated with secondary immunodeficiency

There have been case reports documenting HPV infection in the context of other diseases causing secondary immunosuppression. For example, intestinal lymphangiectasia, which results in impaired CMI due to a cell-losing enteropathy, has been associated with extensive plane and plantar warts.[132,175] An EV-like eruption has also been described in two African sisters with lepromatous leprosy, which is commonly associated with a generalized depression of CMI.[73] EV-like features have been reported in a patient with primary lymphatic dysplasia who also had evidence of depressed CMI and developed periungual carcinoma *in situ* of the thumb from which HPV 16 was isolated.[110] In a similar patient, extensive periungual, subungual, and anogenital warts underwent transformation into microinvasive squamous cell carcinoma.[143]

10.3.5 PUVA therapy

Psoralen and UVA photochemotherapy is associated with a dose-dependent increased risk of non-melanoma skin cancer in patients treated for psoriasis.[160] Like UVB radiation, PUVA is both mutagenic and immunosuppressive and may thus act as a complete carcinogen.[81,104,167,182] However, a cofactor role for HPV infection has been suggested.[176] Our group has analysed a series of benign and malignant lesions from patients receiving PUVA for psoriasis, eczema, and cutaneous T-cell lymphoma.[64] HPV DNA sequences were found in 15/20 (75%) non-melanoma skin cancers, 7/17 (41%) dysplastic PUVA keratoses, 4/5 (80%) cutaneous warts, and 4/12 (33%) PUVA-exposed normal skin samples. The majority of HPV-positive lesions contained EV HPV types, including HPV 5, 20, 21, 23, 24, and 38. Mixed infection with EV, cutaneous and/or mucosal types was present in 6/30 (20%) of all HPV-positive lesions. HPV 41 and 16/18 have previously been found in other PUVA-associated squamous cell carcinomas in smaller studies.[68,133,176] However, the interpretation of these findings has been further complicated by the apparent over-representation of EV HPV types in psoriatic skin,[40] independent of PUVA therapy.[177] Nonetheless, it remains possible that the cutaneous and systemic immunosuppression induced by PUVA may predispose to HPV-associated cutaneous malignancies.

10.4 ORGAN TRANSPLANTATION

Immunodeficiency predisposing to HPV infection may occur in a range of disorders in which long-term immunosuppressive drug regimens are used. The largest group of patients falling into this category is organ transplant recipients (OTRs), who require lifelong immunosuppression to maintain their grafts. This immunosuppression was initially achieved with azathioprine and prednisolone, but since 1984 cyclosporin has also been used and, more recently, other immunosuppressive agents have been introduced.[121] In addition to widespread viral warts, these patients are at markedly increased risk of both anogenital and cutaneous malignancies.[86] There has been considerable interest in recent years in attempting to define the role of HPV in the pathogenesis of transplant-associated non-melanoma skin cancer.[63,96,123]

10.4.1 Cutaneous warts in transplant recipients

Clinicopathological features

Extensive cutaneous and genital warts are a common problem, causing significant morbidity in OTRs. Studies of the first 3 years post-transplant in adult OTRs have reported rates of between 25% and 42%, whereas up to 92% of patients transplanted for over 5 years are affected (reviewed in reference 53). Warts are also a common problem in pediatric OTRs.[70] The rapid resolution of warts after graft rejection and withdrawal of immunosuppression highlights the contribution of immunosuppressive drugs to this tendency, although it has yet to be established whether different drugs vary in their ability to predispose to warts.[27] In addition, high UVR exposure is likely to increase the predisposition to HPV infection.[20]

In the early post-transplant years, warts are usually of the common or palmoplantar type, and tend to be large, numerous, and difficult to treat.[52] With increasing time after transplantation, increasing age, and higher levels of sun exposure, patients are more likely to have flat warts on sun-exposed sites, which may become confluent, particularly over the dorsum of the hands and forearms. In some instances, hyperkeratotic papules on sun-exposed surfaces may be difficult to classify as either viral warts, verrucous or actinic keratoses. Histologically, such warts often show cytological atypia, most frequently of the basal layer,[15,50,122] and it is from such areas that squamous cell carcinomas often arise. EV lesions have also been reported,[89,134] although such appearances are probably rarer than the literature might suggest.[97]

HPV types found in transplant warts

Problems of HPV DNA detection and genotyping in the skin

Studies of HPV types present in cutaneous warts from OTRs have produced remarkably variable results. There are a number of explanations for these apparent discrepancies,[123] including differences in the type of tissues analysed (e.g., DNA obtained from formalin-fixed specimens may produce suboptimal results), and the types of patients included (e.g., patients may be highly selected, such as individuals with multiple squamous cell carcinomas). However, the major source of variability is likely to result from the different experimental approaches used to detect and genotype HPV DNA. Earlier techniques were based on DNA hybridization, with inevitable problems due to relatively low sensitivity and cross-hybridization between HPV types; the prevalence of HPV DNA detected in warts was often less than 60%, suggesting that significant numbers of HPV types were undetected by these techniques.[49,135,137,160] More sensitive polymerase chain reaction (PCR) techniques have largely superseded these methods, but inconsistencies in published data still occur, and are likely to be the consequence of differences in the PCR approach used.[163] Some investigators have used type-specific primers, which are highly sensitive but only capable of detecting a limited range of HPV types, whereas others have used broader spectrum consensus primers, but these have often been designed for the detection of anogenital rather than cutaneous or EV HPV types. More recently, PCR using degenerate nested primers has proved useful.[140] Degenerate primers are essentially mixtures of many primers with nucleotide differences at several positions rendering them complementary to the target DNA of multiple HPV types at the expense of reduced sensitivity, and this has been overcome by using nested primers.[13] Nonetheless, the spectrum of HPV types detected is still limited by the primer sets used.[163] In order to address this problem, we have recently developed a degenerate and nested PCR technique using multiple primer pairs which has proved capable of detecting a broad spectrum of HPV types to a high sensitivity, including mixed infections within single lesions.[65]

HPV types found in cutaneous warts from OTRs

Despite methodological differences between studies, it is useful to review the available data on HPV types reported in OTR warts in order to interpret data relating to non-melanoma skin cancer. Over 20 case reports or series have included such data. Of those employing DNA hybridization techniques, many have reported the presence of common cutaneous HPV types, particularly HPV 2 and 4 and, to a lesser extent, HPV 1, 3, and 10, findings broadly similar to those for the immunocompetent population.[34,49,135,169] Some studies have found EV-related[9,16,88,106,134,135,169] or mucosal HPV types.[38,49] Mixed infections with two or more different HPV types also emerge as being relatively common.[106,135,169] Using PCR-based techniques, it is now clear that transplant warts may actually be associated with a rather more diverse range of HPV types than that found in the general population. In one series, HPV DNA was detected in 11 of 18 warts (61%), and mucosal HPV types were found more frequently.[152] In contrast, 3 of 18 (17%) warts were found to contain HPV 5/8 and the remainder of the positive lesions were found to contain cutaneous or low-risk mucosal types in another series.[155] Shamanin et al. used two pairs of degenerate primers to analyse 47 viral warts; HPV DNA was identified in 60% of warts, the majority of which contained cutaneous HPV types (HPV 10, 27, 28, 57, and 77). Six of the 28 HPV-positive lesions (21%) contained five putatively novel EV HPV types.[142] Our group has recently reported a series of 51 warts from 23 renal transplant recipients.[65] HPV DNA was detected in all lesions, with cutaneous types in 84.3%, EV types in 80.4%, and mucosal types in 27.4%. In addition, two or more distinct HPV types were co-detected in 94.1% of lesions. In contrast, single cutaneous HPV types were detected in all but one of 20 warts from 15 immunocompetent individuals.[65] Thus, OTR warts appear to be characterized by a high prevalence of EV HPV types and multiple infections, compared with the immunocompetent population.

10.4.2 Non-melanoma skin cancer in transplant recipients

Clinicopathological features

OTRs have a well-documented increased risk of malignancy, and of virus-associated tumors in particular. Non-Hodgkin's lymphoma (Epstein–Barr virus), anogenital cancer (HPV 16

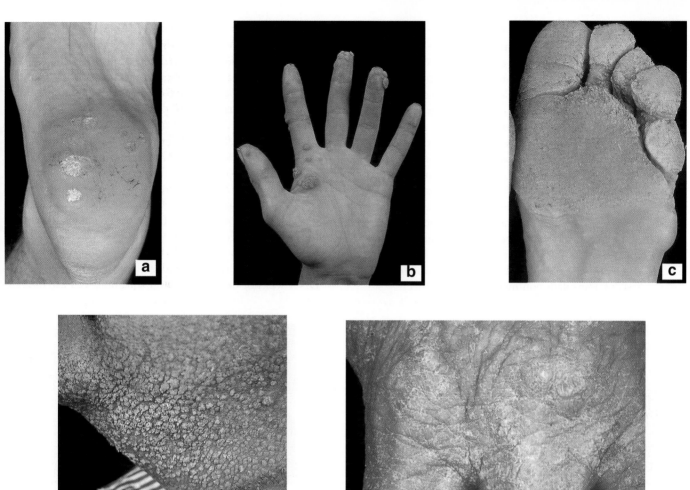

Figure 10.1

Benign HPV infection in renal transplant recipients: (a) extensive mosaic warts over the heel; (b) multiple common hand warts; (c) confluent mosaic warts covering most of the forefoot; (d) multiple plane warts over sun-exposed areas of the neck; (e) a mixture of confluent plane warts and dysplasia over the dorsum of the hand.

and 18), and Kaposi's sarcoma (human herpesvirus 8) occur 50–1000 times more frequently than in the general population.[14] Overall, non-melanoma skin cancers are the most common malignancy, and the risk of cutaneous squamous cell carcinoma is increased 50–100-fold. The cumulative incidence of skin cancer is between 27% and 44% after 20–25 years of immunosuppression.[52,60,61,86] In contrast to the immunocompetent population, in whom the ratio of basal to squamous cell carcinoma is approximately 4:1, squamous cell carcinomas predominate in OTRs, leading to a reversal in this ratio.[144,174] These tumors occur 20–30 years earlier, behave more aggressively, and lead to a greater morbidity and mortality than in the immunocompetent population.[52] Over 90% of transplant squamous cell carcinomas occur on chronically sun-exposed sites, often in areas of diffuse warty change.[52] They may be atypical in appearance, sharing both clinical and histological features in common with viral warts. Thus, some squamous cell carcinomas have an overall verrucous architecture and may retain features of hypergranulosis and perinuclear vacuolation, whereas transplant warts may be associated with dysplasia sufficient to confer a diagnosis of intraepidermal carcinoma.[15,50]

Etiological factors

The major factors contributing to the high rates of non-melanoma skin cancer in transplant recipients are UVR and drug-induced immunosuppression, but immunogenetic factors and infection with HPV may also play an important role. As in the immunocompetent population, UVR exposure is critical; tumors develop on sun-exposed sites and are more common in individuals with high cumulative sun exposure and fair skin.[20,53] Not only is UVR directly mutagenic to epidermal keratinocytes, but it also has immunosuppressive effects, both properties potentially contributing to carcinogenesis. In general terms, immunosuppressive therapy may impair the immunosurveillance mechanisms responsible for the control of malignant progression. More specifically, the active metabolite of azathioprine, 6-thioguanine, may also have direct effects on tumor initiation or promotion.[165] In addition, there is emerging evidence that patients receiving cyclosporin may be at greater risk of developing non-melanoma skin cancer, although this remains controversial;[51] there is also preliminary evidence for a direct carcinogenic role for this drug.[69]

Epidemiology of HPV and OTR non-melanoma skin cancer (Figure 10.2)

An association between warts and skin cancer in OTRs was first noted in Australia,[174] and this, together with the clinico-pathological features of transplant squamous cell carcinoma outlined above which indirectly support progression of warts through increasingly dysplastic squamous lesions to invasive squamous cell carcinoma, has prompted research into a possible role for HPV in transplant non-melanoma skin cancer. However, epidemiological data from over 25 studies have, until recently, shown little consistency in either the frequency or spectrum of HPV types detected. As already discussed, much of this variation may be method-ological. With the use of degenerate PCR techniques by several investigators,[13,33,63,66,142,163] the current consensus is that EV HPV types predominate and may be relevant to the pathogenesis of transplant non-melanoma skin cancer.

Early studies using DNA hybridization techniques focused on HPV 5 and 8 in an attempt to establish the degree of similarity between EV and transplant cancers. Thus, HPV 5 was demonstrated in a transplant squamous cell carcinoma[89] and HPV 5/8 was subsequently found in two of three squamous cell carcinomas.[137] In a larger study which included 25 squamous cell carcinomas from four patients, HPV 5/8 was detected in 15 (60%) squamous cell carcinomas by dot-blot hybridization and HPV 4 in one lesion, although only probes for these three HPV types were used.[9] EV HPV 5 and 8 were also found in squamous cell carcinomas by some other,[126] but not all,[135,153] researchers, whereas a preponderance of mucosal or cutaneous types has been reported by others.[38]

Initial reports using PCR-based detection methods also failed to clarify matters. Indeed, in several studies, HPV DNA was not detected at all in squamous cell carcinomas,

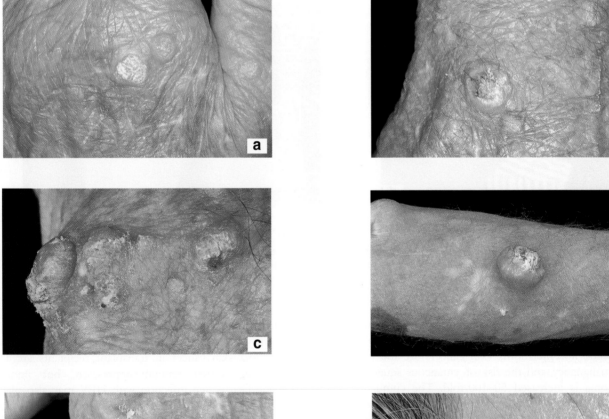

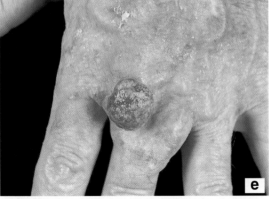

Figure 10.2

Pre-malignant and malignant skin lesions in renal transplant recipients: (a) histologically this wart showed severe epidermal dysplasia; (b) an early invasive squamous cell carcinoma which histologically showed features consistent with HPV infection; (c) multiple squamous cell carcinomas co-localizing on the dorsum of the forearm with several benign warts; (d) a slowly growing, well-differentiated squamous cell carcinoma on the forearm; (e) a rapidly growing, poorly differentiated squamous cell carcinoma on the dorsum of the hand; (f) a moderately differentiated squamous cell carcinoma arising on the forehead.

although all were series in which paraffin-embedded samples were used.[35,44,95,151] Subsequently, Shamanin et al.[141] detected HPV DNA in 11 of 20 (55%) transplant squamous cell carcinomas using two pairs of degenerate primers and Southern blotting. Cutaneous types HPV 41 and HPV 77 were found in four positive lesions, and the remaining seven positive lesions were uncharacterized. In this study, HPV DNA was found in only 60% of warts, suggesting perhaps that some HPV types were not being detected. Using 16 less degenerate primer pairs, the same group reported 13 (65%) of the 20 squamous cell carcinomas and 3 of 5 (60%) basal cell carcinomas to be HPV DNA positive.[142] Only 20% of the HPV types were EV associated; the majority consisted of either high-risk mucosal types (HPV 16, 51, 54, 56, 61, and 69) or cutaneous types (HPV 41 and 60). This study also included 25 squamous cell carcinomas from immunocompetent patients, of which 32% were HPV DNA positive and amongst which several EV types were identified. In contrast, another group[13,31] designed nested degenerate PCR primers capable of detecting EV HPV types and detected EV or EV-related viruses in 49 of 61 (80%) transplant squamous cell carcinomas, 4 of 8 (50%) basal cell carcinoma, 14 of 15 (93%) actinic keratoses, and 2 of 5 (40%) in situ carcinomas; approximately 40% of lesions contained two or more HPV types. These discrepancies are again likely to reflect the methodology employed. Confirmation of this is provided by a separate study in which lesions were initially analysed using the PCR primer panel described by Shamanin et al.[142] and were shown to contain predominantly cutaneous types, whereas additional EV HPV types were detected when the same lesions were reassessed using the nested primer pair of Berkhout et al.[33] The method which our group has described[65] combines features of both approaches. We have recently compared transplant and immunocompetent non-melanoma skin cancer.[66] HPV DNA was detected in 37 of 44 (84.1%) squamous cell carcinomas, 18 of 24 (75%) basal cell carcinomas, and 15 of 17 (88.2%) pre-malignant skin lesions from the immunosuppressed group, compared with 6 of 22 (27.2%) squamous cell carcinomas, 11 of 30 (36.7%) basal cell carcinomas and 6 of 11 (55%) pre-malignancies in the immunocompetent group. EV HPV types prevailed in all lesion types from both groups of patients. In immunosuppressed individuals, cutaneous HPV types were also identified at high frequency, and co-detection of multiple HPV types within single tumors was commonly observed. Thus, there is a very high prevalence of HPV DNA in transplant tumors and a lower prevalence in immunocompetent tumors. EV HPV types predominate in malignancies from both groups, and within the two populations the prevalence and spectrum of HPV types do not appear to differ in squamous cell carcinoma, basal cell carcinoma or pre-malignancies.

Further support for a possible role for EV HPV in transplant skin cancer has come from a different experimental approach. Stark et al.[156] have evaluated the prevalence of antibodies directed against the native L1 epitopes exposed on the surface of HPV 8 virus-like particles. In OTRs (n = 185), antibody prevalence was 21.1%, compared with 7.6% in healthy controls and 6.8% of patients with Hodgkin's lymphoma. Interestingly, 42.9% of PUVA-treated patients and 45.9% of immunocompetent individuals with non-melanoma skin cancer were seropositive. These data largely

accord with the data from HPV DNA prevalence studies, although the particularly high positivity rate in the immunocompetent patients with non-melanoma skin cancer is intriguing and has potential implications for the pathogenesis of non-melanoma skin cancer generally, as well as in immunosuppressed populations.

HPV in normal skin and hair from OTRs

Over the past 3 years, data have become available concerning the prevalence of HPV DNA in normal skin and hair follicles from both immunosuppressed and immunocompetent individuals. Boxman et al.[18] found 45 of 49 (92%) hair samples from immunosuppressed patients and from 20 of 38 (53%) immunocompetent controls harbored EV HPV types irrespective of non-melanoma skin cancer status. The same group has extended this study using HPV 5 type-specific primers and report the presence of HPV 5 in hair from 14/31 (45%) OTRs and 21/135 (16%) immunocompetent controls; no correlation with non-melanoma skin cancer status was observed.[19] The same group has reported a rather lower HPV DNA prevalence of 35% in normal skin from OTRs,[12] closer to that reported in immunocompetent individuals.[4] Our group has recently analysed a series of normal skin samples from transplant and immunocompetent patients (unpublished data). Overall, 18 of 52 (35%) samples from immunocompetent patients were positive, with EV types found in 44% and cutaneous types in 61% of positive cases. In contrast, 56 of 64 (88%) samples from OTRs were positive, with EV types in 84% and cutaneous types in 50%. There was no difference in samples from UVR-exposed versus non-UVR-exposed sites in either group. The interpretation of these results awaits evaluation of localization and viral load of the HPV types found, but these data suggest that HPV DNA, perhaps in latent form, is commonly present in clinically normal skin and hair from immunosuppressed individuals, and is also present at lower levels in the immunocompetent population.

Role of HPV in transplant skin cancers

In both anogenital cancer and EV-associated skin cancer there is a specific association of certain HPV types with transformation. The diverse spectrum of HPV types identified in transplant tumors and the presence of multiple different HPV types in a single tumor, together with the findings of a high prevalence of HPV DNA in normal skin from transplant patients, make it difficult to attribute a carcinogenic role to specific HPV types. These epidemiological data do not allow exclusion of the possibility that HPV may be a 'passenger' in these lesions, present in latent form (detectable by the highly sensitive PCR methods used) and perhaps preferentially replicating in malignant lesions, but not actively contributing to carcinogenesis. Nonetheless, it is plausible that HPV may play an important role, either by a direct transforming capacity or as a cofactor in tumor promotion. In support of a direct transforming role, investigators from our group have, for example, shown that E7 of HPV 77 is capable of transforming both established and primary rodent cells in culture. HPV 77 was first identified in warts and squamous cell carcinomas from OTRs.[141] As a cofactor, various HPVs may act in a general way without encoding direct transforming potential; for example, the ability of HPV to stimulate cell replication and suppress apoptosis may fix DNA mutations induced by UV radiation or other carcinogens, leading to the accumulation of UV-induced mutations and loss of chromosomal stability. Consistent with this hypothesis, investigators from our group have recently shown that certain EV and cutaneous HPV types found in transplant tumors inhibit apoptosis in response to UV damage[72] and one mechanism responsible for this may be degradation of the pro-apoptotic protein BAK.[72a] Interactions between HPV and other cellular proteins such as p53 may also be more complex than was previously appreciated, as two recent studies from our group have highlighted. In the first, we reported that two common polymorphic variants of p53, p53Pro and p53Arg, are not equally susceptible to inactivation mediated by the E6 protein.[158] Our results suggested that, because the Arg form was more easily inactivated by E6 than the Pro form, there might be an excess of the Arg form relative to the Pro form retained in HPV-associated cancers. Our pilot study in HPV-associated anogenital as well as cutaneous cancers suggested that this was the case, but larger studies in genetically diverse populations are required before the significance of these observations can be clearly interpreted. In a second study, investigators from our group demonstrated that the regulatory region of HPV 77 contains a sequence with close homology to a p53-binding consensus.[125] This HPV 77 sequence confers p53 binding and up-regulation of viral gene expression in a p53-dependent manner. The HPV 77 promoter/enhancer is also up-regulated by UV, an effect abolished by mutation of p53. Whether polymorphisms in other tumor suppressor genes have a bearing on the maintenance or progression of lesions containing HPV remains to be elucidated and, similarly, whether other viruses identified in skin cancers also share the regulatory activity of HPV 77 by p53, or whether they are regulated by UVR through other mechanisms, remain outstanding questions. Finally, it also conceivable that extensive HPV infection in many transplant recipients may itself contribute to a local immunosuppressive effect mediated, for example, by viral-induced cytokine changes, and this, together with UV-induced local immunosuppression and the effects of systemic immunosuppression, could facilitate tumor growth.

10.4.3 Anogenital HPV infection in transplant recipients

As in HIV-positive individuals, benign and malignant anogenital HPV infection is observed with increased frequency in OTRs compared with the normal population. In a recent study of over 1000 OTRs, external anogenital warts were identified in 2.3% of patients, and, as with lesions occurring on sun-exposed skin, histological dysplasia was common.[39] The incidence of anogenital malignancy is increased up to 20-fold overall.[146] In one of the first series published, based on information collected by the Cincinnati Transplant Tumor Registry on 2150 patients,[116] 65 patients were affected (3%), of whom 9 subsequently died of anogenital malignancy. In several females, a field effect was observed with multiple tumors of the squamous epithelium of the anogenital area, vagina or cervix. In a series of 105 renal transplant recipients (RTRs) and matched immunocompetent controls,[59] HPV infection was 17-fold greater in the RTRs and cervical neoplasia nine times greater, and multiple

sites of involvement were again found to be common. In another case-controlled study of 49 RTRs and 69 immunocompetent controls,[1] the prevalence of CIN was significantly higher in the women with transplants (49%) than in controls (10%). Although the overall rate of detection of HPV DNA did not differ significantly between the two groups, there was a significantly higher rate of detection of HPV 16/18 in the transplant recipients. Many of the women in this series were found to have widespread HPV infection and intraepithelial neoplasia throughout the anogenital tract, and co-existing cervical and vulvar disease has been confirmed in other studies.[119] A high prevalence of CIN has been confirmed in a more recent, uncontrolled study in which CIN was detected in 20 of 48 (42%) of OTRs.[111] Not all studies have confirmed this high prevalence of HPV positivity and CIN, and some authors have proposed that sexual behavior is more relevant in this regard than immunosuppression.[103] In established CIN, however, Petry et al.[120] have shown that progression and recurrence after destructive treatment were more common in transplant recipients than in controls. Interestingly, there may be an association between susceptibility to cutaneous malignancy and the development of aggressive anogenital carcinomas.[3] Anal intraepithelial neoplasia is also more common than in the normal population. In a case-controlled study[108] involving 133 patients and 145 immunocompetent controls, 26 (19.5%) of transplant recipients were found on anoscopy and biopsy to have AIN grades I–III, and one had anal cancer. This contrasted with only one subject with AIN in the control group. HPV 16 DNA was detected by PCR in 47% of anal biopsies from the transplant recipients, compared with 12.4% of controls, and all patients with anal disease had evidence of HPV infection. Finally, as in the skin, anogenital lesions in the transplant and HIV-positive populations are associated with an increased number and diversity of HPV types compared to the immunocompetent population.[22,24,161]

10.5 MANAGEMENT OF HPV INFECTION IN IMMUNOSUPPRESSED PATIENTS

In view of the widespread nature of HPV infection and the significant risk of HPV-associated mucocutaneous malignancies, a number of general points emerge with respect to strategies for intervention and the treatment of HPV infection in immunosuppressed individuals.

10.5.1 Control rather than cure of warts

The complete eradication of warts is unlikely to be achieved in the majority of patients, unless the immunosuppressed state is in some way reversible. Emphasis is therefore best placed on control of the spread of infection and relief of symptoms, rather than on attempting to cure infection. In this respect, standard treatment methods for warts as described elsewhere in this volume may prove useful, although in refractory cases more interventional treatment with, for example, systemic retinoid therapy, intralesional bleomycin, or intralesional/systemic interferon may be justified. New therapies with the potential to revolutionize the treatment of HPV in immunosuppressed patients may not be too far away. For example, imiquimod is an immune enhancer[154] that has been demonstrated to be highly effective in eradicating genital warts in immunocompetent patients;[36] However, to date, no studies of its efficacy in immunocompromised individuals have been reported.

10.5.2 Regular surveillance of skin and anogenital tract

Regular monitoring of the skin and anogenital tract to facilitate early detection and removal of malignant and premalignant lesions is an important part of the management of HPV infection in this patient population.

Cutaneous surveillance

The distinction between benign warts and warty dysplasia is often very subtle clinically, so experienced dermatological supervision is required.[52,84] For example, in our unit, renal transplant recipients are seen soon after transplantation to assess the degree of pre-existing sun damage and to give advice on strict sun avoidance, protective clothing, and the use of high sun protection factor sunscreens. Thereafter, annual examination, with prompt surgical removal of suspicious lesions, is usually sufficient in most patients, although as dysplasia and non-melanoma skin cancer develop, closer supervision is essential.[52] Progression of dysplastic lesions may be controlled by the long-term use of topical or systemic retinoids or topical 5-fluorouracil.[17,38,52,131,145] Prophylactic excision and grafting of the dorsum of the hands may occasionally be a useful maneuver in certain individuals with multiple non-melanoma skin cancers at this site.[52] Oral lesions require a similar level of vigilance.[80]

Anogenital surveillance

Given the high incidence and multifocal nature of anogenital HPV infection in immunosuppressed individuals, screening for HPV-related diseases should be a routine part of healthcare provision for this population. All women should be offered regular cervical cytology screening, and preferably colposcopic examination of the cervix, in view of documented high rates of false-negative cervical smear tests.[1,92] Screening guidelines issued by the Center for Disease Control and Prevention for cervical disease in HIV-positive women recommend routine screening with cervical cytology at the time of initial evaluation and, if negative, a repeat smear after 6 months. If the latter is also negative, the woman may be followed by annual cervical smear cytology.[139] Aggressive treatment and careful follow-up for evidence of treatment failure or disease recurrence are particularly important in view of the apparent increased potential for rapid progression of pre-malignancy and recurrence after treatment.[48,90,120,180] However, dysplasia of the lower genital tract may be multifocal and so extensive that complete clearance of dysplasia may be extremely difficult to achieve. There is also a good case for annual cytobrush sampling of the anal epithelium, particularly in HIV-infected homosexual males.[56] Although it has yet to be established whether similar screening anal examination are required in OTRs, the potential progression to invasive anal cancer justifies regular review of those individuals with anal pre-malignancy.

10.5.3 Modulation of immunosuppression

Although a reduction in the dose of immunosuppressive drugs may help to control the extent of HPV infection and the progression of dysplastic lesions, this is not always possible without jeopardizing graft survival. In this respect, an objective means of assessing the actual degree of immunosuppression achieved in a given individual would be of great value, but is unfortunately not readily available.

10.6 CONCLUSIONS

Human papillomavirus infection is associated with significant morbidity and mortality in immunosuppressed individuals, particularly those with abnormalities of cell-mediated immunity. Mucocutaneous manifestations may range from extensive common warts to conditions simulating EV. Whilst HPV is undoubtedly the most important etiological factor responsible for the increased prevalence of anogenital malignancies observed in many immunosuppressed states, there is mounting evidence that it may also contribute to the development of skin malignancies, although there are, as yet, only limited mechanistic data to support a functional role for HPV. Finally, with the steady rise in numbers and expected life-span of immunosuppressed individuals, the scale of the problem caused by HPV infection will inevitably escalate. It will therefore become increasingly important for clinicians to be familiar with the spectrum and significance of the clinicopathological manifestations of HPV infection, and to optimize strategies for the prevention, detection, and treatment of these conditions in the context of immunosuppression.

REFERENCES

1. Alloub MI, Barr BBB, McLaren KM, Smith IW, Bunney MH, Smart GE. (1989) Human papillomavirus infection and cervical intraepithelial neoplasia in women with renal allografts. *BMJ* **298**: 153–6.
2. Arany I, Yen A, Tyring SK. (1997). p53, WAF1/CIP1 and mdm2 expression in skin lesions associated with human papillomavirus and human immunodeficiency virus. *Anticancer Res* **17**: 1281–5.
3. Arends MJ, Benton EC, McLaren KM, Stark LA, Hunter JAA, Bird CC. (1997) Renal allograft recipients with high susceptibility to cutaneous malignancy have an increased prevalence of human papillomavirus DNA in skin tumours and a greater risk of anogenital malignancy. *Br J Cancer* **75**: 722–8.
4. Astori G, Lavergne D, Benton C, *et al.* (1998) Human papillomaviruses are commonly found in normal skin of immunocompetent hosts. *J Invest Dermatol* **110**: 752–5.
5. Ateenyi-Agaba C. (1995) Conjunctival squamous-cell carcinoma associated with HIV infection in Kampala, Uganda. *Lancet* **345**: 695–6.
6. Aynaud O, Piron D, Barasso R, Poveda J-D. (1998) Comparison of histological and virological symptoms of human papillomavirus in HIV-1 infected men and immunocompetent controls. *Sex Transm Inf* **74**: 32–4.

7. Barasch A, Eisenberg E, D'Ambrosio JA, Nuki K, Peterson DE. (1996) Oral verruca vulgaris in a bone marrow transplant patient: A case report and review of literature. *Oral Oncol, Eur J Cancer* **32B**: 137–9.

8. Barnett N, Mak H, Winkelstein JA. (1983) Extensive verrucosis in primary immunodeficiency diseases. *Arch Dermatol* **119**: 5–7.

9. Barr B, Benton E, McLaren K, *et al.* (1989) Human papillomavirus infection and skin cancer in renal allograft recipients. *Lancet* **1**: 124–9.

10. Benton C, Shahidullah H, Hunter JAA. (1992) Human papillomavirus in the immunosuppressed. *Papillomavirus Rep* **2**: 23–6.

11. Berger TG, Sawchuk WS, Leonardi C, Langenberg A, Tappero J, Leboit PE. (1991) Epidermodysplasia verruciformis-associated papillomavirus infection complicating human immunodeficiency virus disease. *Br J Dermatol* **124**: 79–83.

12. Berkhout RJ, Bouwes Bavinck JN, ter Schegget J. (2000) Persistence of human papillomavirus DNA in benign and (pre)malignant skin lesions from renal transplant recipients. *J Clin Microbiol* **38**: 2087–96.

13. Berkhout RJM, Tieben LM, Smits HL, Bouwes-Bavinck JN, Vermeer BJ, ter Schegget J. (1995) Nested PCR approach to detection and typing of epidermodysplasia verruciformis-associated human papillomavirus types in cutaneous cancers from renal transplant recipients. *J Clin Microbiol* **115**(33): 690–5.

14. Birkeland SA, Storm HH, Lamm LU, *et al.* (1995) Cancer risk after renal transplantation in the Nordic countries, 1964–1986. *Int J Cancer* **60**: 183–9.

15. Blessing K, McClaren KM, Benton EC, *et al.* (1989) Histopathology of skin lesions in renal allograft recipients: an assessment of viral features and dysplasia. *Histopathology* **14**: 129–39.

16. Blessing K, McLaren KM, Morris R, *et al.* (1990) Detection of human papillomavirus in skin and genital lesions of renal allograft recipients by in situ hybridisation. *Histopathology* **16**: 181–3.

17. Bouwes Bavinck JN, Tieben LM, Van Der Woude FJ, *et al.* (1995) Prevention of skin cancer and reduction of keratotic skin lesions during acitretin therapy in renal transplant recipients: a double-blind, placebo-controlled study. *J Clin Oncol* **13**: 1933–8.

18. Boxman ILA, Berkhout RJM, Mulder LHC, *et al.* (1997) Detection of human papillomavirus DNA in plucked hairs from renal transplant recipients and healthy volunteers. *J Invest Dermatol* **108**: 712–15.

19. Boxman ILA, Mulder LHC, Russell A, Bouwes Bavinck JN, Green A, ter Schegget J. (1999) Human papillomavirus type 5 is commonly present in immunosuppressed and immunocompetent individuals. *Br J Dermatol* **141**: 246–9.

20. Boyle J, McKie R, Briggs J, Junor BJR, Aitchison TC. (1984) Cancer, warts and sunshine in renal transplant recipients: a case control study. *Lancet* **1**: 702–5.

21. Broderson I, Genner J, Brodthagen H. (1974) Tuberculin sensitivity in BCG vaccinated children with common warts. *Acta Dermatol-Venereol (Stockh)* **54**: 291.

22. Broker TR, Jin G, Richardson M, *et al.* (1997) Molecular epidemiology of HPV infections of the female genital tract, identified by a novel PCR/restriction/sequencing analysis of renal transplant candidates and recipients and of HIV-positive patients. Abstract 16th International Papillomavirus Conference, Siena, Italy, September 1997.

23. Brooks EG, Schalmalstieg FC, Wirt D, *et al.* (1990) A novel X-linked combined immunodeficiency disease. *J Clin Invest* **86**: 1623–31.

24. Brown DR, Bryan JT, Cramer H, Katz BP, Handy V, Fife KH. (1994) Detection of multiple human papillomavirus types in condyloma acuminata from immunosuppressed patients. *J Infect Dis* **170**: 759–65.

25. Bryan JT, Stoler MH, Tyring SK, McClowry T, Fife KH, Brown DR. (1998) High-grade dysplasia in genital warts from two patients infected with the human immunodeficiency virus. *J Med Virol* **54**: 69–73.

26. Bundino S, Zina AM, Bernengo MG. (1978) Dyskeratosis congenita with epidermodysplasia verruciformis of Lewandowsky and Lutz. *Dermatologica* **156**: 15–23.

27. Bunney MH, Benton EC, Barr BBB, Smith IW, Anderton JL, Hunter JAA. (1990) The prevalence of skin disorders in renal allograft recipients receiving cyclosporin A compared with those receiving azathioprine. *Nephrol Dial Transplant* **5**: 379–82.

28. Castro K, Ward J, Slutsker L, *et al.* (1992) 1993 revised classification system for HIV infection and expanded surveillance case definition for AIDS among adolescents and adults. *MMWR* **41**: 1–19.

29. Chiasson MA, Ellerbrock TV, Bush TJ, Sun XW, Wright TC. (1997) Increased prevalence of vulvo-vaginal condyloma and vulvar intraepithelial neoplasia in women infected with the human immunodeficiency virus. *Obstet Gynecol* **89**: 690–4.

30. Chopra KF, Tyring SK. (1997) The impact of the human immunodeficiency virus on the human papillomavirus epidemic. *Arch Dermatol* **133**: 629–33.

31. de Jong Tieben LM, Berkhout RJM, Smits HL, *et al.* (1995) High frequency of detection of epidermodysplasia verruciformis-associated human papillomavirus DNA in biopsies from malignant and premalignant skin lesions from renal transplant recipients. *J Invest Dermatol* **105**: 367–71.

32. de Villiers E-M. (1989) Prevalence of HPV 7 papillomas in the oral mucosa and facial skin of patients with human immunodeficiency virus. *Arch Dermatol* **125**: 1590.

33. de Villiers E-M, Lavergne D, Mclaren K, Benton EC. (1997) Prevailing papillomavirus types in non-melanoma carcinomas of the skin in renal allograft recipients. *Int J Cancer* **73**: 356–61.

34. Dyall-Smith D, Trowell H, Dyall-Smith MA. (1991) Benign human papillomavirus infection in renal transplant recipients. *Int J Dermatol* **30**: 785–9.

35. Dyall-Smith D, Trowell H, Mark A, Dyall-Smith MA. (1991) Cutaneous squamous cell carcinoma and papillomaviruses in renal transplant recipients: a clinical and biological study. *J Dermatol Sci* **2**: 139–46.

36. Edwards L, Ferenczy A, Eron L, *et al.* (1998) Self-administered topical 5% imiquimod cream for external anogenital warts. HPV Study Group. Human Papillomavirus. *Arch Dermatol* **134**: 25–30.

37. Ellerbrock TV, Chiasson MA, Bush TJ, *et al.* (2000) Incidence of cervical squamous intraepithelial lesions in

human immunodeficiency virus infected women. *JAMA* **283**: 1031–37.

38. Euvrard S, Chardonnet Y, Pouteil-Noble C, *et al.* (1993) Association of skin malignancies with various and multiple carcinogenic and non-carcinogenic human papillomaviruses in renal transplant recipients. *Cancer* **72**: 2198–206.

39. Euvrard S, Kanitakis J, Chardonnet Y, *et al.* (1997) External anogenital lesions in organ transplant recipients – a clinicopathologic and virologic assessment. *Arch Dermatol* **133**: 175–8.

40. Favre M, Orth G, Majewski S, Baloul S, Pura A, Jablonska S. (1998).Psoriasis: a possible reservoir for human papillomavirus type 5, the virus associated with skin carcinomas of epidermodysplasia verruciformis. *J Invest Dermatol* **110**: 311–17.

41. Feldman JG, Chirgwin K, Dehovitz JA, Minkoff H. (1997) The association of smoking and risk of condyloma acuminata in females. *Obstet Gynecol* **89**: 346–50.

42. Feldman SB, Sexton M, Glenn JD, Lookingbill DP. (1989) Immunosuppression in men with Bowenoid papulosis. *Arch Dermatol* **125**: 651–4.

43. Fennema JSA, van Ameijden EJC, Coutinho RA, van den Hoek JAR. (1995) HIV, sexually transmitted diseases and gynecologic disorders in women: increased risk for genital herpes and warts among HIV-infected prostitutes in Amsterdam. *AIDS* **9**: 1071–8.

44. Ferrandiz C, Fuente MJ, Ariza, A, Ribera M, Paradelo C. (1998) Detection and typing of human papillomavirus in skin lesions from renal transplant recipients and equivalent lesions from immunocompetent patients. *Arch Dermatol* **134**: 381–2.

45. Flaitz CM, Nichols M, Adler-Storthz K, Hicks MJ. (1995) Intraoral squamous cell carcinoma in human immunodeficiency virus infection. *Oral Surg Oral Med Oral Path Oral Radiol Endod* **80**: 55–62.

46. Forman AB, Prendiville JS. (1988) Associations of human immunodeficiency virus seropositivity and extensive perineal condylomata acuminata in a child. *Arch Dermatol* **124**: 1010–11.

47. Frazer IH, Medley G, Crapper RM, Brown TC, Mackay IR. (1986) Association between anorectal dysplasia, human papillomavirus, and human immunodeficiency virus infection in homosexual men. *Lancet* **2**: 657–60.

48. Fruchter RG, Maiman M, Sedlis A, Bartley L, Camilien L, Arrastai C. (1996) Multiple recurrences of cervical intraepithelial neoplasia in women with the human immunodeficiency virus. *Obstet Gynecol* **87**: 338–44

49. Gassenmaier A, Fuchs P, Scell H, Pfister H. (1986) Papillomavirus DNA in warts of immunosuppressed renal allograft recipients. *Arch Derm Res* **278**: 219–23.

50. Glover M, Cerio R, Corbett M, Leigh IM, Hanby AM. (1995) Cutaneous squamoproliferative lesions in renal transplant recipients – differentiation from lesions in immunocompetent patients. *Am J Dermatopathol* **17**: 551–4.

51. Glover MT, Deeks JJ, Raftery MJ, Cunningham J, Leigh IM. (1997) Immunosuppression and risk of non-melanoma skin cancer in renal transplant recipients. *Lancet* **349**: 398.

52. Glover MT, Niranjan N, Kwan JTC, Leigh IM. (1994). Non-melanoma skin cancer in renal transplant recipients: the extent of the problem and a strategy for management. *Br J Plastic Surg* **47**: 86–9.

53. Glover MT, Proby CM, Leigh IM. (1993) Skin cancer in renal transplant patients. *Cancer Bull* **45**: 220–4.

54. Goedert JJ, Cote TR, Virgo P, *et al.* (1998) Spectrum of AIDS associated malignant disorders. *Lancet* **351**: 1833–9.

55. Goldes JA, Filipovich AH, Neudorf SM, *et al.* (1984) Epidermodysplasia verruciformis in a setting of common variable immunodeficiency. *Pediatr Dermatol* **2**: 136–9.

56. Goldie SJ, Kuntz KM, Weinstein ML, Freedberg KA, Welton ML, Palefsky JM. (1999) The clinical effectiveness of screening for anal squamous intraepithelial lesions in homosexual and bisexual HIV positive men. *JAMA* **281**: 1822–9.

57. Greenspan D, de Villiers E-M, Greenspan JS, de Souza YG, zur Hausen H. (1988) Unusual HPV types in oral warts associated with HIV infection. *J Oral Pathol* **17**: 482–7.

58. Gross G, Ellinger K, Roussaki A, Fuchs PG, Peter H-H, Pfister H. (1988) Epidermodysplasia verruciformis in a patient with Hodgkin's disease: characterisation of a new papillomavirus type and interferon treatment. *J Invest Dermatol* **91**: 43–8.

59. Halpert R, Fruchter RG, Sedlis A, Butt K, Boyce JG, Sillman F. (1986) Human papillomavirus and lower genital tract neoplasia in renal transplant patients. *Obstet Gynecol* **68**: 251–8.

60. Hardie IR, Strong RW, Hartley LC. (1989) Skin cancer in Caucasian renal allograft recipients living in a subtropical climate. *Surgery* **87**: 177–83.

61. Hartevelt MM, Bavinck JN, Kootte AMM, Vermeer BJ, Vandenbroucke JP. (1990) Incidence of skin cancer after renal transplantation in the Netherlands. *Transplantation* **49**: 506–9.

62. Harwood CA, Lacey CJN. (1998) Human papillomavirus disease in HIV infection. *AIDS Target Inform* **12**: R47–9.

63. Harwood CA, McGregor JM, Proby CM, Breuer J. (1999) Human papillomavirus and the development of non-melanoma skin cancer. *J Clin Pathol* **52**: 249–53.

64. Harwood CA, Spink PJ, Surentheran T, *et al.* (1998) Detection of human papillomavirus DNA in PUVA-associated non-melanoma skin cancers. *J Invest Dermatol* **111**: 123–7.

65. Harwood CA, Spink PJ, Surentheran T, *et al.* (1999) Degenerate and nested PCR; a highly sensitive and specific method for the detection of human papillomavirus infection in cutaneous warts. *J Clin Microbiol* **37**: 3545–55.

66. Harwood CA, Surentheran T, McGregor JM, *et al.* (2000) Human papillomavirus infection and non-melanoma skin cancer in immunosuppressed and immunocompetent individuals. *J Med Virol* **61**: 289–97.

67. Hillemanns P, Ellerbrock TV, McPhillips S, *et al.* (1996) Prevalence of anal human papillomavirus infection and anal cytologic abnormalities in HIV-seropositive women. *AIDS* **10**: 1641–7.

68. Hirt L, Hirsch-Behnam A, de Villiers E-M. (1990) Nucleotide sequence of human papillomavirus (HPV)

type 41: an unusual HPV type without typical E2 binding site consensus sequence. *Virus Res* **18**: 179–90.

69. Hojo M, Morimoto T, Maluccio M, *et al.* (1999) Cyclosporine induces cancer progression by cell-autonomous mechanism. *Nature* **397**: 530–4.

70. Ingelfinger JR, Grupe WE, Topor M, Levey RH. (1977) Warts in a pediatric renal transplant population. *Dermatologica* **155**: 7–12.

71. International Agency for Research on Cancer. (1995) Monographs on the evaluation of the carcinogenic risk to humans [No. 64]. *Human papillomaviruses.* Lyons, International Agency for Research on Cancer, 196–212.

72. Jackson S, Storey A. (2000) E6 proteins from diverse cutaneous HPV types inhibit apoptosis in response to UV damage. *Oncogene* **19**: 592–8.

72a. Jackson S, Harwood C, Thomas M, Banks L, Storey A. (2000) Role of BAK in UV-induced apoptosis in skin cancer and abrogation by HPV E6 proteins. *Genes Dev* **14**: 3065–73.

73. Jacyk WK, Lechner W. (1984) Epidermodysplasia verruciformis in lepromatous leprosy. *Dermatologica* **168**: 202–5.

74. Jacyk WK, Hazelhurst JA, Dreyer L, Coccia-Portugal MA. (1993) Epidermodysplasia verruciformis and malignant thymoma. *Clin Exp Dermatol* **18**: 89–91.

75. Johansson E, Pyrhönen S, Rostila T. (1977) Warts and wart virus antibodies in patients with systemic lupus erythematosus. *BMJ* **1**: 74–6.

76. Johnstone FD, McGoogan E, Smart GE, Brettle RP, Prescott RJ. (1994) A population-based, controlled study of the relation between HIV infection and cervical neoplasia. *Br J Obstet Gynaecol* **101**: 986–91.

77. Kang S, Fitzpatrick TB. (1994) Debilitating verruca vulgaris in a patient infected with the human immunodeficiency virus. *Arch Dermatol* **130**: 294–6.

78. Kent C, Samuel M, Winkelstein W. (1987) The role of anal/genital warts in HIV infection *JAMA* **258**: 3385–6.

79. Kenyon E, Loveland L, Kilpatrick R, Barbosa P. (1998) Epidemiology of plantar verrucae in HIV-infected individuals (1998) *J Acq Imm Defic Synd* **17**: 94–5.

80. King GN, Healy CM, Glover MT, *et al.* (1995) Increased prevalence of dysplastic and malignant lip lesions in renal transplant recipients. *N Engl J Med* **332**: 1052–7.

81. Kripke ML, Morison WL, Parrish JA. (1983) Systemic suppression of contact hypersensitivity in mice by psoralen plus UVA radiation (PUVA). *J Invest Dermatol* **81**: 87–92.

82. Laraque D. (1989) Severe anogenital warts in a child with HIV infection. *New Engl J Med* **320**: 1220–1.

83. Leigh IM, Buchanan JAG, Harwood CA, Cerio R, Storey A. (1999) Role of human papillomaviruses in cutaneous and oral manifestations of immunosuppression. *J AIDS* **21** (Suppl. 1) : S49–S57.

84. Leigh IM, Glover MT. (1995) Cutaneous warts and tumours in immunosuppressed patients. *J R Soc Med* **88**: 61–2.

85. Lobo DV, Chu P, Grekin RC, Berger TG. (1992) Non melanoma skin cancers and infection with the human immunodeficiency virus. *Arch Dermatol* **128**: 623–7.

86. London NJ, Farmery SM, Will EJ, Davison AM, Lodge JPA. (1995) Risk of neoplasia in renal transplant patients. *Lancet* **346**: 403–6.

87. Lookingbill DP, Kreider JW, Howett MK, Olmstead PM, Conner GH. (1987) Human papillomavirus type 16 in bowenoid papulosis, intraoral papillomas, and squamous cell carcinoma of the tongue. *Arch Dermatol* **123**: 363–8.

88. Lutzner M, Croissant O, Ducass M-F, Kreiss H, Crosnier J, Orth G. (1980) A potentially oncogenic human papillomavirus (HPV-5) found in two renal allograft recipients. *J Invest Dermatol* **75**: 353–6.

89. Lutzner MA, Orth G, Dutronquay V, Ducasse MF, Kreis H, Crosnier J. (1983) Detection of human papillomavirus type 5 DNA in skin cancer of an immunosuppressed renal allograft recipient. *Lancet* **ii**: 422–4.

90. Maiman M, Fruchter RG, Serur E, Levine PA, Arrastia CD, Sedlis A. (1993) Recurrent cervical intraepithelial neoplasia in human immunodeficiency virus-serposi-tive women. *Obstet Gynecol* **82**: 170–4.

91. Maiman M, Fruchter RG, Serur E, Remy JC, Feuer G, Boyce J. (1990) Human immunodeficiency virus and cervical neoplasia. *Gynecol Oncol* **38**: 377–82.

92. Maiman M, Tarricone N, Vieira J, Suarez J, Serur E, Boyce J. (1991) Colposcopic evaluation of human immunodeficiency virus-seropositive women. *Obstet Gynecol* **78**: 84–8.

93. Majewski S, Jablonska S. (1995) Epidermodysplasia verruciformis as a model of human papillomavirus-induced genetic cancer of the skin. *Arch Dermatol* **131**: 1312–18.

94. Maurer TA, Vin Christian K, Kerschmann RL, *et al.* (1997) Cutaneous squamous cell carcinoma in human immunodeficiency virus-infected patients. A study of epidemiologic risk factors, human papillomavirus, and p53 expression. *Arch Dermatol* **133**: 577–83.

95. McGregor JM, Farthing A, Crook T, *et al* (1994) Post-transplant skin cancer: a possible role for p53 gene mutation but not for oncogenic human papillomaviruses. *J Am Acad Dermatol* **30**: 701–6.

96. McGregor JM, Proby CM. (1996) The role of papillomaviruses in human non-melanoma skin cancer. In *Cancer Surveys; Vol. 26 Skin cancer*, eds IM Leigh, JA Newton Bishop, ML Kripke. Plainview, NY, Cold Spring Harbour Laboratory Press, 219–36.

97. McGregor JM, Proby CM, Leigh IM. (1996) Virus infection and cancer risk in transplant recipients. *Trends Microbiol* **4**: 2–3.

98. Milburn PB, Brandsma JL, Goldsman CI, Teplitz ED, Heilman EI. (1988) Disseminated warts and evolving squamous cell carcinoma in a patient with acquired immuno- deficiency syndrome. *J Am Acad Dermatol* **19**: 401–5.

99. Misbah SA, Spickett GP, Zeman A, *et al.* (1992) Progressive multifocal leucoencephalopathy, sclerosing cholangitis, bronchiectasis and disseminated warts in a patient with primary combined immune deficiency. *J Clin Path* **45**: 624–7.

100. Mohanty KC, Roy RB. (1984) Thymus derived lymphocyte (T-cells) in patients with genital warts. *Br J Vener Dis* **60**: 186–8.

101. Morison WL. (1975) Cell-mediated immune responses in patients with warts. *Br J Dermatol* **93**: 553–6.

102. Morison WL. (1975) Survey of viral warts, herpes

zoster and herpes simplex in patients with secondary immune deficiencies and neoplasms. *Br J Dermatol* **93**: 8–19.

103. Morrison EA, Dole P, Sun XW, Stern L, Wright TC. (1996) Low prevalence of human papillomavirus infection of the cervix in renal transplant recipients. *Nephrol Dial Transplant* **11**: 1603–6.

104. Nataraj AJ, Wolf P, Cerroni L, Ananthaswarmy HN. (1997) p53 mutation in squamous cell carcinomas from psoriasis patients treated with psoralen + UVA (PUVA). *J Invest Dermatol* **109**: 238–43.

105. Obalek S, Favre M, Jablonska S, Szymanczyk J, Orth G. (1988) Human papillomavirus type 2-associated basal cell carcinoma in two immunosuppressed patients. *Arch Dermatol* **124**: 930–4.

106. Obalek S, Favre M, Szymanczyk J, Misiewicz, Jablonska S, Orth G. (1992) Human papillomavirus types specific of epidermodysplasia verruciformis detected in warts induced by HPV 3 or HPV 3-related types in immunosuppressed patients. *J Invest Dermatol* **98**: 936–41.

107. Obalek S, Glinski W, Haftek M, Orth G, Jablonska S. (1980) Comparative studies on cell-mediated immunity in patients with different warts. *Dermatologica* **161**: 73–83.

108. Ogunbiyi OA, Scholefield JH, Raftery AT, *et al.* (1994) Prevalence of anal human papillomavirus infection and intraepithelial neoplasia in renal allograft recipients. *Br J Surg* **81**: 365–7.

109. Orth G. (1986) Epidermodysplasia verruciformis: a model for understanding the oncogenicity of human papillomaviruses. *Ciba Found Symp* **120**: 157–74.

110. Ostrow RS, Manias D, Mitchell AJ, Stawowy, Faras AJ. (1987) Epidermodysplasia verruciformis: a case associated with primary lymphatic dysplasia, depressed cell-mediated immunity, and Bowen's disease containing human papillomavirus 16 DNA. *Arch Dermatol* **123**: 1511–16.

111. Ozsaran AA, Ates T, Dikmen Y, *et al.* (1999) Evaluation of the risk of cervical intraepithelial neoplasia and human papillomavirus infection in renal transplant patients receiving immunosuppressive therapy. *Eur J Gynaecol Oncol* **20**: 127–30.

112. Palefsky JM. (1997) Cutaneous and genital HPV-associated lesions in HIV-infected patients. *Clin Dermatol* **15**: 439–47.

113. Palefsky JM, Gonzales J, Greenblatt RM, Ahn DK, Hollander H. (1990) Anal intraepithelial neoplasia and anal papillomavirus infection among homosexual males with group IV HIV disease. *JAMA* **263**: 2911–16.

114. Palefsky JM, Holly EA, Ralston ML, *et al.* (1998) Anal squamous intraepithelial lesions in HIV positive and HIV negative homosexual and bisexual men: prevalence and risk factors. *J AIDS Hum Retrovirol* **17**: 320–6.

115. Payne D, Newman C, Tyring S. (1995) Human papillomavirus DNA in nonanogenital keratoacanthoma and squamous cell carcinoma of patients with HIV infection. *J Am Acad Dermatol* **33**: 1047–9.

116. Penn I. (1986) Cancers of the anogenital region in renal transplant recipients: analysis of 65 cases. *Cancer* **58**: 611–16.

117. Penneys NS. (1995) Cutaneous viral disease in AIDS. In *Skin manifestations of AIDS*, 2nd edn, ed. NS Penneys. London, Martin Dunitz. 84–91.

118. Perry TL, Marman JL. (1974) Warts in disease with immune defects. *Cutis* **13**: 359–62.

119. Petry KU, Kochel H, Bode U, *et al.* (1996) Human papillomavirus is associated with the frequent detection of warty and basaloid high-grade neoplasia of the vulva and cervical neoplasia among immunocompromised women. *Gynecol Oncol* **60**: 30–4.

120. Petry KU, Scheffel D, Bode U, *et al.* (1994) Cellular immunodeficiency enhances the progression of human papillomavirus-associated cervical lesions. *Int J Cancer* **57**: 836–40.

121. Pouteil-Noble C. (1998) Immunosuppressive treatments. In *Skin diseases after organ transplantation*, eds S Euvrard, J Kanitakis, A Claudy. Montrouge, France, Eurotext, 17–28.

122. Price M, Tidman M, Fagg N, Palmer T, MacDonald D. (1987) Distinctive epidermal atypia in immunosuppression-associated cutaneous malignancy. *Histopathology* **13**: 89–94.

123. Proby C, Storey A, McGregor J, Leigh I. (1996) Does human papillomavirus infection play a role in non-melanoma skin cancer? *Papillomavirus Rep* **7**: 53–60.

124. Prose NS, von Knebel-Doeberitz C, Miller S, Milburn PB, Heilman E. (1990) Widespread flat warts associated with human papillomavirus type 5: a cutaneous manifestation of human immunodeficiency virus infection. *J Am Acad Dermatol* **23**: 978–81.

125. Purdie KJ, Pennington J, Proby CM, *et al.* (2000) The promoter of a novel human papillomavirus (HPV-77) associated with skin cancer displays UV responsiveness which is mediated through a consensus p53 binding sequence. *EMBO* **18**: 5359–69.

126. Purdie KJ, Sexton CJ, Proby CM, *et al.* (1993) Malignant transformation of cutaneous lesions in renal allograft patients: a role for human papillomavirus. *Cancer Res* **53**: 5328–33.

127. Ramoz N, Rueda L-A, Montoya L-S, Bouadjar B, Favre M, Orth G. (1999) A susceptibility locus for epidermodysplasia verruciformis, an abnormal predisposition to infection with the oncogenic human papillomavirus type 5, maps to chromosome 17qter in a region containing a psoriasis susceptibility locus. *J Invest Dermatol* **112**: 259–63.

128. Ramoz N, Taïeb A, Rueda LA, Bouadjar B, Favre M, Orth G. (2000) Evidence for a nonallelic heterogeneity of epidermodysplasia verruciformis with two susceptibility loci mapped to chromosome regions 2p21-p24 and 17q25. *J Invest Dermatol* **114**: 1148–53.

129. Regezi JA, Greenspan D, Greenspan JS, Wong E, Macphail LA. (1994) HPV-associated epithelial atypia in oral warts in HIV positive patients. *J Cutan Pathol* **21**: 217–23.

130. Reid TMS, Fraser NG, Kernohan IR. (1976) Generalized warts and immune deficiency. *Br J Dermatol* **95**: 559–64.

131. Rook AH, Jaworsky C, Nguyen T, *et al.* (1995) Beneficial effect of low-dose systemic retinoid in

combination with topical tretinoin for the treatement and prophylaxis of premalignant and malignant skin lesions in renal transplant recipients. *Transplantation* **59**: 714–19.

132. Ross IN, Chesner I, Thompson RA, Parker RG, Asquith P. (1982) Cutaneous viral infection as a presentation of intestinal lymphangiectasia. *Br J Dermatol* **107**: 357–64.

133. Rubben A, Baron JM, Grussendorf-Conen E-I. (1996) Demonstration of human papillomavirus type 16-related DNA and absence of detectable p53 gene mutations in widespread cutaneous squamous cell carcinomas after oral psoralen with UV-A treatment. *Arch Dermatol* **132**: 1257–9.

134. Rudlinger R, Bunney MH, Smith IW, Hunter JAA. (1988) Detection of human papillomavirus type 5 DNA in a renal allograft patient from Scotland. *Dermatologica* **177**: 280–6.

135. Rudlinger R, Grob R. (1989) Papillomavirus infection and skin cancer in renal allograft recipients. *Lancet* **1**: 1132–3.

136. Rudlinger R, Grob R, Buchmann P, Christen D, Steiner R. (1988) Anogenital warts of the condyloma acuminatum type in HIV-positive patients. *Dermatologica* **176**: 277–81.

137. Rudlinger R, Smith IW, Bunney MH, Hunter JA. (1986) Human papillomavirus infections in a group of renal transplant recipients. *Br J Dermatol* **115**: 681–92.

138. Schulz TF, Boshoff CH, Weiss, RA. (1996) HIV infection and neoplasia. *Lancet* **348**: 587–91.

139. Sexually transmitted diseases treatment guidelines. (1993) *MMWR* **42** (No. RR-14): 90–1.

140. Shamanin V, Delius H, de Villiers E-M. (1994) Development of a broad spectrum PCR assay for papillomaviruses and its application in screening lung cancer biopsies. *J Gen Virol* **75**: 1149–56.

141. Shamanin V, Glover M, Rausch C, *et al.* (1994) Specific types of human papillomavirus found in benign proliferations and carcinomas of the skin in immunosuppressed patients. *Cancer Res* **54**: 4610–13.

142. Shamanin V, zur Hausen H, Lavergne D, *et al.* (1996) HPV infections in non-melanoma skin cancers from renal transplant recipients and non-immunosuppressed patients. *J Natl Cancer Inst* **88**: 802–11.

143. Shelley WB, Wood MG. (1981) Transformation of the common wart into squamous cell carcinoma in a patient with primary lymphedema. *Cancer* **48**: 820–4.

144. Shiel A, Flavel S, Disney A, Mathew T. (1985) Cancer development in patients progressing to dialysis and renal transplantation. *Transplant Proc* **17**: 1685–8.

145. Shuttleworth D, Marks R, Griffin PJA, Salaman JR. (1988) Treatment of cutaneous neoplasia with etretinate in renal transplant recipients. *Q J Med* **68**: 717–24.

146. Sillman F, Sentovich S. (1997) Ano-genital neoplasia in renal transplant patients. *Ann Transplant* **2**: 59–66.

147. Sillman F, Stanek A, Sedlis A, *et al.* (1984) The relationship between human papillomavirus and lower genital intraepithelial neoplasia in immunosuppressed women. *Am J Obstet Gynecol* **150**: 300–8.

148. Silverman S, Migliorati CA, Lozada-Nur F, Greenspan D, Conant MA. (1986) Oral findings in people with or

at high risk for AIDS: a study of 375 homosexual males. *J Am Dental Assoc* **112**: 187–92.

149. Six C, Heard I, Bergeron C, *et al.* (1998) Comparative prevalence, incidence and short-term prognosis of cervical squamous intraepithelial lesions amongst HIV-positive and HIV-negative women. *AIDS* **12**: 1047–56.

150. Smith KJ, Skelton HG, Yeager J, Angritt P, Wagner KF. (1993) Cutaneous neoplasms in a military population of HIV-1-positive patients. *J Am Acad Dermatol* **29**: 400–6.

151. Smith SE, Davis IC, Leshin B, Fleischer AB, White WL, Feldmann SR. (1993) Absence of human papillomavirus in squamous cell carcinomas of nongenital skin from immunocompromised renal transplant patients. *Arch Dermatol* **129**: 1585–8.

152. Soler C, Chardonnet Y, Allibert P, Euvrard S, Schmitt D, Mandrand B. (1993) Detection of mucosal human papillomavirus types 6/11 in cutaneous lesions from transplant recipients. *J Invest Dermatol* **101**: 286–91.

153. Soler C, Chardonnet Y, Euvrard S, Chignol MC, Thivolet J. (1992) Evaluation of human papillomavirus type 5 on frozen sections of multiple lesions from transplant recipients with in situ hybridisation and non-isotopic probes. *Dermatology* **184**: 248–53.

154. Stanley MA. (1999) Mechanism of action of Imiquimod. *Papillomavirus Rep* **10**: 23–9.

155. Stark LA, Arends MJ, McLaren KM, *et al.* (1994) Prevalence of human papillomavirus DNA in cutaneous neoplasms from renal allograft recipients supports a possible viral role in tumour promotion. *Br J Cancer* **69**: 222–9.

156. Stark S, Petridis AK, Ghim S-J, *et al.* (1998) Prevalence of antibodies against virus-like particles of Epidermodysplasia Verruciformis-associated HPV8 in patients at risk of skin cancer. *J Invest Dermatol* **111**: 696–701.

157. Stevens DA, Ferrington RA, Merigan TC, Marinkovich VA. (1975). Randomized trial of transfer factor treatment of human warts. *Clin Exp Immunol* **21**: 520–4.

158. Storey A, Thomas M, Kalita A, *et al.* (1998) Role of a p53 polymorphism in the development of human papillomavirus-associated cancer. *Nature* **393**: 229–34.

159. Stritzler C, Sawitzsky A, Stritzler R. (1971) Bittner's syndrome. *Arch Dermatol* **103**: 548–9.

160. Studniberg HM, Weller P. (1993) PUVA, UVB, psoriasis and nonmelanoma skin cancer. *J Am Acad Dermatol* **29**: 1013–22.

161. Sun X-W, Ellerbrock TV, Lungu O, Chaisson MA, Bush TJ, Wright TC. (1995) Human papillomavirus infection in human immunodeficiency virus-seropositive women. *Obstet Gynecol* **85**: 680–6.

162. Sun X-W, Kuhn L, Ellerbrock TV, Chiasson MA, Bush TJ, Wright TC. (1997) Human papillomavirus infection in women infected with the human immunodeficiency virus. *N Engl J Med* **337**: 1343–9.

163. Surentheran T, Harwood CA, Spink PJ, *et al.* (1998) Detection and typing of human papillomaviruses in mucosal and cutaneous biopsies from immunosuppressed and immunocompetent patients and patients with epidermodysplasia verruciformis: a unified diagnostic approach. *J Clin Path* **51**: 606–10.

164. Tanigaki T, Kanda R, Sato K. (1986) Epidermodyspla-

sia verruciformis (L-L,1922) in a patient with systemic lupus erythematosus. *Arch Derm Res* **278**: 247–8.

165. Taylor A, Shuster S. (1992) Skin cancer after renal transplantation: the causal role of azathioprine. *Acta Derm Venereol* **72**: 115–19.

166. Tornosello ML, Buonaguro FM, Beth-Giraldo E, Giraldo G. (1993) Human immunodeficiency virus type 1 *tat* gene enhances human papillomavirus early gene expression. *Intervirology* **36**: 57–64.

167. Ullrich SE. (1991) Systemic immunosuppression of cell-mediated immune reactions by a monofunctional psoralen plus ultraviolet A radiation. *Photodermatol Photoimmunol Photomed* **8**: 116–22.

168. Valle S-L. (1987) Dermatologic findings related to human immunodeficiency virus infection in high-risk individuals. *J Am Acad Dermatol* **17**: 951–61.

169. Van der Leest RJ, Zachow KR, Ostrow RS, Bender M, Pass F, Faras AJ. (1987) Human papillomavirus heterogeneity in 36 renal transplant recipients. *Arch Dermatol* **123**: 354–7.

170. Vernon, SD, Hart CE, WC, Icenogle JP. (1993) The HIV-tat protein enhances E2-dependent human papillomavirus 16 transcription. *Virus Res* **27**: 133–45.

171. Viraben R, Aquilina C, Brousset P, Bazex J. (1996) Focal epithelial hyperplasia (Heck disease) associated with AIDS. *Dermatology* **193**: 261–2.

172. Volter C, He Y, Delius H, *et al.* (1996) Novel HPV types present in oral papillomatous lesions from patients with HIV infection. *Int J Cancer* **66**: 453–6.

173. Waddell KM, Lewallen S, Lucas SB, Atenyi-Agaba C, Herrington CS, Liomba G. (1996) Carcinoma of the conjunctiva and human immunodeficiency virus infection in Uganda and Malawi. *Br J Ophthalmol* **80**: 503–8.

174. Walder BK, Robertson MR, Jeremy D. (1971) Skin cancer and immunosuppression. *Lancet* **ii**: 1282–3.

175. Ward M, LeRoux A, Small WP, Sircus W. (1977) Malig-

nant lymphoma and extensive viral wart formation in a patient with intestinal lymphangiectasia and lymphocyte depletion. *Postgrad Med J* **53**: 753

176. Weinstock MA, Coulter S, Bates J, Bogaars HA, Larson PI, Burmer GC. (1995) Human papillomavirus and widespread cutaneous carcinoma after PUVA photochemotherapy. *Arch Dermatol* **131**: 701–4.

177. Weissenborn SJ, Höpfl R, Weber F, Smola H, Pfister HJ, Fuchs PG. (1999) High prevalence of a variety of epidermodysplasia verruciformis-associated human papillomaviruses in psoriatic skin of patients treated or not treated with PUVA. *J Invest Dermatol* **113**: 122–6.

178. Williams AB, Darragh TM, Vranizan K, Ochia C, Moss AR, Palefsky JM. (1994) Anal and cervical human papillomavirus infection and risk of anal and cervical epithelial abnormalities in human immunodeficiency virus-infected women. *Obstet Gynecol* **83**: 205–11.

179. Wright TC, Ellerbrock RV, Chiasson MA, Sun X-W, Van Devanter N. (1994) The New York Cervical Disease Study: CIN in women infected with HIV: prevalence, risk factor, and validity of Papanicolaou smears. *Obstet Gynecol* **84**: 591–7.

180. Wright TC, Koulos J, Schnoll F, *et al.* (1994) Cervical intraepithelial neoplasia in women infected with the human immunodeficiency virus: outcome after loop electrosurgical excision. *Gynecol Oncol* **55**: 253–8.

181. Yell JA, Burge SM. (1993) Warts and lupus erythematosus. *Lupus* **2**: 21–3.

182. Young AR. (1990) Photocarcinogenicity of psoralens used in PUVA treatment: present status in mouse and man. *J Photochem Photobiol B: Biol* **6**: 237–47.

183. Zaia JA. (1990) Viral infections associated with bone marrow transplantation. *Hematol Oncol Clin N Am* **4**: 603–23.

184. Zinn K-H, Belohradsky BH. (1977) Wiskott–Aldrich–Syndrom mit verrucae vulgares. *Hautartz* **28**: 664–7.

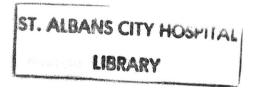

Part IV

Future prospects: treatment and basic research

11

Antivirals

Isobel Greenfield and Scott Cuthill

11.1 INTRODUCTION

Human papillomaviruses (HPVs) are associated with a spectrum of epithelial proliferative disorders in humans such as common cutaneous and anogenital warts and cervical dysplasia which can progress to carcinoma. It is estimated that about 1% of the sexually active population have overt anogenital warts and this is anticipated only to be the 'tip of the iceberg' of genital HPV infection.[53]

Although the incidence of HPV infections is extremely high and advances have been made with the diagnosis of these infections, progress with the development of therapeutic agents has not been significant, due mainly to the difficulty in studying the biology and life cycle of these viruses. There is no readily available *in vitro* assay to propagate HPV, which requires terminally differentiating epithelial cells for full virus maturation to occur. HPVs encode only eight proteins, six of which are non-structural (early) proteins, namely E1, E2, E4, E5, E6, and E7, and two are structural (late) proteins, L1 and L2. Details of the biological functions of each of these proteins can be found elsewhere in this volume but, briefly, the early proteins are involved with viral replication and induction of cellular proliferation, whereas the late proteins are capsid proteins (for review, see reference 69). As described below, with the exception of the E1 protein, all the HPV proteins perform their functions via macromolecular interactions within infected cells, making antiviral strategies difficult to design. This review concentrates chiefly on current and future therapies for anogenital papillomavirus infections; lesions at other anatomical sites are referred to where relevant.

Spontaneous regression of warts occurs in some patients, whereas in others untreated lesions frequently increase in size and may spread to other anatomical sites.[66] Persistent lesions can cause the patient physical discomfort and emotional trauma. An ideal therapy would result in the resolution of symptoms and in elimination of the virus from the host, preventing the recurrence of lesions. Treatment should also be economical, rapid, and painless. Unfortunately, advances in therapeutic approaches have not been dramatic and most current therapies are non-specific, fairly crude, and largely inadequate; none eliminates the virus from the host. Generally speaking, the type of therapy used is determined by the anatomical site of the infection, the type of virus involved (low or high-risk) and the patient's therapeutic history. Commonly used therapeutic agents target macroscopically visible lesions and fall into three broad categories: cytotoxic agents, physically ablative therapies, and immunomodulators. There is no therapy for latent or subclinical infections.[85]

11.2 CURRENT THERAPIES

11.2.1 Cytotoxic Agents

These agents are topically applied and kill cells on contact, regardless of HPV status, by antiproliferative or chemodestructive mechanisms of action. Cytotoxic agents may be patient administered and show variable efficacy (Table 11.1). Adverse local reactions can be fairly severe and recurrence rates are high (Table 11.1). These are generally the cheapest and most convenient therapeutic approaches as clinic visits

Table 11.1

Clearance and recurrence rates for current therapies for external genital warts

Treatment	Clearance rates (%)	Recurrence rates (%)
Podophyllotoxin	42–88	10–91
Podophyllin	22–79	11–74
TCA	50–81	36
5-FU	10–97	0–13
LEEP	72–90	51
Cryotherapy	63–96	0–39
Surgical excision	89–93	0–29
Laser therapy	27–97	7–45
IFNα, intralesional	19–63	0–33
Imiquimod	53	13

Data taken from references 8 and 10.

are kept to a minimum; however, it may take some time (weeks) for lesions to resolve. Cytotoxic agents are primarily used on visible, accessible, low-grade anogenital lesions.[85]

Podophyllin/Podophyllotoxin

Since the 1940s, the most commonly used treatment for genital warts has been the topical application of podophyllin, a crude mixture of cytotoxic materials from the root of the May apple plant (*Podophyllum hexandrum Royle)* or from *P. peltatum*.[48] One of the major problems associated with this agent is that it is not pure, nor is it standardized. It contains a number of active components – lignans (alpha-peltatin and beta-peltatin and 4-dimethylpodophyllotoxin) as well as carcinogenic flavenoids (quercitin and kaempherol). The standard formulation, a 20–25% solution in an alcohol solvent, contains 2–10% podophyllotoxin and 0.5–2.5% of other active components. The pharmacological effect of this agent occurs via binding of lignans to intracellular micrototubule proteins, leading to the arrest of cell division in metaphase. This results in localized tissue necrosis and, over a number of weeks, the warty lesion sloughs off. Systemic and local adverse reactions, including ulceration and severe irritation, may occur. Consequently, podophyllin is only applied in the clinic and is not used during pregnancy. Clearance rates vary from 22 to 79%, but recurrence may be as high as 74% (Table 11.1).[8,10,64,94]

To decrease the number and severity of adverse tissue reactions, to minimize the drug dose, and to increase efficacy, von Krogh formulated the concept of a standardized pharmacologically stable solution of 0.5% podophyllotoxin in ethanol or cream as a therapeutic agent. This new formulation eliminated the variability and lack of stability associated with podophyllin. In the clinic, efficacy of podophyllotoxin is at least as good as that seen with podophyllin,[51] and some studies suggest that it is more effective and results in faster resolution than podophyllin.[24,61] Due to an enhanced safety profile, podophyllotoxin is self-administered, which dramatically reduces the cost of therapy as fewer clinic visits are required.[51] However, recurrence rates are high with both preparations (Table 11.1).

Trichloroacetic acid

Trichloroacetic acid (TCA) is a caustic agent which is applied weekly by a practitioner to anogenital lesions as an 80–90%

solution. The acid causes chemical coagulation of lesions, which slough off with time. TCA may be used during pregnancy as there is no systemic toxicity, although its use may be painful, with ulceration, scarring, and secondary infections occurring in rare cases. TCA is effective, and less harmful in mucous membrane lesions as the acid is neutralized by epithelial moisture.[59] As with most cytotoxic therapies, recurrences may be frequent (Table 11.1).[36]

5-Fluorouracil

5-Fluorouracil (5-FU) has been used as a therapeutic agent for HPV lesions but is not approved for this indication in the USA. It inhibits cell growth via inhibition of the thymidine salvage pathway by blocking the transport of extracellular thymidine. It has also been shown to be immunostimulatory and elicits local sensitivity.[19,75] Treatment with 5% 5-FU cream may be effective in refractory disease, either alone or in combination with surgical removal of the lesion. It has been effective in cases of multiple, small, non-keratinizing lesions and in vaginal condylomas and vaginal intraepithelial neoplasias.[55] Although it has been proven to be efficacious in the treatment of genital warts, with low recurrence rates (Table 11.1), it is highly irritant, with some patients unable to tolerate therapy.[54] 5-FU is a known teratogen and its use is contraindicated during pregnancy.

Cantharidin

Cantharidin is a chemical extract from the blister beetle which acts as a mitochondrial poison to cause acantholysis and cell death. When applied to the skin, suprabasal blistering occurs, and care has to be taken to apply it only to visible warts. Cantharidin is used only for the treatment of cutaneous warts and is often given in combination with podophyllin and salicylic acid.[76] Salicylic acid softens the affected skin, podophyllin kills the wart cells, and cantharidin causes blistering which helps removal of the wart. Extensive blistering can result, but this heals rapidly. Multiple treatments may be necessary.

Cytotoxic agents: summary

The use of cytotoxic agents in the treatment of warts is common-place; however, these therapies are not without side-effects, are associated with high recurrence rates, and in many cases require application by a physician. Importantly, these approaches are not antiviral and do not address the underlying HPV infection. In future, more specific therapies will replace cytotoxic agents as first-line therapies for genital warts and other HPV diseases.

11.2.2 Ablative therapies

Surgical excision

Anogenital warts are effectively eliminated by surgical excision. They may be removed individually and accurately without damaging underlying tissue; bleeding is easily dealt with.[37,45] Disease recurrence occurs in about 20% of patients after surgical treatment, a lower frequency than in those treated with podophyllin.[45,50] This approach is effective if disease is limited and the lesions are isolated. The major drawback is one of cost, which includes physician's time, anesthesia, and operating theater visits.

Electrosurgery

Electrosurgical techniques are widely used in the treatment of anogenital lesions such as cervical intraepithelial neoplasia (CIN), vulval intraepithelial neoplasia (VIN), and genital warts. These methods use high-frequency current to destroy the diseased tissue and include techniques such as electrodesiccation, electrocautery, and loop electrosurgical excisional procedure (LEEP). LEEP has become the electrosurgical method of choice as it can be used to electroexcise most lesions irrespective of grade, size, or distribution.[31] LEEP involves the excision of the diseased tissue and marginal surrounding tissue with a thin electrical wire loop under local anesthetic, although general anesthesia may be required in some circumstances.[99] In general, loops are used which remove tissue to a depth of 6–7mm, limiting the amount of tissue removed and the incidence of postoperative bleeding. Success rates are typically around 70% for LEEP and recurrence rates have been reported to be relatively low (Table 11.1).[29]

Cryotherapy

Cryotherapy using liquid nitrogen sprayed directly on to lesions or via a cryoprobe is a common treatment for genital and cutaneous warts, especially where the disease is not extensive. Cryotherapy freezes the wart and leads to tissue destruction, and the size and thickness of the lesion determine the number of treatments required for resolution. However, most lesions resolve after fewer than three treatments. Side-effects include pain, discomfort, edema, necrosis, ulceration, and blister formation. Cryotherapy has been used for a number of years and has been shown to be more effective than podophyllin in treating lesions of the outer genitalia.[21,34]

Laser therapy

Carbon dioxide laser therapy is widely used, with high success rates for the treatment of genital warts, although recurrence rates are highly variable (Table 11.1).[6,12,28] Targeted tissue is destroyed by immediate vaporization and delayed necrosis, but, because the laser can be used with a high degree of precision, surrounding normal tissue is not harmed. Care has to be taken to avoid exposure to the smoke plumes that arise during this procedure as they have been shown to contain HPV.[30] Side-effects may result from thermal damage and include pain, itching, and swelling, but these are less of an issue in the hands of a skilled operator. The procedure is expensive and local or general anesthesia is required.

Ablative therapies: summary

Physically ablative therapies are often highly effective in clearing genital warts, but recurrence rates are also often high as only the visible lesion is removed, and in many cases the viral infection remains. These procedures often require specialist equipment and skilled operators, making them expensive. They are often painful and some form of anesthesia is usually required. Current Center for Disease Control (CDC) guidelines suggest that patients are given a self-applied therapy (podophyllotoxin or imiquimod, see below) as a first-line therapy, which, if unsuccessful, is followed by a surgical or other physician-administered therapy. A safe and effective antiviral agent would replace the need for expensive surgical techniques for the treatment of genital HPV disease.

11.2.3 Light therapies

Photodynamic therapy

The combination of light and chemicals to treat skin diseases is widely accepted. Recently, photodynamic therapy (PDT) has emerged as a promising modality for the management of various tumors and non-malignant diseases. Its mode of action is by activation of a photosensitizer by light, resulting in the generation of highly reactive intermediate oxygen radicals which lead to tissue destruction. The most commonly used photosensitizer is dihematoporphrynether (DHE) administered intravenously 48–72 hours before therapy. The drug exhibits no systemic toxicity apart from generalized photosensitivity for 4–8 weeks after treatment.[56] The only commercially available pharmacological photosensitizing agent is Photofrin, which has been used off-label to treat dermatological disease. This agent is given intravenously and produces longlasting cutaneous photosensitivity. PDT is a novel approach for the treatment of HPV disease and is particularly appropriate for accessible lesions such as laryngeal papillomas, CIN, VIN, or condyloma.

Shikowitz and colleagues[77] have used PDT to treat recurrent respiratory papillomatosis (RRP) for a number of years. A randomized prospective study involving 81 patients was undertaken to compare the efficacy of PDT with DHE and traditional therapy. Patients receiving DHE experienced a significantly larger decrease in the rate of papilloma growth compared to conventional therapy. A 3-year follow-up of a subset of patients confirmed that this improvement was maintained.

Dermatological procedures generally involve topical application of a photosensitizer, usually a precursor of aminolevulinic acid (ALA). However, other porphyric derivatives, phthalocyanines, chlorins, and porphycenes, are being studied. The goal of such research is to find compounds that are selective, have shorter half-lives, are non-carcinogenic, react to visible light, and do not damage the healthy epidermis. Topical application of ALA in concentrations of 0.05–0.2 g cm^{-2} avoids detectable systemic effects and excitation (at 695 nm) is usually achieved with an argon or gold vapor laser. Wierrani and colleagues[98] conducted a study of the efficacy of PDT with ALA in 20 patients with CIN 2 and 3. 5-ALA (12% w/v) was applied topically via a cervical cap 8 hours before exposure to light. Preliminary results of follow-up visits at 1, 3, 6, and 9 months post-therapy showed a cytological improvement in the grading of the Pap smears in 19/20 patients (95%) and the eradication of cervical HPV in 80%. These data show that PDT may be used as an effective therapy for ectocervical dysplasia.

Hillemanns and colleagues[42] investigated the clinical response to PDT with 5-ALA in patients with VIN. Twenty-five patients with 111 lesions of VIN 1–3 were topically sensitized with 10 ml of a 20% solution of 5-ALA and treated with 57 cycles of laser light. Seventy (63%) of the 111 VIN lesions regressed after PDT. A complete response was achieved in 13 patients (52%) with 27 lesions. All patients with VIN 1 and monofocal and bifocal VIN 2–3 showed complete clearance. However, a complete response could be achieved in only 4 (27%) of 15 women with multifocal VIN

2–3. These data show that PDT with 5-ALA has promise as an alternative treatment modality for VIN. It is easy to perform and has the advantage of minimal tissue destruction, low side-effects, and excellent cosmetic results. However, multifocal VIN disease with pigmented and hyperkeratotic lesions remains difficult to treat.

Photochemotherapy

Photochemotherapy involves treatment with a photosensitizing chemical followed by electromagnetic non-ionizing radiation. The most commonly used form of photochemotherapy is the combination therapy of the photosensitizing agent 8-methoxypsoralen (8-MOP) and subsequent exposure to a source of high-intensity UVA radiation (PUVA). This therapeutic approach is widely used in dermatology with some adaptations such as the psoralen or UV source used, the dose, and the number of treatments given.[56] Recent studies have been directed at trying to optimize the efficacy of PUVA while minimizing acute side-effects and the risk of cutaneous carcinogenesis, believed to be independently related to the cumulative dose of UVA and the total number of treatments.

Photochemotherapy with 8-MOP and modest doses of UVA have been shown to stimulate T-helper (Th1) cytokine production such as interferon-gamma (IFNγ) from T-lymphocytes.[88] Whilst this approach has not been approved for the treatment of HPV infection, several studies have shown that spontaneously regressing warts do so via a CD4+ T-cell-mediated event which is consistent with a Th1 immune response.[18,32] Because photochemotherapy with 8-MOP is thought to induce apoptosis and a Th1 immune response, there is a good rationale for its use as a potential treatment of HPV disease.

Phototherapy

Phototherapy is the therapeutic use of exposure to non-ionizing radiation. It may arise as a result of exposure to natural light, UVA or UVB radiation, or a combination of all three. The inhibitory effect of UV radiation on DNA synthesis may be one of the mechanisms of action that is effective in the treatment of proliferating skin diseases. In addition, phototherapy alters cytokine profiles, changes the cytotoxic inmmune response in the skin, and kills diseased cells by apoptosis (programmed cell death).[35]

Light therapies: summary

The data presented here show that PDT, in particular, is an exciting new treatment modality that is effective for the treatment of HPV disease. However, the present arsenal of photosensitive molecules is limited as is clinical data on their use in the treatment of HPV infections. Future research could focus on the generation of clinical data with currently available agents, the discovery and development of molecules with increased specificity, shorter half-lives, and the ability to be activated by a desired wavelength of light.

11.2.4 Immunomodulators

The immune system plays an important role in clearing HPV infection and, generally speaking, disease occurs when immunosurveillance fails. HPVs employ a number of strategies to bypass immunosurveillance, so it seems rational that an agent that stimulates the immune system and, in particular, the response to HPV may be an effective agent for the treatment of HPV disease. Further evidence to support this statement has come from the observation that the incidence of infection and progression to malignancy of HPV-associated lesions are increased in immunocompromised individuals.[46,62,71] Also, histopathological studies in spontaneously regressing genital warts strongly indicate that regression involves a Th1 cell-mediated immune response.[18,32]

Interferon

The use of IFNs has been an attractive therapeutic approach for genital wart therapy because of their immunostimulatory and antiproliferative activities. Only IFNα has been approved for genital wart therapy and is usually given by direct injection into warts or by topical application. Clearance of warts is variable (negligible in the case of topical application) and recurrence rates are in the order of 30% (Table 11.1).[8] Intralesional injection is often very painful and is commonly associated with side-effects such as flu-like symptoms, but it allows maximal drug delivery to the site of infection. IFN therapy is expensive and requires frequent physician visits for multiple local injections (See Table 11.1).[8,97] Current indications for IFNs in papillomavirus infections include recalcitrant genital and cutaneous warts refractory to other treatments, disseminated disease recurring after conventional therapy, and extensive disease where conventional therapy is not practical. Trials of IFN therapy in anogenital lesions have been carried out with systemic delivery, intralesion injection, and topical application.[86] Topical administration of IFN in a gel formulation is attractive as it minimizes adverse effects and systemic toxicity.

Systemic IFN is administered subcutaneously or intramuscularly. Variable efficacy in the treatment of recurrent or refractory warts has been observed. Response rates vary from 0% to 71% and recurrence rates are high.[95] Further studies are required to determine optimum dosing regimes for maximal efficacy. IFN may be more effective if used in combination with an antiviral agent. Improvements have been made in the formulation and preparation of IFN. The most successful of these is pegylated IFNα, which is a chemically modified form of IFNα in which a polyethylene glycol moiety has been covalently attached to the parent molecule. It is more stable and efficacious than current forms of IFN and may lead to improvements in the efficacy of IFN therapy of genital warts.

The data generated on the response to IFN therapy are variable. This may be due to the fact that HPV 16 E7 has been shown to inhibit the induction of IFNα-inducible genes. Expression of E7 correlates with the loss of formation of the IFN-stimulated transcription complex. This may provide a means by which HPV can avoid the innate immune system.[7] Recently, Chang and colleagues used a microarray analysis to examine the global changes in gene expression induced by high-risk HPV 31. The basal level of expression of several IFN-responsive genes was found to be down-regulated in HPV 31 cells.[14] When cells were treated with IFNα or IFNγ, expression of IFN-inducible genes was impaired. At high doses of IFN, the effects were less pronounced. Among the genes repressed by HPV 31 was the signal transducer and activator of transcription, which plays a major role in mediating the IFN response. Thus, it would seem logical that any therapeutic approach that could overcome these blocks to the IFN response pathway may stimulate the host immune defenses against HPV and facilitate elimination of the virus.[14]

In addition to impairment of the IFN response pathway, HPV seems to abrogate antigen presentation by down-regulation of the transporter associated with antigen presentation (TAP-1). In laryngeal papilloma tissue biopsies and cell culture of primary explants, there was a statistically significant correlation between reduction of TAP-1 expression and rapid recurrence of disease. Data suggest that HPV may evade immune recognition by down-regulating class I major histocompatibility complex (MHC) cell surface expression via decreased TAP-1 levels, and that expression of TAP-1 could be used for prognostic evaluation of disease severity. IFNγ was able to restore class I MHC expression at the surfaces of laryngeal papilloma cells in culture. This up-regulation of class I MHC antigen at the cell surface potentially allows the infected cell to become a target for the immune system again. This finding provides some promise for the non-surgical treatment of laryngeal papillomas.[91]

Imiquimod

The immune response modifier imiquimod was approved first in the USA in 1997 as a self-applied topical cream for the treatment of genital warts. The precise mechanism of action of imiquimod is not known, but there is compelling preclinical and clinical evidence to support its action as a modulator of both innate and cell-mediated immunity due to its ability to induce a variety of cytokines from monocytes and macrophages *in vitro*.[5,63,72] The major cytokines induced are IFNα, interleukin (IL) -1, 6, 8, and 12, and tumor necrosis factor α (TNFα). Imiquimod is believed indirectly to activate T-cells via IFNα and IL-12 which stimulate Th1 cytokine production (IFNγ and IL-2). These cytokine changes are similar to those measured during spontaneous wart regression and are consistent with regression being mediated by a Th1 immune response.[18,32] In addition to Th1 cytokine production, imiquimod has been shown to inhibit Th2 cytokine production, e.g., IL-4 and IL-5. The cytokines produced in imiquimod-treated warts are consistent with this proposed mechanism of action.[5] It remains to be shown if clearance results in the long-term resolution of warts.

Imiquimod is applied as a 5% cream to the wart area three times a week until warts have resolved or for a maximum of 16 weeks. In trials, clearance of warts was shown to be higher in female than in male patients (72% versus 33%) and recurrence rates were reported to be relatively low, although the follow-up period was only 3 months.[25] Therapy is well tolerated but is not without side-effects, which are generally mild and limited to the area of warts. Side-effects include burning (22%), itching (13%), pain (6%), erythema (61%), and erosion (30%).

Cimetidine

Cimetidine is a type 2 histamine receptor (H2) antagonist commonly used for the treatment of gastric ulcers; however, at high doses (40 mg/kg/day) it has also found use in the treatment of common cutaneous warts. The mechanism of action is not proven, but it is believed that cimetidine blocks H2 receptors on suppressor T-cells thus enhancing cell-mediated immune responses.[49] Controlled studies with large

numbers of patients have not been performed with cimetidine and the small studies which have been carried out in a variety of wart types have generated conflicting data.[17] Nevertheless, cimetidine treatment has enjoyed widespread anecdotal success, especially in the treatment of cutaneous warts, with clearance rates as high as 81%.[68] Cimetidine was recently shown to be highly effective in a case of life-threatening recurrent respiratory papillomatosis previously shown to be resistant to other therapies.[40] Clearly, cimetidine is not a first-line therapy for warts and its acceptance as such awaits further trials.

Immunomodulators: summary

Immunomodulators comprise an important approach to the treatment of HPV disease. They show some success as therapeutic agents due to their antiviral activity and, in addition, they may be able to overcome the mechanisms by which HPVs evade the host immune system. Further understanding of the immune response to HPV will enable more effective use and design of immunomodulators in the treatment of this virus. However, immunomodulators may yet show most promise when used in combination with other treatments, for example with an antiviral – this approach has been used in the treatment of hepatitis C virus (HCV).[96]

11.3 FUTURE PROSPECTS

As there is no known agent that eliminates HPV infection, the primary aim of treatment for HPV disease is the removal of the lesion. This relieves symptoms such as pain, itching, and bleeding, and may reduce transmission of the virus. Currently, such an approach is not very successful and, in future, treatment schedules will be designed to remove the visible lesion and eliminate the virus, preventing its transmission and the recurrence of lesions.

11.3.1 Combination therapy

The treatment of human immunodeficiency virus (HIV) has established the approach of using a combination of specific antiviral therapies for the treatment of a viral disease.[93] The use of combination therapy to treat HIV is effective in that the therapies act synergistically, leading to improved efficacy and a reduced incidence of resistance. As specific antiviral agents are not yet available for the treatment of HPV disease, combination therapy with antivirals has not yet been used in the clinic. However, preliminary studies using combinations of different treatment modalities that are currently available for papillomavirus disease have been documented.[13,22] Such approaches have involved the use of an ablative therapy such as surgery to remove the lesion followed by a cytotoxic agent or immunomodulator to prevent recurrence.

Cardamakis and colleagues[13] assessed the effectiveness of carbon dioxide laser (vaporization), 5-FU topical application, and IFNα-2a for the therapy of penile intraepithelial neoplasia (PIN) in 208 patients. The best treatment modalities, irrespective of grade of lesion, were found to be the triple combination of 5-FU plus carbon dioxide laser vaporization plus IFNα-2a (with a response rate of 96.15%). The combination of 5-FU plus carbon dioxide laser vaporization gave a response rate of 87.09% and the combination of carbon dioxide laser vaporization plus IFNα-2a gave a response rate of 80%. It was concluded that IFNα-2a can be used as first-line treatment in combination with 5-FU in patients with PIN 2 and as an adjuvant treatment in patients with recurrent PIN 1 and PIN 3.

Preliminary data obtained from studies on cervical carcinoma cell lines have shown that IFN and retinoic acid may act synergistically to reduce cell proliferation. Whilst this is still early *in vitro* work, it may hold promise in the clinic.[90].

In future, a more targeted approach toward the elimination of HPV disease could combine the use of an antiviral agent with an immunomodulator. The rationale behind such an approach is that the antiviral agent would abrogate HPV replication and the immunomodulator would activate the host immune system to eliminate the virus and prevent recurrence.

11.3.2 Antiviral therapies

HPV Targets

As discussed in the introduction, none of the currently available therapies for HPV disease is directly antiviral in action, resulting in generally high recurrence rates. Traditionally, antiviral therapies target critical viral enzyme functions such as polymerases and proteases;[26] however, HPVs encode only one enzyme, the E1 helicase, which makes traditional antiviral approaches limited. The remaining non-structural HPV-encoded proteins, namely E2, E4, E5, E6, and E7, largely function by macromolecular interactions with host/viral proteins or DNA, which are much less attractive drug targets. Technologies such as yeast-two-hybrid analysis have been and are continuing to be used to identify cellular proteins that interact with HPV proteins and some of these interactions may identify potential therapeutic targets for intervention in HPV disease. Some of the interactions that have been identified for HPV proteins and that may represent antiviral targets are discussed below.

E1 helicase

The 72 kDa E1 protein, as stated above, encodes the only enzymatic function of HPV, making it an attractive antiviral target. E1 is an adenosine triphosphate (ATP) dependent helicase and is the most highly conserved HPV protein, suggesting that an inhibitor will have broad activity against many HPV types, although this remains to be shown. It acts as an initiator of HPV replication by causing unwinding of DNA at the origin of replication (ori).[87] E1 has only a weak affinity for its DNA binding site within the ori and requires the higher affinity binding of E2 to localize it there. Once localized to the ori, the E1 is believed to form hexameric complexes and E2 is released; host cellular replication factors such as DNA polymerase α, DNA primase, proliferating cell nuclear antigen (PCNA), and topoisomerases are then recruited and replication initiated.[87] Disruption of the interactions between E1 and any of these proteins could potentially be achieved by small-molecule inhibitors; however, it remains to be seen how accessible these interactions are to this approach.

E2

The HPV E2 protein, in addition to acting as an anchor for E1 at the ori during the initiation of replication, has been

shown to be a regulator of HPV transcription. The 50 kDa E2 protein homodimerizes and interacts with a palindromic DNA element found in multiple copies within the non-coding regions of HPV genomes. Given the central role of E2 in the control of HPV replication and transcription, E2 is an attractive antiviral target. Indeed, small-molecule inhibitors of E2 binding to DNA have been identified,[39] although it remains to be seen if such a molecule will inhibit HPV replication or can be developed to have drug-like characteristics.

E6

The E6 proteins of high-risk mucosal HPV types, such as HPV 16 and 18, in particular, have been intensively studied and have been shown to cooperate with high-risk E7 proteins to transform primary human cells.[41] The best-characterized activity of E6 is its ability to interact with the tumor suppressor protein p53 and to cause its degradation via ubiquitin-dependent proteolysis.[74] However, the E6 proteins of several other HPVs have been reported either not to interact with p53 or, as with HPV 6 and 11 E6, to bind only weakly.[74] This suggests that p53-mediated degradation is not a generic function of E6 and indeed may be of significance only for high-risk virus types. Yeast-two-hybrid studies with E6 proteins have identified host proteins which interact with E6 and which could potentially be therapeutic targets (Table 11.2),[69] although E6-protein interactions have yet to be identified for HPV 6 and 11 E6 proteins. The significance of these macromolecular interactions to the completion of the HPV life cycle remains to be elucidated, and the design of small-molecule inhibitors which disrupt these interactions is likely to be much more difficult than that of traditional enzyme inhibitors. However, inhibitors of pathways downstream of the E6 interaction may be more tractable drug targets.

E7

The E7 protein of high-risk HPV types is a small nuclear phosphoprotein which can immortalize primary human cells in cooperation with E6.[41] Similar to E6, E7 has been shown to interact with a number of host cellular proteins (Table 11.3), the best characterized of which is its interaction with the retinoblastoma family of proteins (pRb). pRb is a critical regulator of cell-cycle progression at the G1/S boundary, and disruption by E7 leads to loss of control of proliferation and expression of enzymes that are required for replication and HPV DNA synthesis.[52] As with E6, the inhibition of the E7–protein interactions described in Table 11.3 is a theoretical inhibition of therapeutic option for HPV disease. Once again, however, such an approach is less attractive than inhibition of viral enzymes because a disruption in the association between viral and cellular proteins could block essential cellular functions and thus result in toxicity.

Table 11.2

Host cellular proteins shown to interact with HPV E6

Protein	Proposed consequence	Reference
p53	Cell proliferation	74
E6-AP	Degradation of p53	43,44
E6-BP (ERC55)	Unknown	15
hDLG	Unknown	52
Paxillin	Unknown	89

Table 11.3
Host cellular proteins shown to interact with HPV E7

Protein	Proposed consequence	Reference
pRb family	Deregulated cell growth	23,27
	Increased expression of cell-cycle-dependent genes	
p21	Deregulated cell growth	33
p27	Deregulated cell growth	47
AP-1	Altered transcriptional regulation	4
TAF-1	Altered transcriptional regulation	70
TBP	Altered transcriptional regulation	60
S4 proteasome subunit	Unknown	9

HPV targets: summary

The paucity of HPV enzymes makes traditional antiviral drug design difficult for HPV-induced disease. A wealth of information is available detailing mechanisms of action of HPV proteins; however, it is clear that the macromolecular interactions that mediate these functions are not readily amenable to drug design and/or high throughput screening. The identification of appropriate HPV protein–host interactions which are accessible to small-molecule inhibitors is crucial to the discovery of anti-HPV therapies.

11.3.3 Novel approaches

This section describes therapeutic approaches that are in, or are approaching, clinical trials for the treatment of HPV-induced disease.

Reticulon

Reticulon, originally developed in the 1930s as an immuno-stimulant therapy for influenza, is a preparation of peptide and nucleic acid which has been shown to inhibit the replication of HIV *in vitro*, presumably via its ability to induce IFN γ. Subsequently, clinical trials in HIV-infected patients showed stimulation of the Th1 arm of the cellular immune response with sustained improvements in CD4 and CD8 cell counts. Reticulon is reported to be in clinical trials for the treatment of HPV disease. The rationale for this approach is obvious as spontaneous regression of genital warts has been shown to be mediated by a Th1-type response[18,32] in which IFNγ has a key role.

PEN 203

PEN 203 belongs to a class of compounds called papirines which are analogs of 2',5'-oligoadenylate (2',5'A), an intracellular mediator of IFN response.[82] Classically, IFN induces the expression of 2',5'-oligoadenylate synthetases which, in the presence of viral double-stranded RNA, induce the polymerization of ATP into 2',5'-linked oligomers of adenosine. 2',5'A then activates RNaseL which leads to the degradation of both cellular and viral single-stranded RNA.[82] Thus, PEN 203 should show antiviral activity due to activation of this arm of the IFN response. In Russian phase II trials, PEN 203 has reportedly shown positive results when applied topically to cutaneous and genital warts,[1] and trials are underway in the USA and Europe for the treatment of external genital warts.

Cidofovir

Originally developed as an antiherpetic, cidofovir is a cytidine nucleotide analog which exhibits its antiviral activity via its ability to inhibit herpes virus DNA polymerase.[73] It is approved for the treatment of cytomegalovirus (CMV) induced retinitis and a topical formulation is in development for the treatment of genital herpes. In pre-clinical studies cidofovir has shown antiviral activity against a number of viruses including CMV, herpes simplex virus (HSV) 1 and 2, varicella zoster virus (VZV), Epstein–Barr virus (EBV), human herpes virus (HHV) 6 and 8, adenoviruses, human poxviruses and HPV.[73] The rationale for the use of cidofovir in the treatment of HPV disease is not clear as HPVs do not encode their own polymerase, but recent clinical studies have reinforced the potential of this drug in this area. For example, intralesional or topical application of cidofovir has shown promise in the treatment of a number of HPV diseases, including recurrent laryngeal papillomatosis,[81,92] anogenital warts in immunocompromised and immunocompetent patients[67,78,80] and, more recently, in CIN 3.[79] In a double-blind, placebo-controlled trial of 31 immunocompetent patients with anogenital warts, cidofovir was applied topically as a 1% gel. Eighty percent of patients had a complete or partial response, with only one of the complete responders having a recurrence within 6 months of follow-up.[78] Cidofovir has well-characterized toxicity when administered systemically. Side-effects include nephrotoxicity, neutropenia, and metabolic acidosis; however, no evidence of systemic toxicity has been noted after topical cidofovir application.

As mentioned above, the mechanism of action of cidofovir against HPV is not clear, but it appears to be cytotoxic, preferentially in HPV-infected tissue over surrounding normal tissue[79] via its ability to induce apoptosis.[3] Clinical research on the efficacy and safety of cidofovir is ongoing. If the early promise shown in the above studies is confirmed in larger trials, then topical cidofovir may become an approved therapy for HPV lesions in the next few years.

Antisense therapy

Antisense technology offers the potential of totally rational antiviral therapy as oligonucleotides may be designed which specifically recognize and inhibit the normal processing of critical viral mRNAs.

Antisense oligonucleotides block the translation of target mRNAs by forming untranslatable double-stranded hybrids and by inducing intracellular degradation by RNaseH.[84] Successful antiviral therapy using antisense oligonucleotides has been acheived as Vitravene was approved for CMV-induced retinitis by the FDA in 1998. Pre-clinical studies have shown that antisense molecules designed against a number of HPV targets such as E1, E2, E6, and E7 have activity against HPV replication or HPV-induced proliferation and immortalization.[2,16,20,83] Antisense therapy was seen a few years ago to be the most promising new technology for the development of specific antiviral agents. However, with the exception of an antisense agent for the treatment of CMV retinitis in acquired immunodeficiency syndrome (AIDS) patients by direct intraocular injection, the realization of antisense molecules as therapeutics has yet to occur and requires further development in chemistry to overcome issues such as stability, toxicity, and delivery.

Vaccines

A great deal of effort has been directed toward the design of both prophylactic and therapeutic vaccines for the treatment of genital warts and cervical dysplasia and vaccines offer great hope for the prevention and treatment of these diseases in years to come. This area is vast and is covered in a Chapter 12 in this volume.

Retinoids

Another potential therapeutic option for HPV disease is the use of retinoids. Retinoids are a class of natural or synthetic compounds that are related to vitamin A (comprising all-*trans*-retinoic acid, 13-*cis*-retinoic acid, and the aromatic retinoids). They have proven efficacy in a number of dermatological indications, including invasive cancers and premalignant lesions of the skin, cervix, and vulva associated with papillomavirus infection. Retinoids are antiproliferative and modify keratinocyte differentiation. The basis of their anti-papillomavirus activity resides with their ability to disrupt keratinocyte differentiation, thus abrogating viral gene expression.[11,38,58]

Narayanan and colleagues[65] studied the effects of all-*trans*-retinoc acid and 9-*cis* retinoic acid on E6–E7 transcription, cell proliferation, cell-cycle distribution, and p53 expression in CaSki cells (a cell line derived from cervical carcinoma containing 600 copies of the HPV 16 genome). Both the all-*trans* and 9-*cis* forms of retinoic acid may act on highly proliferating tumor cells by arresting DNA synthesis and inducing cells to remain in the G1 phase of the cell cycle. In addition, retinoids may also induce a p53-dependent cell-cycle arrest and thus they may have a cytostatic effect rather than a cytotoxic effect on CaSki cells. The increase in expression of p53 coupled with an inhibition of E6–E7 transcription after treatment with these retinoids indicate the potential role of all-*trans* and 9-*cis* retinoic acid as antiviral agents.

11.4 SUMMARY

Many therapies are available for the treatment of HPV disease, especially anogenital warts. However, conventional therapies are aimed at removing the warts themselves rather than eliminating the underlying HPV infection and, as a result, current treatments are generally inadequate, having high recurrence rates. Future therapies will be directly or indirectly antiviral as they will target HPV protein functions or enhance the ability of the immune system to resolve infection. The way forward lies in the use of combinations of treatment modalities to eliminate the lesion and prevent recurrence. Successful therapeutic approaches for HPV-induced disease will require further understanding of the critical interactions required between HPV and host proteins for the completion of the HPV life-cycle and of the host immune response that controls or eliminates HPV disease.

REFERENCES

1. Ackerman S, Monath TP, Budowsky EI. (1998) Controlled clinical trial of PEN203 in treatment of HPV-associated genital and cutaneous warts. 8th International Congress for Infectious Diseases, 15 May, 200–1.

2. Alvarez-Salas LM, Arpawong TE, DiPaolo JA. (1999) Growth inhibition of cervical tumor cells by antisense oligodeoxynucleotides directed to the human papillomavirus type 16 E6 gene. *Antisense Nuc Acid Drug Dev* **9**: 441–50.

3. Andrei G, Snoeck R, de Clercq E. (1998) Detection of soluble nuclear matrix protein (NMP) released from apoptotic nuclei of human papillomavirus (HPV) positive cell lines treated with cidofovir. Abstracts of the 11th International Conference on Antiviral Research, San Diego, California, USA, 5–10 April 1998. *Antiviral Res* **37**: A47.

4. Antimore MJ, Birrer MJ, Patel D, Nader I, McCance DJ. (1996) The human papillomavirus type 16 E7 gene product interacts with and transactivates the AP1 family of transcription factors. *EMBO J* **15**: 1950–60.

5. Arany I, Tyring SK, Stanley MA, *et al.* (1999) Enhancement of the innate and cellular immune response in patients with genital warts treated with topical imiquimod cream 5%. *Antiviral Res* **43**: 55–63.

6. Baggish MS. (1980) Carbon dioxide laser treatment for condyloma acuminata venereal infections. *Obstet Gynecol* **55**: 711–15.

7. Barnard P, McMillan NA. (1999) The human papillomavirus E7 oncoprotein abrogates signaling mediated by interferon-alpha. *Virology* **259**: 305–13.

8. Barrasso R. (1998) Treatment of genital warts: an overview. *J Obstet Gynecol* **18**(Suppl. 2): S70–1.

9. Berezutskaya E, Bagchi S. (1997) The human papillomavirus E7 oncoprotein functionally interacts with the S4 subunit of the 26S proteasome. *J Biol Chem* **272**: 30135–40.

10. Beutner K. (1997) Therapeutic approaches to genital warts. *Am J Med* **102**: 28–37.

11. Bollag W. (1991) Retinoids and interferon: a new promising combination? *Br J Haematol* **79**: 87–91.

12. Calkins JW, Masterson BJ, Magrina JF, Capen CV. (1982) Management of condyloma acuminata with the carbon dioxide laser therapy. *Obstet Gynecol* **59**: 105–8.

13. Cardamakis E, Relakis K, Ginopoulos P, *et al.* (1997) Treatment of penile intraepithelial neoplasia (PIN) with interferon alpha-2a, CO₂ laser (vaporization) and 5-fluorouracil 5% (5-FU). *Eur J Gynaecol Oncol* **18**: 410.

14. Chang YE, Laimins LA. (2000) Microarray analysis identifies interferon-inducible genes and stat-1 as major transcriptional targets of human papillomavirus type 31. *J Virol* **74**: 4174–82.

15. Chen JJ, Reid CE, Band V, Androphy EJ. (1995) Interaction of papillomavirus E6 oncoproteins with a putative calcium-binding protein. *Science* **269**: 529–31.

16. Clark PR, Roberts ML, Cowsert LM. (1998) A novel drug screening assay for papilloma specific antiviral activity. *Antiviral Res* **37**: 97–106.

17. Coker K. (1998) Cimetidine in the treatment of warts. *Can Pharm J* **131**: 44–9.

18. Coleman N, Birley H, Renton AM, *et al.* (1994)

Immunological events in regressing genital warts. *Am J Clin Pathol* **102**: 768–74.

19. Cowsert LM. (1994) Treatment of papillomavirus infections: recent practice and future approaches. *Intervirology* **37**: 226–30.

20. Cowsert LM, Fox MC, Zon G, Mirabelli CK. (1993) In vitro evaluation of phosphorothioate oligonucleotides targeted to the E2 mRNA of papillomavirus: potential treatment for genital warts. *Antimicrob Agents Chemother* **37**: 171–7.

21. Damstra RJ, van Vloten WA. (1991) Cryotherapy in the treatment of condyloma acuminata: a controlled study of 64 patients. *J Dermatol Surg Oncol* **17**: 273–6.

22. Davis BE, Noble MJ. (1992) Initial experience with combined interferon alpha and carbon dioxide laser for the treatment of condyloma acuminata. *J Urol* **197**: 627–9.

23. Dyson N, Howley PM, Munger K, Harlow E. (1989) The human papillomavirus-16 E7 oncoprotein is able to bind to the retinoblastoma gene product. *Science* **243**: 934–7.

24. Edwards A, Atma-Ram A, Thin RN. (1988) Podophyllotoxin 0.5% v podophyllin 20% to treat penile warts. *Genitourin Med* **64**: 263–5.

25. Edwards L, Ferenczy A, Eron L, et al. (1998) Self-administered topical 5% imiquimod cream for external anogenital warts. *Arch Dermatol* **134**: 25–30.

26. Elion GB, Furman PA, Fyfe JA, et al. (1977) Selectivity of an anti-herpetic agent, 9-(2-hydroxyethoxymethyl) guanine. *Proc Natl Acad Sci USA* **74**: 5711–20.

27. Farnham PJ, Slansky JF, Kollmar R. (1993) The role of E2F in the mammalian cell cycle. *Biochim Biophys Acta* **1155**: 125–31.

28. Ferenczy A. (1984) Laser therapy of genital condyloma acuminata. *Obstet Gynecol* **63**: 703–7.

29. Ferenczy A, Behelak Y, Haber G, Wright TC, Richart RM. (1995) Treating vaginal and external anogenital condylomas with electrosurgery vs CO_2 laser ablation. *J Gynecol Surg* **11**: 41–50.

30. Ferenczy A, Bergeron C, Richart RM. (1990) Human papillomavirus DNA in CO_2 laser-generated plume of smoke and its consequences to the surgeon. *Obstet Gynecol* **75**: 114–18.

31. Ferenczy A, Choukroun D, Arseneau J. (1996) Loop electrosurgical excision procedure for squamous intraepithelial lesions of the cervix: advantages and potential pitfalls. *Obstet Gynecol* **87**: 332–7.

32. Fierlbeck G, Schiebel U, Muller C. (1989) Immunohistology of genital warts in different stages of regression after therapy with interferon gamma. *Dermatologica* **179**: 191–5.

33. Funk JO, Waga S, Harry JB, Espling E, Stillman B, Galloway D. (1997) Inhibition of CDK activity and PCNA-dependent DNA replication by p21 is blocked by interaction with the HPV16 E7 oncoprotein. *Genes Dev* **11**: 2090–10.

34. Ghosh AK. (1977) Cryosurgery of genital warts in cases in which podophyllin treatment failed or was contraindicated. *Br J Vener Dis* **53**: 49–53.

35. Godar DE. (1999) Light and death: photons and apoptosis. *J Invest Dermatol Symp Proc* **4**: 17–23.

36. Godley MJ, Bradbeer CS, Gellan M, Thin RN. (1987)

37. Gollock JM, Slatford K, Hunter JM. (1982) Scissor excision of anogenital warts. *Br J Vener Dis* **58**: 400–1.

38. Gross G, Pfister H, Hagedorn M, Stahn W. (1983) Effect of oral aromatic retinoid (Ro 10-95319) on human papillomavirus-2-induced common warts. *Dermatologica* **166**: 48–53.

39. Hadjuk PJ, Dinges J, Miknis GF, et al. (1997) NMR-based discovery of lead inhibitors that block DNA binding of the human papillomavirus E2 protein. *J Med Chem* **40**: 3144–50.

40. Harcourt JP, Worley G, Leighton SEJ. (1999) Cimetidine treatment for recurrent respiratory papillomatosis. *Int J Ped Otorhinolaryngol* **51**: 109–13.

41. Hawley-Nelson P, Vousden K, Hubbert NL, Lowy DR, Schiller JT. (1989). HPV16 E6 and E7 proteins cooperate to immortalize human foreskin keratinocytes. *EMBO J* **8**: 3905–10.

42. Hillemanns P, Untch M, Dannecker C, et al. (2000) Photodynamic therapy of vulvar intraepithelial neoplasia using 5-aminolevulinic acid. *Int J Cancer* **85**: 649–53.

43. Huibregtse JM, Scheffner M, Howley PM. (1991) A cellular protein mediates association of p53 with the E6 oncoprotein of human papillomavirus types 16 or 18. *EMBO J* **10**: 4129–35.

44. Huibregtse JM, Scheffner M, Howley PM. (1993) Localization of the E6-AP regions that direct human papillomavirus E6 binding, association with p53 and biquitination of associated proteins. *Mol Cell Biol* **13**: 4918–27.

45. Jensen SL. (1985) Comparison of podophyllin application with simple surgical excision in clearance and recurrence of perianal condylomata acuminata. *Lancet* **ii**: 1146–8.

46. Johnson JC, Burnett AF, Willett GD, Young MA, Doniger J. (1992) High frequencies of latent and clinical human papillomavirus cervical infections in immuno-compromised human immunodeficiency-virus-infected women. *Obstet Gynecol* **79**: 321–7.

47. Jones DL, Alani RM, Munger K. (1997) The human papillomavirus E7 oncoprotein can uncouple cellular differentiation and proliferation in human keratinocytes by abrogating p21Cip1-mediated inhibition of cdk2. *Genes Dev* **11**: 2101–11.

48. Kaplan IW. (1942) Condyloma acuminata. *New Orleans Med Surg J* **94**: 388–90.

49. Karabulut AA. (1997) Is cimetidine effective for non-genital warts: a double blind placebo-controlled study. *Arch Dermatol* **133**: 533–4.

50. Khawaja HT. (1989) Podophyllin versus scissor excision in the treatment of perianal condyloma acuminata: a prospective study. *Br J Surg* **76**: 1067–8.

51. Kinghorn GR, McMillan A, Mulcahy F, Drake S, Lacey C, Bingham JS. (1993) An open comparative study of the efficacy of 0.5% podophyllotoxin lotion and 25% podophyllin solution in the treatment of condyloma acuminata in males and females. *Int J STD AIDS* **4**: 194–9.

52. Kiyono T, Hiraiwa A, Fuijita M, Hayashi Y, Akiyama T, Ishibashi M. (1997) Binding of high risk human papillomavirus E6 oncoproteins to the human homolog of the

Cryotherapy compared with trichloroacetic acid in treating genital warts. *Genitourin Med* **63**: 390–2.

Drosophila disc large tumor suppressor protein. *Proc Natl Acad Sci USA* **94**: 11612–16.

53. Koutsky L. (1997) Epidemiology of genital human papillomavirus infection. *Am J Med* **102**: 3–8.

54. Krebs HB. (1987) The use of topical 5-fluorouracil in the treatment of genital condylomas. *Obstet Gynecol North Am* **14**: 559–68.

55. Krebs HB. (1991) Treatment of genital condyloma with 5-fluorouracil. *Dermatol Clin* **9**: 333–41.

56. Ledo E, Ledo A. (2000) Phototherapy, photo-chemotherapy and photodynamic therapy: unapproved uses and indications. *Clin Dermatol* **18**: 77–86.

57. Lee SS, Weiss RS, Javier RT. (1997) Binding of human virus oncoproteins to hDlg/SAP97, a mammalian homolog of the *Drosophila* disc large tumor suppressor protein. *Proc Natl Acad Sci USA* **94**: 6670–5.

58. Lutzner MA, Blanchet-Bardon C. (1980) Oral retinoid treatment of human papillomavirus-type-5-induced epidermodysplasia verruciformis. *N Engl J Med* **302**: 1091–3.

59. Malvija VK, Deppe G, Plusczynski R, *et al.* (1987) Trichloroacetic acid in the treatment of human papillomavirus infection of the cervix without associated dysplasia. *Obstet Gynecol* **70**: 72–4.

60. Massimi P, Pim D, Storey A, Banks L. (1996) HPV-16 E7 and adenovirus E1a complex formation with TATA box binding protein is enhanced by casein kinase II phosphorylation. *Oncogene* **12**: 2325–30.

61. Mazurkiewicz W, Jablonska S. (1986) Comparison between the therapeutic efficacy of 0.5% podophyllotoxin preparations and 20% podophyllin ethanol solution in condyloma acuminata. *Z Hauttkr* **61**: 1387–95.

62. Melbye M, Palefsky J, Gonzales J, *et al.* (1990) Immune status as a determinant of human papillomavirus detection and its association with anal epithelial abnormalities. *Int J Cancer* **46**: 203–6.

63. Miller RL, Gerster GF, Owens ML, Slade HB, Tomai MA. (1999) Imiquimod applied topically: a novel immune response modifier and new class of drug. *Int J Immunopharmacol* **21**: 1–14.

64. Murphy M, Bloom GD. (1991) Podophyllin or podophyllotoxin as treatment for condyloma acuminata. *Papillomavirus Rep* **2**: 87–9.

65. Narayanan BA, Holladay EB, Nixon DW, Mauro CT. (1998) The effect of all-trans and 9-cis retinoic acid on the steady state level of HPV16 E6/E7 mRNA and cell cycle in cervical carcinoma cells. *Life Sci* **63**: 565–73.

66. Oriel JD. (1971) Natural history of genital warts. *Br J Vener Dis* **47**: 1–13.

67. Orlando G, Fasolo MM, Beretta R, *et al.* (1999) Intralesional or topical cidofovir (HPMPC, VISTIDE) for the treatment of recurrent genital warts in HIV-1-infected patients. *AIDS* **13**: 1978–80.

68. Orlow SJ, Paller A. (1993) Cimetidine therapy for multiple viral warts in children. *J Am Acad Dermatol* **28**: 794–6.

69. Phelps WC, Barnes JA, Lobe DC. (1998) Molecular targets for human papillomaviruses: prospects for antiviral therapy. *Antiviral Chem Chemother* **9**: 359–77.

70. Phillips AC, Vousden KH. (1997) Analysis of the interaction between human papillomavirus type 16 E7 and the TATA binding protein, TBP. *J Gen Virol* **78**: 905–9.

71. Porreco R, Penn I, Droegemueller W, Greer B, Makowski E. (1975) Gynecological malignancies in immunosuppressed organ homograft recipients. *Obstet Gynecol* **45**: 359–64.

72. Richwald GA. (1999) Imiquimod. *Drugs of Today* **35**: 497–511.

73. Safrin S, Cherrington J, Jaffe HS. (1997) Clinical uses of cidofovir. *Rev Med Virol* **7**: 145–56.

74. Scheffner M, Werness BA, Huibregtse JM, Levine AJ, Howley P. (1990) The E6 oncoprotein encoded by human papillomavirus types 16 and 18 promotes the degradation of p53. *Cell* **63**: 1129–36.

75. Schwartz PM, Milstone LM. (1989) Dipyridamole potentiates the growth-inhibitory action of methotrexate and 5-fluorouracil in human keratinocytes in vitro. *J Invest Dermatol* **93**: 523–7.

76. Seigfried EC. (1997) Warts and molluscum on children – an approach to therapy. *Dermatol Ther* **2**: 51–67.

77. Shikowitz MJ, Abramson AL, Freeman K, Steinberg BM, Nouri M. (1998) Efficacy of DHE photodynamic therapy for respiratory papillomatosis: immediate and long-term results. *Laryngoscope* **108**: 962–7.

78. Snoeck R, Andrei G, Gerard M, *et al.* (1998) A double-blind placebo-controlled study of cidofovir gel for human papillomavirus (HPV)-associated genital warts. Abstracts of the 11th International Conference on Antiviral Research, San Diego, California, USA, 5–10 April 1998. *Antiviral Res* **37**: A47.

79. Snoeck R, Noel J-C, Muller C, de Clercq E, Bossens M. (2000) Cidofovir, a new approach for the treatment of cervix intraepithelial neoplasia grade III (CIN III). *J Med Virol* **60**: 205–9.

80. Snoeck R, van Ranst M, Andrei G, *et al.* (1995) Treatment of anogenital papillomavirus infections with an acyclic nucleoside phosphonate analogue. *N Engl J Med* **333**: 943–4.

81. Snoeck R, Wellens W, Desloovere C, *et al.* (1998) Treatment of severe laryngeal papillomatosis with intralesional injections of cidofovir [(S)-1-(3-hydroxy-2-phosphonylmethoxyprophyl) cytosine]. *J Med Virol* **54**: 219–25.

82. Stark GR, Kerr IM, Williams BRG, Silverman RH, Schreiber D. (1998) How cells respond to interferons. *Annu Rev Biochem* **67**: 227–64.

83. Steele C, Cowsert LM, Shillitoe EJ. (1993) Effects of human papillomavirus type-18 specific antisense oligonucleotides on the transformed phenotype of human carcinoma cell lines. *Cancer Res* **53**: 2330–7.

84. Stein CA, Cheng Y-C. (1993) Antisense oligonucleotides as therapeutic agents – is the bullet really magical? *Science* **261**: 1004–12.

85. Steinberg JL, Cibley LJ, Rice PA. (1993) Genital warts: diagnosis, treatment and counseling for the patient. *Curr Top Inf Dis* **13**: 99–122.

86. Strander H. (1989) The action of interferons on virus associated human neoplasms. *Cancer Surv* **8**: 755–91.

87. Titolo S, Pelletier A, Sauve F, *et al.* (1999) Role of the ATP-binding domain of the human papillomavirus type 11 helicase in E2-dependent binding to the origin. *J Virol* **73**: 5282–93.

88. Tokura YJ. (1999) Modulation of cytokine production by 8-methoxypsoralen and UVA. *Dermatol Sci* **19**: 114–22.

89. Tong X, Howley PM. (1997) The bovine papillomavirus E6 oncoprotein interacts with paxillin and blocks its interaction with vinculin and the focal adhesion kinase. *J Biol Chem* **272**: 33373–6.

90. Um SJ, Kim EJ, Hwang ES, Kim SJ, Namkoong SE, Park JS. (2000) Antiproliferative effects of retinoic acid/interferon in cervical carcinoma cell lines: cooperative growth suppression of IRF-1 and p53. *Int J Cancer* **85**: 416–23.

91. Vambutas A, Bonagura VR, Steinberg BM. (2000) Altered expression of TAP-1 and major histocompatibility complex class I in laryngeal papillomatosis: correlation of TAP-1 with disease. *Clin Diagn Lab Immunol* **7**: 79–85.

92. van Cutsem E, Snoeck R, van Ranst M, *et al.* (1995) Successful treatment of a squamous papilloma of the hypopharynx by local injections of (s)-1-(3-hydroxy-2-phosphonylmethoxypropyl)cytosine. *J Med Virol* **45**: 230–5.

93. Vella S, Palmisano L. (2000) Antiretroviral therapy: state of the HAART. *Antiviral Res* **45**: 1–7.

94. Webb DG, King SJ. (1994) Management of external genital warts: a comparison of podophyllin and podophyllotoxin. *Pharm J* **252**: 291–3.

95. Weck PK, Buddin DA, Whisnant JK. (1988) Interferons in the treatment of genital human papillomavirus infections. *Am J Med* **85**: 159–64.

96. Weiland O. (2000) Interferon and ribavirin combination therapy: indications and schedules. *Forum* **10**: 22–8.

97. Wielander LE, Homesley HD, Smiles KA, Peets EA. (1990) Intralesional interferon alpha-2β for the treatment of genital warts. *Am J Obstet Gynecol* **162**: 348–54.

98. Wierrani F, Kubin A, Jindra R, *et al.* (1999) 5-aminolevulinic acid-mediated photodynamic therapy of intraepithelial neoplasia and human papillomavirus of the uterine cervix – a new experimental approach. *Cancer Detect Prev* **23**: 351–5.

99. Wright T Jr, Gaghon S, Ferenczy A, *et al.* (1991) Excising CIN lesions by loop electroexcisional procedure. *Contemp Obstet Gynecol* **36**: 56–74.

12

Vaccines

Stephen C. Inglis and Terence O'Neill

12.1 TARGETS FOR HPV VACCINATION

From the discovery some 15 years ago of the link between human papillomavirus (HPV) and the development of cervical cancer,[20] the idea that humans could be vaccinated against this virus group has steadily gathered momentum. Over 70 different types of HPV have now been recognized, but the emergence of strong epidemiological evidence that a small subset of these types can cause malignant anogenital disease, together with the recognition that certain other HPV types are entirely responsible for one of the most prevalent and fastest growing sexually transmitted diseases world-wide, have focused attention primarily on these viruses as targets for vaccine development.

While the causative relationship between HPV 6 and 11 and genital warts is immediately obvious, the link between HPV and malignant disease is less direct. Cervical cancer occurs only in a very small proportion of those infected, even with the 'high-risk' oncogenic HPV types such as HPV 16 and 18, and may take many years to develop. Malignancy is preceded, however, by a pre-cancerous abnormality of the cervix, cervical dysplasia, which is also the result of HPV infection and which, though not in itself a clinical problem for the affected individual, presents a valid and rather more accessible target for vaccination.

Proof of principle that papillomavirus infection can be prevented by prophylactic vaccination has been firmly established in animal models. However, HPV vaccine development has received a further major boost from the increasing recognition that therapeutic vaccination against chronic virus infection, i.e., elimination of pre-existing disease by active immunization, is a realistic possibility and that the natural history of HPV makes it a prime candidate for this kind of approach. These factors, complemented by important recent advances in our understanding of the structure and molecular genetics of human papillomaviruses made possible through the application of recombinant DNA technology, have accelerated dramatically the pace of HPV vaccine development in recent years, to the point where clinical trials for both therapy and prophylaxis are underway, with a growing optimism that success is not only possible but likely.

12.2 HPV VACCINE DESIGN

Papillomaviruses are exquisitely species specific. Thus, although several animals, including primates, are naturally infected with their own papillomaviruses, none can be used to test directly the efficacy of HPV vaccine candidates, and this represents a major difficulty for would-be vaccine developers. Nevertheless, information gleaned from testing animal papillomavirus vaccines, coupled with a growing understanding of the immunological mechanisms which underlie the remarkable success of other virus vaccines in humans, and a detailed knowledge of HPV molecular biology, provide a solid theoretical framework for the prediction of vaccine strategies that are likely to be successful.

The chief aim of prophylactic vaccination against HPV is to induce protective immune responses against the virus so that, when natural infection occurs, it does not result in disease. A more valuable, but considerably more challenging, goal is to block infection of the host altogether. This has the advantage that transmission of HPV to further hosts will be interrupted and so benefit will be conferred on the population as well as the individual. Therapeutic vaccination can similarly be viewed at two levels. The simplest aim is to induce an immune response that can attack the pre-existing infection and ameliorate disease symptoms locally, while a higher goal is to eliminate infection from the body altogether.

There are two main elements to the immune response against virus infection. The first is through the humoral immune system, i.e., the production of specific antibodies that are capable of attaching to the surface of the virus particle to neutralize its infectivity, and the second is through the induction of antigen-specific T-cells that can recognize and destroy cells already infected with the virus.

12.2.1 Humoral immunity

To be completely effective, neutralizing antibodies must be available at the site of entry of the virus at sufficient concentration to deal with all of the input virus. Below this level, they may still be useful for limiting the extent of initial infection and the spread of virus within the host, provided that during passage from cell to cell virus particles become available for antibody binding. In the case of HPV, however, the disease lesion consists of a mass of epithelial cells derived from one or a small number of initial infected cells in the basal layer that have been driven into cell division by the presence of the virus. Fully assembled virus particles that might be targets for neutralizing antibody are only evident in the upper, keratinized layers of the lesion.

A further important point relating specifically to HPV vaccine development is that the virus infects its host via the mucosal epithelium and persists at that site only. Thus, neutralizing antibody needs to remain available at the mucosa to provide continued protection. The body manufactures a specific class of antibody, immunoglobulin (Ig) A, designed especially for secretion at mucosal surfaces, and so it may be that a preventative vaccine will have to induce strong HPV-specific IgA responses in order to be effective. IgG can also be found in mucosal secretions, however, so this point remains unclear.

12.2.2 T-cell immunity

The second important element of the immune response against virus infection is the generation of cell-mediated immunity, through the activation of specific T-cells. Whilst antibodies generally recognize virus particles, antigen-specific T-cells have the capacity to recognize cells infected with virus.[23] This is achieved through the recognition of peptide fragments of virus-specific proteins that are displayed on the surface of the cell in conjunction with host-encoded major histocompatibility complex (MHC) molecules. Two main classes of T-cell are currently defined. Cytotoxic T-lymphocytes (CTL) carrying the CD8 surface marker can destroy virus-infected cells through binding to complexes of MHC class I with virus peptides derived from within the infected cell cytoplasm. Helper T-cells (Th) carrying the CD4 surface marker recognize peptide fragments complexed with MHC class II molecules, and function to provide accessory signals for promoting both specific antibody production and CTL, though they may also be able in some circumstances to exert direct antiviral effects. In recent years, a further refinement of Th cell definition has been introduced. Th1 cells appear to promote primarily the production of CTL and are characterized by production of the cytokines interferon-gamma (IFNγ) and interleukin-2 (IL-2), while Th2 cells promote antibody production and produce IL 5 and IL 10. The balance maintained between these two types of Th cell may thus be important in determining the nature of the immune response to a particular antigen.

The nature of the T-cell antigen-recognition mechanism means that the virus peptides likely to be targets for T-cells are not easily identifiable. Any protein encoded by the virus, whether part of the virion structure or only produced within the infected cell, could provide peptides that might be recognized by T-cells. Furthermore, the protein targets are not restricted to surface components, and so proteins involved solely in intracellular events (for example the early HPV proteins) may be effective antigens. Furthermore, extensive polymorphism of MHC molecules in the human population means that the precise set of peptides capable of MHC binding and hence becoming available for T-cell recognition is very likely to differ from individual to individual.

12.2.3 Immune responses required for the control of HPV

For prophylaxis, the ideal HPV vaccine would protect completely against infection at the site of virus entry, i.e., the genital mucosa, and clearly the critical immune component for achieving this would be neutralizing antibody, whether of the IgG or the IgA subclass. This is an extremely difficult target, however, and it is generally accepted that most existing vaccines, although highly successful in providing disease protection, are not capable of preventing infection altogether. Because HPV infection, once established, can result in cell proliferation and hence disease without assembly of neutralizable virions, it would therefore seem prudent to include components designed to stimulate T-cell immunity also in order to deal with infected cells resulting from virus breakthrough.

Successful therapeutic vaccination against HPV, on the other hand, is likely to require primarily a T-cell-based immune response. Interestingly, studies of naturally regressing genital warts have suggested that the majority of the T-cells infiltrating the regressing lesions are CD4+ T-cells,[15] implying that, for wart therapy, induction of this kind of response may be very important. For the elimination of HPV-associated tumor cells, however, it is widely believed that virus-specific CD8+ CTL cells will be required, though a potential role for CD4+ T-cells cannot be excluded.[58]

12.2.4 Vaccine delivery

It is quite clear that the method by which antigens are delivered to the body has a critical influence on the strength, duration, and type of immune response produced. In general, protein-based subunit vaccines are administered in combination with an adjuvant to improve immunogenicity. Currently, the only adjuvants licensed for human use are those based on aluminum salts, and these have proved satis-factory for promoting good neutralizing antibody responses in humans, but are less effective stimulators of T-cell immunity, especially CTLs. However, the responses generated using vaccines adjuvanted with aluminum salts often depend on the nature of the antigen. For example, good T-cell proliferative responses were generated in people vaccinated with an HPV 6 L2E7 recombinant fusion protein vaccine adjuvanted with Alhydrogel®. This was probably due to the particulate nature of the fusion protein.[57] Several new adjuvants are currently being tested, however, and the indications from animal model studies and from early human trials are that these are likely to offer significant advantages.[60]

Where the aim is to induce a strong CD8-mediated CTL response against virus antigens, the mechanism of T-cell recognition dictates that the vaccine antigen is introduced into the host in such a way that the appropriate peptide epitopes can gain access to the host cell MHC class I in order that proper presentation can take place. This has fundamental implications for vaccine design and delivery.

Formation of recognizable MHC class I–peptide complexes can be achieved in several different ways. The first is by introducing into the cells of the host a gene encoding the selected target antigen; the gene product will then be synthesized naturally in the cell cytoplasm and presented appropriately to T-cells via the host MHC. The most obvious way to achieve this is to vaccinate the host with a virus vector engineered to carry the selected gene and which is therefore naturally equipped to deliver the target gene effectively. A more direct approach which has attracted a great deal of interest recently is through direct injection of plasmid DNA encoding the target gene. This strategy has also proved successful in generating CTL responses.[18]

An alternative approach is to deliver the virus antigen as a protein product, but in combination with an additional component that can promote uptake of the protein into the host cell cytoplasm and hence correct processing and MHC presentation. Many laboratories are currently attempting to develop antigen formulations that can achieve this goal and some success has been reported, although as yet these studies have not been confirmed in humans. One of the most promising approaches involves the use of microparticles, which comprise tiny beads of defined size into which antigen can be loaded. Several groups have shown that vaccines based on such formulations are capable of inducing strong CTL responses in mice.[38,40]

Finally, there has been considerable interest in a strategy that aims to deliver 'pre-processed' T-cell recognition targets to the body in a form that can gain direct access to host MHC class I molecules without the need to go through the normal processing and presentation pathway.[2] In this case, potential target antigens are analysed to identify peptide sequences that can bind to particular molecular species of MHC class I and thus act as recognition elements for CTL. These peptides are then synthesized chemically and delivered to the host, usually coupled to an additional peptide sequence designed to provide CTL 'help' and, optionally, a carrier molecule to promote cellular uptake.

12.3 PROPHYLACTIC VACCINES

12.3.1 Vaccine candidates

Whole virions
There is now considerable optimism that the successful prevention of HPV-associated disease can be achieved by vaccination based on experience with animal papillomaviruses. As early as 1935, Shope was able to protect rabbits against cottontail rabbit papillomavirus (CRPV) using a vaccine based on infected rabbit tissue,[54] and vaccines based on whole bovine papillomavirus (BPV) virions are also effective in cattle.[27] Perhaps the most significant of all the animal model studies, however, showed that a vaccine based on formalin-inactivated canine oral papillomavirus (COPV) could protect dogs not only from experimental challenge, but also in a large field trial where infection was transmitted naturally.[4] This gives clear encouragement that preventative vaccination may also be effective in humans.

However, the use of an equivalent approach in humans is impractical for two reasons. First, at present at least, the virus cannot be propagated except under highly specialized conditions that would not be appropriate for vaccine production. Second, even if this problem were soluble, the oncogenicity associated with certain types of HPV would almost certainly preclude the use of a whole virus vaccine on safety grounds. For these reasons, therefore, attention has focused on the use of HPV components produced by recombinant DNA techniques.

Recombinant protein-based vaccines
The major and minor capsid proteins, L1 and L2 respectively, together make up the virus coat which mediates penetration of the virus into susceptible cells. They therefore represent the most obvious targets for neutralizing antibody, and several studies have confirmed this supposition. Pilacinski and colleagues first showed that protection of cattle against BPV2 could be achieved using a bacterial fusion protein containing sequences from the L1 capsid protein.[41] Jarrett et al.[28] confirmed these findings and further showed that an L2-containing bacterial fusion protein could also provide protection. A similar picture has emerged from studies using CRPV.[35]

These vaccines were based, however, on conformationally inaccurate capsid protein fragments which seemed unlikely to be able to induce neutralizing antibodies as effectively as whole virions. The work of Zhou et al.[64] and Kirnbauer et al.[29] showing that self-assembled structures resembling whole virions (virus-like particles or VLPs) could be produced by expression of L1 protein using virus vectors in mammalian cells thus generated considerable interest. These VLPs are highly immunogenic,[29] and VLP vaccines based on BPV, CRPV and COPV can provide effective protection against disease in the appropriate animal models.[9,26,30,56] Furthermore, it has been shown that VLP vaccines can be effectively delivered by mucosal routes.[19,47] Consequently, HPV VLPs are now the major focus of attention for the development of human prophylactic vaccines. All the most important HPV types have now been successfully produced as VLPs and it is clear that they can be generated not only in mammalian cells, but also in yeast[26] and even in bacteria.[62] This work has progressed rapidly to the point where at least three different VLP-based human vaccine trials are now underway. Initial results from the study conducted by a group from the National Cancer Institute (NCI) have recently been reported.[50] This trial showed that L1 VLPs were safe and generated good antibody responses in healthy subjects without the need for an adjuvant.

Though VLPs can be generated from L1 protein alone, co-expression of L1 and L2 leads to the formation of particles containing both antigens.[31,64] As L2 can be effective as a vaccine in its own right,[28,35] it may therefore be that VLPs comprising both antigens could provide better protection than a vaccine based on a single antigen, though it remains to be seen whether this will be necessary.

The capsid proteins are not, however, the only possible components of a prophylactic HPV vaccine. From a theoretical standpoint, it would be advantageous to induce not only neutralizing antibodies to block initial infection, but also a strong T-cell-based response to destroy any infected cells resulting from virus 'breakthrough.' While L1/L2-based vaccines may generate effective T-cell responses as well as antibody, the fact that cells during the initial stages of papillomavirus vaccines express only early proteins has highlighted the possibility of including one or more of these proteins also. It may therefore be that a combination of capsid protein-based VLPs together with one or more of the early proteins offers the best opportunity for vaccination currently available, and in this regard it is interesting that VLPs consisting of L1 or L2 fused to E7 can be constructed successfully and can induce protective cell-mediated immune responses against E7-bearing tumor cells.[24,39,49]

Genetic vaccines

Delivery of genes that encode protective antigens offers an alternative strategy for vaccine development that has some potential advantages over conventional protein-based approaches. In particular, genetic vaccination allows synthesis of the target antigen within the cells of the vaccinee, and hence presentation to the immune system in a form which should provoke strong CTL responses as well as antibody.

Success has been achieved using variants of this approach in animal models of papillomavirus infection. Protection against CRPV disease was obtained using a recombinant vaccinia virus engineered to express the L1 protein[35] and by direct injection of DNA comprising the CRPV L1 gene[55] or a mixture of the E1, E2, E6, and E7 genes.[25] A naked DNA vaccine encoding the COPV L1 protein was also successful in a dog model of disease.[17] Plasmid-based DNA vaccines against other infectious diseases have shown considerable promise in model systems[18] and have now progressed to human trials. They are relatively simple to produce and are likely to be very stable, and so, provided they are able to match the effectiveness of more traditional approaches, which is as yet unproven, they could offer considerable practical advantages for large-scale vaccination.

12.3.2 Vaccine testing

There is currently considerable optimism that the success of vaccination against animal papillomaviruses can be translated to the human situation. There is, however, no direct way to carry out pre-clinical efficacy testing of actual human vaccine candidates, because HPV does not cause disease in animals. The lack of a robust cell culture system for HPV also presents a major hurdle, because it is currently difficult to measure antibody responses against test vaccines using a direct virus-neutralization assay. This problem is being circumvented in several ways. Certain HPV types will agglutinate red blood cells and hence this can provide a test for antibodies that can block agglutination.[45] This is a very convenient assay, but has the drawback that the viral determinants for red-cell binding may not necessarily be the same as those required for true infectivity. Rose et al.[48] reported the use of a more direct but much more complex system for measuring virus neutralization using human skin xenografts that can be infected with HPV 11. An alternative approach is through the construction of pseudotype particles comprising the genome of BPV encased in the capsid proteins of HPV,[44] which can successfully infect a BPV-sensitive line, but which should be sensitive to HPV-specific neutralizing antibodies. If successful, this could prove to be the method of choice for the screening of serological responses to vaccination in large-scale field trials.

The development of assays for measuring immunological responses is only one of many challenges that face the testing of HPV vaccines in humans. One of the fundamental questions that has to be resolved is the precise endpoint for assessing vaccine success. In the case of genital warts, the effectiveness of a vaccine can be measured directly by comparing rates of disease acquisition in vaccinated versus control groups, and the attack rates in certain 'at-risk' populations are sufficiently high[10] that trial design should be relatively straightforward.

Vaccination to prevent cervical cancer, however, presents a much more complex problem. Clearly, the ultimate measure of success will be a reduced incidence of cancer in the vaccinated population, but as there may be a 20–30-year lag between infection with HPV and the development of malignant disease, this is an unrealistic endpoint. It seems reasonable to suggest that the link with cervical cancer is sufficiently well established that the prevention of infection by high-risk HPV types offers an alternative endpoint. This is fraught with difficulty, however, for a variety of reasons. First, the prevention of infection is likely to be an extremely difficult target: most successful vaccines are generally recognized to prevent disease incidence but not necessarily infection. Second, detection of the incidence of infection is not straightforward. Monitoring infection by seroconversion is not feasible, because many individuals do not mount a measurable immune response following natural infection. In any case, it is likely to be very difficult to distinguish between responses against the vaccine and subsequent natural infection. The alternative, detection of HPV directly in the genital tract by DNA-based analyses, is possible, but would require regular monitoring of vaccinees, is technically quite demanding, and may actually prove to be oversensitive, because the presence of DNA does not necessarily mean the presence of active infection.

The most promising endpoint for vaccine trials would appear to be the incidence of cervical dysplasia following vaccination. It is widely accepted that this is a precursor to the development of malignant disease, and there are well-established screening procedures for the detection of dysplasia on a large scale. The problem here is that dysplasia can be caused by a variety of different HPV types, some of which are not associated with malignant disease and thus would not be targets for a cervical cancer vaccine. It seems, therefore, that the best option for measuring vaccine efficacy following vaccination will be to combine monitoring of cervical dysplasia incidence with DNA analysis to establish, in those cases where dysplasia is detected, the type of virus involved.

The fact that several different virus types are responsible for disease presents a further complication for vaccine design. For genital warts, once again the situation is fairly straightforward. About three-quarters of cases appear to be caused by HPV 6, and the remaining fraction by HPV 11. The two viruses are closely related, however, and there is evidence for a degree of immunological cross-reactivity,[46] and so either virus type could provide the basis for a generally applicable vaccine.

By contrast, several different HPV types are associated with the development of cervical cancer, and these are clearly immunologically distinct. HPV 16 and HPV 18 account for about 75% of cervical cancers, and so these viruses are likely to represent the core elements of a prophylactic vaccine, but there are a number of other virus types, such as HPV 31, 33, 35, 39, and 45, which could also be candidates for inclusion. While this appears quite feasible experimentally, developing such a multicomponent vaccine would present a tremendous challenge from the perspective of manufacturing and clinical development.

12.4 THERAPEUTIC VACCINES

The concept of therapeutic vaccination against a virus-associated disease appears at first sight somewhat illogical. If the immune system has failed to eliminate disease thus far, why should vaccination now improve the situation? This view, however, is predicated on the assumption that immune responses against viruses are always optimal. It ignores the obvious point that pathogens, particularly those leading to chronic or persistent infections, have, almost by definition, evolved strategies to avoid provoking effective immune responses. Armed with this understanding and a much greater awareness of the mechanisms by which immune responses are mounted and regulated, it should therefore be possible, through carefully designed vaccine strategies, to exceed the natural responses mounted against infection, opening the way to the development of vaccines that may be effective against pre-existing infection.

The natural history of HPV makes it a prime target for therapeutic vaccination. The virus is highly specific for epithelial tissue and does not spread systemically. This highly restricted tissue tropism may explain why the presence of infection often does not provoke a strong immune response and why HPV lesions can persist, sometimes for very long periods. It is clear, however, that the immune system is capable of controlling HPV disease. Wart virus infections and HPV-associated tumors are much more frequent in those receiving immunosuppressive therapy.[3] Furthermore, it is well established that spontaneous wart regression can often occur in humans who have had disease for considerable periods of time, and that this regression is driven by a vigorous cell-mediated immune response.[15] This implies that the immune system failed to respond initially

not through any inherent incapacity, but through what might be described as 'immunological ignorance'.

12.4.1 Treatment of wart virus infections

Over the past 40 years, there have been several reports that warts could be treated successfully using autogenous vaccines derived from patients' own lesions,[1,6,36,61] but until recently the idea of developing a general therapeutic vaccine against warts attracted relatively little interest. Today, however, the theoretical arguments in favor of the concept allied with the availability of modern tools for vaccine design have strongly rekindled interest in the approach.

Confidence in its potential success has been bolstered by experimental data from animal models. Jarrett et al.[28] reported that vaccination of cattle with an alum-formulated fusion protein containing the BPV L2 sequence was capable of inducing early regression of BPV-induced alimentary papillomas, and similar studies have been reported using the CRPV model.[52] Immunological analysis of regressing lesions in each case revealed the presence of a strong T-cell infiltrate,[32,53] consistent with the observations from regressing genital warts in humans.[15]

This has led directly to the development of equivalent therapeutic vaccines for human disease. The most advanced of these is designed to treat genital warts and consists of the HPV 6 L2 and E7 sequences expressed as a single fusion protein in bacteria. The purified protein is delivered in conjunction with an adjuvant in order to induce strong HPV-specific T-cell responses against both early-stage and late-stage infected cells. Phase I human studies have shown the vaccine to be safe and immunogenic,[57] and early phase II studies, though conducted on an open-label basis, provided encouragement that the vaccine may be effective in preventing wart recurrence,[33] a major drawback with existing therapies.[5] More recently, results have been reported from a vaccine study in genital wart patients conducted in China using unadjuvanted HPV 6 VLPs based on the L1 protein.[63] The authors presented data showing both specific antibodies and a delayed-type hypersensitivity response against L1 and suggested that the vaccine may have accelerated wart regression.

Vaccines based on a similar rationale are also being developed for the treatment of cervical dysplasia, though their clinical development is less advanced. Phase I trials are underway in women with high-grade disease (cervical intraepithelial neoplasia 1/2) using a fusion protein comprising the HPV 16 E7 protein linked to the *Mycobacterium bovis* heat shock protein Hsp65. This approach is based on pre-clinical studies showing that vaccination of mice with the protein, in the absence of adjuvant, is capable of inducing anti-E7 CTLs and can protect against the development of E7-bearing tumor cells.[14]

12.4.2 Malignant Disease

HPV-associated anogenital cancers represent one of the few situations in which tumor cells are marked unambiguously by the presence of tumor-specific antigens, and hence are attractive targets for immunotherapy. Progression from HPV infection to malignancy involves integration of HPV DNA into the host cell chromosome, and it is well established that two virus genes in particular, encoding the E6 and E7 proteins, are consistently retained and expressed by the tumor cell.[51] The E6 and E7 proteins therefore present obvious targets for therapeutic vaccination to induce an anti-tumor immune response, and their location inside the tumor cell rather than on its surface suggests strongly that the most appropriate immune effector mechanism is likely to be the CTL.

Animal model studies, though not exactly reflective of the real situation, have supported the concept of HPV antigen-mediated tumor immunotherapy. Vaccines based on the delivery of genes encoding HPV E6 or E7 genes have provided effective immunity against the growth of tumor cells expressing the equivalent antigens *in vivo*,[11,12,34,37] and analysis of the anti-tumor effect suggested that it is mediated by CTLs.[13]

Human trials are now underway using several different strategies. The most advanced is based on a recombinant vaccinia virus engineered to express the E6 and E7 sequences (modified to eliminate their transforming capability) from both HPV 16 and HPV 18.[8] This vaccine has been tested so far in a small number of advanced cancer patients in the UK and USA, and the results showed that it was safe and capable of stimulating anti-HPV immune responses including, in at least one patient, CTLs.[7] Trials are now underway in patients with less advanced disease who are more likely to benefit from immunotherapy. A second study carried out in Australia involved the use of purified HPV 16 E7 protein administered in conjunction with adjuvant, once again in late-stage patients. Data from this trial again indicated that the vaccine was safe and able to induce E7-specific antibodies and helper T-cell responses, although no specific CTLs were detected.[22] Human trials are also underway based on delivery of specific peptide sequences corresponding to regions of the HPV 16 E7 that are known to complex with the A2 allele of human MHC class I molecules, and hence predicted to be able to induce tumor-specific CTLs in human leukocyte antigen (HLA) A2 patients.[42] The peptides were combined with an unrelated peptide selected to provide T-cell help. Although the therapy was shown to be safe, no specific CTL responses were demonstrated in the end-stage cervical carcinoma patients.[43,59] All patients immunized with the highest dose of the vaccine (1000 μg) showed progressive disease.

There are clearly pitfalls to this kind of immunotherapeutic approach for the treatment of cervical cancer. One obvious difficulty with the initial human studies is that they have so far been confined to late-stage patients, who have very advanced disease, who are often immunocompromised as a direct result of their disease status or previous therapy,[21] and who are consequently less than ideal subjects. It seems clear that the highest chance of success will be earlier-stage patients whose prognosis is better and who are fully immunocompetent. There is also a question as to whether tumors might develop resistance to destruction by HPV-specific CTLs. It has been reported that some cervical tumors, particularly those at an advanced stage, may have defects in expression of MHC class I molecules,[16] which could compromise the effectiveness of immunotherapy in certain cases. Cervical cancer treatment has not advanced significantly over the past 20 years, however, and there remains a clear need for improvement, even on an incre-

mental basis. Indeed, it seems generally likely that cancer immunotherapy will find its place not as a stand-alone therapy, but rather as an adjunct to conventional methods of treatment, with the aim of eradicating minimal residual disease and hence lessening the chance of subsequent recurrence. As recurrent cervical cancer has an extremely poor prognosis, this would be an eminently worthwhile clinical goal.

REFERENCES

1. Abcarian H, Sharon N. (1982) Long term effectiveness of the immunotherapy of anal condyloma acuminata. *Dis Colon Rectum* **25**: 648–51.
2. Alexander J, Ruppert J, Page DM, *et al*, (1995) Antigen analogs as therapeutic agents. *Adv Exp Med Biol* **386**: 109–18.
3. Barr BB, Benton EC, McLaren K, *et al.* (1989) Human papillomavirus infection and skin cancer in renal allograft recipients. *Lancet* **1**: 124–9.
4. Bell JA, Sunberg JP, Ghim SJ, *et al.* (1994) A formalin-inactivated vaccine protects against mucosal papillomavirus infection: a canine model. *Pathobiology* **62**: 194–8.
5. Beutner K, Ferenczy A. (1997) Therapeutic approaches to genital warts. *Am J Med*, **102**(5A): 28–37.
6. Biberstein H. (1944) Immunization therapy of warts. *Arch Dermatol Syph* **50**: 12.
7. Borysiewicz LK, Fiander A, Nimako M, *et al.* (1996) A recombinant vaccinia virus encoding human papillomavirus types 16 and 18, E6 and E7 proteins as immunotherapy for cervical cancer. *Lancet* **347**: 1523–7.
8. Boursnell MEG, Rutherford E, Hickling JK, *et al.* (1996) Construction and characterisation of a recombinant vaccinia virus expressing human papillomavirus proteins for immunotherapy of cervical cancer. *Vaccine* **14**: 1485–94.
9. Breitburd F, Kirnbauer R, Hubbert NL, *et al.* (1995) Immunisation with virus-like particles from cottontail rabbit papillomavirus (CRPV) can protect against experimental CRPV infection. *J Virol* **69**: 3959–63.
10. Carter JJ, Wipf GC, Hagensee ME, *et al*, (1995) Use of human papillomavirus type 6 capsids to detect antibodies in people with genital warts. *J Infect Dis* **172**: 11–18.
11. Chen CH, Ji H, Suh KW, *et al*, (1999) Gene gun-mediated DNA vaccination induces antitumor immunity against human papillomavirus type 16 E7-expressing murine tumour metastases in the liver and lungs. *Gene Ther* **12**: 1972–81.
12. Chen L, Kinney Thomas E, Hu S-L, *et al.* (1991) Human papillomavirus type 16 nucleoprotein E7 is a tumor rejection antigen. *Proc Natl Acad Sci USA* **88**: 110–14.
13. Chen LP, Mizuno MT, Singhal MC, *et al.* (1992) Induction of cytotoxic T lymphocytes specific for a syngeneic tumor expressing the E6 oncoprotein of human papillomavirus type 16. *J Immunol* **148**: 2617–21.
14. Chu NR, Wu HB, Wu TC, *et al.* (2000) Immunotherapy of a human papillomavirus type 16 E7-expressing tumour by administration of fusion protein comprised of *M. bovis* BCG Hsp65 and HPV16 E7. *Clin Exp Immunol* **121**: 216–25.

15. Coleman N, Birley HDL, Renton AM, *et al.* (1994) Immunological events in regressing genital warts. *Am J Clin Path* **102**: 768–74.

16. Connor ME, Stern PL. (1990) Loss of of MHC class 1 expression in cervical carcinomas. *Int J Cancer* **46**: 1029–34.

17. Donnelly JJ, Martinez D, Jansen K, *et al.* (1996) Protection against papillomavirus with a polynucleotide vaccine. *J Infect Dis* **173**: 314–20.

18. Donnelly JJ, Ulmer JB, Shiver JW, *et al.* (1997) DNA vaccines. *Ann Rev Immunol* **15**: 617–48.

19. Dupuy C, Buzoni-Gatel D, Touze A, *et al.* (1999) Nasal immunization of mice with human papillomavirus type 16 (HPV16) virus-like particles or with the HPV16 L1 gene elicits specific cytotoxic T lymphocytes in vaginal draining lymph nodes. *J Virol* **73**: 9063–71.

20. Dürst M, Gissman L, Ikenberg H, *et al.* (1983) A papillomavirus DNA from a cervical carcinoma and its prevalence in cancer biopsy samples from different geographic regions. *Proc Natl Acad Sci USA* **80**: 3812–15.

21. Fiander AN, Adams M, Evans AS, *et al.* (1995) Immunocompetent for immunotherapy? A study of the immunocompetence of cervical cancer patients. *Int J Gynecol Cancer* **5**: 438–42.

22. Frazer IH. (1996) The role of vaccines in the control of STDs: HPV vaccines. *Genitourin Med* **72**: 398–403.

23. Germaine RN, Margulies DH. (1993) The biochemistry and cell biology of antigen processing and presentation. *Annu Rev of Immunol* **11**: 403–50.

24. Greenstone HL, Nieland JD, de Visser KE, *et al.* (1998) Chimeric papillomavirus-like particles elicit antitumor immunity against the E7 oncoprotein in an HPV16 tumor model. *Proc Natl Acad Sci USA* **17**: 1800–5.

25. Han R, Cladel NM, Reed CA, *et al.* (1999) Protection of rabbits from viral challenge by gene gun-based intracutaneous vaccination with a combination of cottontail rabbit papillomavirus E1, E2, E6 and E7 genes. *J Virol* **73**: 7039–43.

26. Jansen KU, Rosolowsky M, Schultz LD, *et al.* (1995) Vaccination with yeast expressed cottontail rabbit papillomavirus (CRPV) virus-like particles protects rabbits from CRPV-induced papilloma formation. *Vaccine* **13**: 1509–14.

27. Jarrett WFH, O'Neil BW, Gaukroger JM, *et al.* (1990) Studies on vaccination against papillomaviruses: the immunity after infection and vaccination with bovine papillomaviruses of different types. *Vet Rec* **126**: 473–5.

28. Jarrett WFH, Smith KT, O'Neil BW, *et al.* (1991) Studies on vaccination against papillomaviruses: prophylactic and therapeutic vaccination with recombinant structural proteins. *Virology* **184**: 33–42.

29. Kirnbauer R, Booy F, Cheng N, *et al.* (1992) Papillomavirus L1 major capsid protein self assembles into virus-like particles that are highly immunogenic. *Proc Natl Acad Sci USA* **89**: 12180–4.

30. Kirnbauer R, Chandrachud LM, O'Neil BW, *et al.* (1996) Virus-like particles of bovine papillomavirus type 4 in prophylactic and therapeutic immunsation. *Virology* **219**: 37–44.

31. Kirnbauer R, Taub J, Greenstone H, *et al.* (1993) Efficient self assembly of human papillomavirus type 16 L1 and L1 plus L2 into virus-like particles. *J Virol* **67**: 6923–36.

32. Knowles G, O'Neill BW, Campo MS. (1996) Phenotypical characterisation of lymphocytes infiltrating regressing papillomas. *J Virol* **70**: 8451–8.

33. Lacey C, Thompson HSG, Monteiro E. *et al.* (1999) Phase IIa safety and immunogenicity of a therapeutic vaccine, TA-GW, in persons with genital warts. *J Infect Dis* **179**: 612–18.

34. Lin KY, Guarnieri FG, Staveley-O'Carroll KF, *et al.* (1996) Treatment of established tumors with a novel vaccine that enhances major histocompatibility class II presentation of tumor antigen. *Cancer Res* **56**: 21–6.

35. Lin Y-L, Borenstein LA, Selvakumar R, *et al.* (1992) Effective vaccination against papillomavirus development by immunization with L1 or L2 structural protrein of cottontail rabbit papillomavirus. *Virology* **187**: 612–19.

36. Malison MD, Morris R, Jones LW. (1982) Autogenous vaccine: therapy for condyloma acuminatum. *Br J Vener Dis* **58**: 62–5.

37. Meneguzzi G, Cerni C, Kieny MP, *et al.* (1991) Immunization against human papillomavirus type 16 tumor cells with recombinant vaccinia viruses expressing E6 and E7. *Virology* **181**: 62–9.

38. Moore A, McGuirk P, Adams S, *et al.* (1995) Immunization with a soluble recombinant HIV protein entrapped in biodegradable microparticles induces HIV-specific CD8+ cytotoxic T lymphocytes and CD4+ Th1 cells. *Vaccine* **13**: 1741–9.

39. Muller M, Zhou J, Reed TD. (1997) Chimeric papillomavirus-like particles. *Virology* **234**: 93–111.

40. Nixon DF, Hioe C, Chen PD, *et al.* (1996) Synthetic peptides entrapped in microparticles can elicit cytotoxic T cell activity. *Vaccine* **14**: 1523–30.

41. Pilacinski WP, Glassman DL, Glassman KF, *et al.* (1986) Immunisation against bovine papillomavirus infection. *Ciba Found Symp* **120**: 136–56.

42. Ressing ME, Sette A, Brandt RM, *et al.* (1995) Human CTL epitopes encoded by human papillomavirus type 16 E6 and E7 identified through in vivo and in vitro immunogenicity studies of HLA-A*0201-binding peptides. *J Immunol* **154**: 5934–43.

43. Ressing ME, van Driel WJ, Brandt RM, *et al.* (2000) Detection of T helper responses, but not of human papillomavirus-specific cytotoxic T lymphocyte responses, after peptide vaccination of patients with cervical carcinoma. *J Immunother* **23**: 255–66.

44. Roden RBS, Greenstone HL, Kirnbauer R, *et al,* (1996) In vitro generation and type-specific neutralization of a human papillomavirus type 16 virion pseudotype. *J Virol* **70**: 5875–83.

45. Roden RBS, Hubbert NL, Kirnbauer R, *et al.* (1995) Papillomavirus L1 capsids agglutinate mouse erythrocytes through a proteinaceous receptor. *J Virol* **69**: 5147–51.

46. Roden RBS, Hubbert NL, Kirnbauer R, *et al.* (1996) Assessment of the serological relatedness of genital human papillomaviruses by hemagglutination inhibition. *J Virol* **70**: 3298–301.

47. Rose RC, Lane C, Wilson S, *et al.* (1999) Oral vaccination of mice with human papillomavirus virus-like particles induces systemic virus-neutralizing antibodies. *Vaccine* **17**: 2129–35.

48. Rose RC, Reichman RC, Bonnez W. (1994) Human papillomavirus (HPV) type 11 recombinant virus-like particles induce the formation of neutralizing antibodies and detect HPV-specific antibodies in human sera. *J Gen Virol* **75**: 2075–9.

49. Schafer K, Muller M, Faath S, *et al.* (1999) Immune response to human papillomavirus 16 L1E7 chimeric virus-like particles: induction of cytotoxic T cells and specific tumor protection. *Int J Cancer* **81**: 881–8.

50. Schiller JT. (2000) Human papillomavirus-like particle vaccines. *Abstract 18,* 3rd Annual Conference on Vaccine Research, April 30–May 2, Washington DC, USA.

51. Schwartz E, Freese UK, Gissman L, *et al.* (1985) Structure and transcription of human papillomavirus sequences in cervical carcinoma cells. *Nature* **314**: 111–14.

52. Selvakumar R, Borenstein LA, Lin Y-L, *et al.* (1995) Immunisation with non-structural proteins E1 and E2 of cottontail rabbit papillomavirus stimulates regression of virus-induced papillomas. *J Virol* **69**: 602–95.

53. Selvakumar R, Schmitt A, Iftner T, *et al.* (1997) Regression of papillomas induced by cottontail rabbit papillomavirus is associated with infiltration of CD8+ cells and persistence of viral DNA after regression. *J Virol* **71**: 5540–8.

54. Shope RE. (1935) Immunisation of rabbits to infectious papillomatosis. *J Exp Med* **65**: 219–31.

55. Sundaram P, Tigelaar RE, Brandsma JL, *et al.* (1997) Intracutaneous vaccination of rabbits with the cottontail rabbit papillomavirus (CPV) L1 gene protects against virus challenge. *Vaccine* **15**: 664–71.

56. Suzich JA, Ghim SJ, Palmer Hill FJ, *et al.* (1995) Systemic immunization with papillomavirus L1 protein completely prevents the development of viral mucosal papillomas. *Proc Natl Acad Sci USA* **92**: 11553–7.

57. Thompson HSG, Davies M, Holding FP, *et al* . (1999) Phase I safety and antigenicity of TA-GW: a recombinant HPV6 L2E7 vaccine for the treatment of genital warts. *Vaccine* **17**: 40–9.

58. van Driel WJ, Ressing ME, Brandt RM, *et al.* (1996) The current status of therapeutic HPV vaccines. *Ann Med* **28**: 471–7.

59. van Driel WJ, Ressing ME, Kenter GG, *et al.* (1999) Vaccination with HPV16 peptides of patients with advanced cervical carcinoma: clinical evaluation of a phase I-II trial. *Eur J Cancer* **35**: 946–52.

60. Vogel FR, Powell MF. (1995) A compendium of vaccine adjuvants and excipients. In *Vaccine design – the subunit and adjuvant approach,* eds MF Powell, MJ Newman. The Language of Science. Pharmaceutical Biotechnology Vol. 6. New York, Plenum Press, 141–227.

61. Wiltz OH, Torregrosa M, Wiltz O. (1995) Autogenous vaccine: The best therapy for perianal condyloma acuminata. *Dis Colon Rectum* **38**: 838–41.

62. Zhang W, Carmichael J, Inglis SC, *et al.* (1998) Expression of human papillomavirus type 16 L1 protein in *Escherichia coli* and denaturation/renaturation and self assembly of virus-like particles in vitro. *Virology* **243**: 423–31.

63. Zhang LF, Zhou J, Chen S, *et al.* (2000) HPV6b virus like particles are potent immunogens without adjuvant in man. *Vaccine* **18**: 1051–8.

64. Zhou J, Sun XY, Stenzel DJ, *et al.* (1991) Expression of vaccinia recombinant HPV 16 L1 and L2 ORF proteins in epithelial cells is sufficient for assembly of HPV virion-like particles. *Virology* **185**: 251–7.

13

Basic research

Stephen K. Tyring

13.1 INTRODUCTION

Vast knowledge has accumulated during the past few years regarding the molecular biology, pathogenesis, and immunology of human papillomaviruses (HPVs). As discussed in the preceding chapters, this knowledge has led to better detection methods for HPV as well as improved methods of therapy and prophylaxis.

Although HPV infections are very prevalent, lack of good *in vitro* systems to grow the virus as well as the fact that HPV does not produce disease in animal models have limited progress in this field. Nevertheless, basic research on the biology of HPV (Chapter 2) and the mechanisms of viral oncogenesis (Chapter 3) has led to a greater understanding of this pathogen. Similarly, basic studies on the immune response to HPV (Chapter 4) have been conducted by observing spontaneously regressing warts as well as warts treated with antiviral and/or immunomodulatory agents. The components of the immune system necessary to control HPV and its associated lesions have been better recognized from investigations involving specimens from patients whose immune systems were compromised toward a spectrum of infectious diseases (Chapter 10), as well as from studies of patients who were highly susceptible to only a few select HPV types (Chapter 9). Much of this knowledge, however, has been accumulated during the past decade and thus has not yet radically changed the treatment of the mucocutaneous manifestations of HPV (Chapters 5, 6, 7, and 8). In fact, in most of these clinical presentations, it is the lesion, not the viral infection, that is being treated. Likewise, the most prevalent method of detecting the presence of oncogenic HPV, i.e., the Pap smear, is indirect because it detects abnormal cytology but not the actual virus.

Over the past 3 years, however, basic science has led to improved immunologic/antiviral interventions for benign lesions (e.g., imiquimod) and is leading to both therapeutic and prophylactic HPV vaccines and to viral typing of cervical smears.

13.2 INTERACTIONS BETWEEN GENETIC AND ENVIRONMENTAL RISK FACTORS FOR HPV-ASSOCIATED MALIGNANCIES

While virological and serological evidence suggests that infection with oncogenic HPV is very common, it is fortunate that only a minority of patients infected with HPV actually develop malignancy. Although cervical cancer in the most studied manifestation of HPV oncogenesis, much remains to be learned regarding the genetic and environmental factors that allow the viral infection to progress to malignancy.

Approximately 500 000 women develop cervical cancer annually world-wide, and 200 000 die of this malignancy each year.[86,114] Although the exact mechanism(s) for the initiation of cervical carcinogenesis is unknown, it is well documented that persistent infection with high-risk HPVs (e.g., HPV 16, and 18) is a major risk factor.[45,104,126] HPV-infected basal cells of the differentiating cervical epithelium may establish low-grade cervical intraepithelial neoplasias (CIN 1), which may regress, persist, or progress.[8,104,127] The likelihood of spontaneous regression of a diagnosed CIN 1 is 50–60%.[8]

High viral loads promote the progression of high-grade CIN (CIN 2–3) to invasive cancer (squamous cell carcinoma, SCC),[128] and p53 inactivation is definitely involved in this process.[8,34] Consequently, a large body of research has elucidated in great detail the molecular biology of HPV function in tumorigenesis.[8] Interestingly, HPV infections are very common in many populations,[74] but infection with high-risk HPVs is frequently found in asymptomatic individuals.[160] Thus,[52,144,147] HPV alone is not sufficient to account for the etiology of cervical cancer and a multifactorial etiology is likely.[60] An important research priority is to identify the additional factors, particularly their interaction with HPV, which may contribute to cervical cancer progression. One factor that requires considerable attention is cigarette smoking, with many epidemiological studies demonstrating a significant increase in relative risk for cervical cancer associated with this exposure.[8,74,75,108] Understanding the precise interactions between these risk factors and cervical cancer will facilitate the implementation of more effective disease-prevention programs.

The factors determining the progression of CIN 2–3 to squamous cell carcinoma are unknown, but are likely to include both environmental and genetic susceptibility influences.[58,100] This is supported by epidemiological evidence for a genetic predisposition to cervical cancer and its precursor forms.[92] After taking HPV into account, smoking is the most significant environmental risk factor for cervical cancer.[17,22,81,117] Smoking has been associated with a 2.6-fold increased risk (confidence interval 1.7–4.0) for CIN 2–3, and the effect was dose dependent ($p = 0.002$).[81] The biologic plausibility of this association is strengthened by the finding of cigarette-derived mutagenic chemicals in cervical mucus,[66] and cigarette smoke-specific DNA adducts in cervical epithelial cells.[134] Using animal models as prototypes, it has been proposed that the etiology of cervical cancers in humans could be an interaction between HPV and tar exposure through cigarette smoking and/or tar-based vaginal douching.[60] On the other hand, the cessation of cigarette smoking has been associated with a size reduction of CIN lesions.[145] Genetic differences in the metabolism of carcinogens may co-determine individual predisposition to cancer.[87,154] Future studies, therefore, will need to investigate polymorphic CYP2E1, mEH, and GSTM1 metabolizing genes that are known to biotransform cigarette smoke chemicals. It should be emphasized that, to date, the role of these genes in the susceptibility to cervical cancer has not been elucidated.

CYP2E1 activates several known tobacco-smoke carcinogens, including N-nitrosamines [e.g., 4-(methylnitrosamino)-1-(3-pyridyl)-1-butanone, NNK), benzene, styrene, butadiene, and urethane.[119] Several investigators[21,61,148,150,158] have shown that a variant form of the gene (CYP2E1*) detected by either Rsa1 or Pst1 enzyme digestion is expressed at higher levels than the wild type, and therefore it has greater ability to activate certain substrates.[21,158] The frequency of this allelic variant is from 6% to 16% among different ethnic groups.[6,40,44,98,164] CYP2E1* has been associated with the development of lung cancer[40,115] and nasopharyngeal carcinoma.[71,72] This allele may also have an important role in cervical carcinogenesis because of the high concentrations of NNK found in the cervical mucus of smokers compared to non-smokers.[118] mEH contributes to the bioac-

tivation of benzo[a]pyrene, a cigarette-smoke constituent, to the highly carcinogenic benzo[a]pyrene-diolepoxide (BPDE).[51] mEH is also a key participant in chemical detoxification pathways, catalysing the hydrolysis of reactive epoxides generated by cytochrome P450 enzymes to more water-soluble dihydrodiol derivatives.[59] Interindividual differences in mEH activity ranging in scale from several to 40-fold[109,129] can be attributed to genetic polymorphisms at two residue positions within the coding region of the gene: residue 113 Tyr/Hist and residue 139 Arg/Hist.[50,58] Substitution at residue 113 has been shown to decrease mEH activity by approximately 40% in vitro.[58] Among Caucasian individuals, about 40% are homozygous for [113]Tyr.[59] Polymorphic variants of mEH have been associated with hepatocellular cancer (His-113 allele), chronic obstructive pulmonary disease (His-113 allele), and ovarian cancer (Tyr-113 allele).[68]

GSTM1 belongs to the glutathione S-transferase family, which represents a major group of detoxification enzymes.[97] GSTM1 plays an important role in detoxification of chemical carcinogens (e.g., benzo[a]pyrene)[51] either by binding them directly or by conjugating glutathione to their reactive electrophilic sites.[97] Approximately 50% of the population have the homozygous deletion of the gene,[13,57,79] and this GSTM1*0 (null) allelic variance may impose susceptibility. An association between the GSTM1*0 genotype and susceptibility to several types of cancer has been reported.[6,11,23,29,39,56,62,73,78,99,161,165]

CYP2E1 acts coordinately with mEH in the bioactivation of several cigarette-derived chemicals, leading to the formation of diol-intermediates[87,135] that are further metabolized by GSTM1.[15,49,54] Some of these reactive metabolites can bind to DNA to initiate a series of events that may lead to tumor formation.[154,163] Therefore, a major need is to determine whether women with an early cancer onset are better identified by certain combinations of the variant alleles from these polymorphic metabolizing genes.

Epidemiological evidence suggests that the presence of HPV, when combined with smoking behaviors, considerably enhances the risk of developing oral, cervical, vulvar, and/or anal carcinomas.[18] The importance of etiologic cofactors like smoking, however, may vary by geographic region,[126] which may be partly determined by the ethnic-dependent distribution of variant metabolizing genes that confer susceptibility to cigarette smoke. Warwick et al.[157] showed that inheritance of GSTM1 null or the combination GSTT1 null/GSTM1 null did not appear to influence susceptibility to CIN or squamous cell carcinoma. However, they did not type for HPV; therefore, interactions between these risk factors were not established. More recently, Chen and Nirunsuksiri[24] have shown that GSTM1 mRNA levels of HPV-transfected human cervical keratinocytes were much lower than those of parental cells, suggesting that HPV infection may down-regulate GSTM1 expression. This observation may explain the lack of association as reported by Warwick et al.[157] On the other hand, CYP2E1 and mEH gene expression was detected in primary and HPV-immortalized oral and cervical epithelial cultures.[43] Although the overall impact of HPV infection on the expression of these systems remains to be fully elucidated, these in vitro findings provide support for examining the association between HPV and genetic susceptibility to smoking in the etiology of cervical cancer.

Among the different types of HPV which infect the cervical epithelial cells, HPV 16 and HPV 18 appear to exert their proliferative and oncogenic effects through an increase in viral oncogene expression (HPV E6),[166] acting primarily on inactivation of the p53 protein.[27,53,116,159] An alternative mode of inactivation of p53 is by somatic gene mutation,[28] from exposure to mutagens such as cigarette-smoke chemicals.[33] Inactivation of p53, whether by HPV E6 or gene mutation, results in the loss of p53 function to cause genomic instability and/or abnormal control of cell proliferation.[25,55] Cervical cancers with mutated p53 have a worse prognosis even without HPV infection.[69] Although mutagenic inactivation of p53 occurs much less frequently than protein inactivation in cervical cancer,[65] the former mechanism appears to be involved in the progression from CIN 2–3 to squamous cell carcinoma, being present in 15% and 30% of the cases, respectively.[34] Among these tumors, however, only a small proportion of cells showed mutagenic p53 inactivation.[34] Therefore, potential interactions between both mutagenic and HPV-E6 inactivation of p53 may occur in the development of cervical cancer.

Other evidence further supports this possibility. For example, in response to DNA damage, at least 11 post-translational modifications (e.g., phosphorylation) of p53 have been identified.[20] It is further postulated that redundant modifications might be necessary to provide a fail-safe mechanism.[20] Therefore, duplicated inactivating mechanisms may be needed to develop cervical cancer, and such a possibility has not been investigated. In addition, tumors are known to be made up of heterogeneous cancer cells, possibly due to their different rates of accumulation of gene mutations.[89] Consequently, some cervical cancers might be made up of cancer cells having p53 that is inactivated by different mechanisms. Women carrying susceptibility metabolizing genes may have an increased burden of cigarette-smoke-induced mutagenic damage. The induced damage may collaborate with the p53 inactivation mechanism to enhance the induction of cervical cancer. To date, there are no data on the potential interactions between the two p53 inactivation mechanisms and genetic susceptibility for early disease onset. Therefore, these interactions should be analysed in patients with varying grades of cervical disease, with potential implications for early diagnosis and prevention.

13.3 INTERACTIONS BETWEEN IMMUNE SUPPRESSION AND PROGRESSION TO MALIGNANCY

Immune suppression may lead to proliferation of HPV-related benign lesions as well as to progression of oncogenic HPV infection to malignancy. Immunosuppression appears in many forms, such as the iatrogenic immunosuppression seen in organ transplant patients and immunosuppression due to infection with human immunodeficiency virus (HIV). Paradoxically, whereas HIV-related morbidity and mortality have declined significantly in most patients taking combination anti-retroviral therapy, cervical dysplasia and carcinoma continue to be major problems in HIV-seropositive women. Most recently, however, significant increases in anal dysplasia

and carcinoma have been reported in HIV-seropositive individuals. HIV and HPV may interact at multiple levels. For example, HIV infection may result in the attenuation of systemic cell-mediated immunity against HPV, and/or HIV proteins could transactive the HPV promoter. The target cell for HIV, however, is different from that for HPV. Furthermore, HPV progression appears to correlate more closely with HIV RNA levels than with CD4 counts. Thus, the lack of systemic immunosurveillance or putative viral–viral interactions does not completely explain the role of HIV in the progression of HPV-associated diseases.

A newly emerging concept is that HIV infection may lead to aberrant cytokine expression at the tissue level, which could modulate HPV gene expression. Indeed, the cytokine microenvironment of the genital mucosa changes significantly in HIV infection and is characterized by the predominance of T-helper (Th2) cytokines.

Several studies have reported that HIV-infected women are approximately four times more likely to be infected with HPV than are women not infected with HIV.[82] These infections are also more likely to persist and be associated with the HPV types that are strongly linked to the development of high-grade squamous intraepithelial lesions (SILs) and invasive cancer,[19,103,143,151] and these persistent infections may explain the increased incidence of cervical dysplasias in women infected with HIV.[14,19,121,130] Moreover, CINs in HIV-positive patients may be of a higher grade than those in HIV-negative patients, with more extensive involvement of the lower genital tract.[95] Data have also demonstrated that HIV infection may cause a more rapid progression of CINs to invasive carcinoma,[1,76] and cervical carcinomas are more aggressive than in their HIV-negative counterparts.[94] Furthermore, HPV-associated lesions may be more difficult to treat in HIV-infected women.[82] Taken together, cervical cancer is an important acquired immune deficiency syndrome (AIDS)-defining illness and may be the most common AIDS-related malignancy in women.[93] It is interesting that HIV infection affects the natural history of anal HPV infection in a similar manner.[26,85,111–113]

HPV infection is under the control of the innate immune system.[47,96,101,138] A low peripheral blood CD4 count is associated with the presence of multiple and oncogenic HPV types in the lower genital tract.[7,77,125,137,151] Also, the incidence of SILs and the progression rate of low-grade SILs to high-grade SILs were significantly higher in HIV-positive individuals with low CD4 counts.[136] A widely accepted explanation is that the increase in HPV-associated lesions seen in HIV-infected individuals might be expected to occur primarily as a result of systemic immunosuppression,[125] in a manner analogous to that seen in organ transplant patients.[110,132,133]

The relationship between HIV infection and HPV-associated disease, however, is probably more complex than it might seem at first glance. A primary means by which HIV infection may influence the pathogenesis of HPV-associated cervical lesions is molecular interaction between HIV and HPV genes. Indeed, up-regulation of HPV early genes by HIV-*tat* has been demonstrated *in vitro*.[146,152] Conversely, HIV has not been detected *in vivo* in keratinocytes,[106] which are primary targets of HPV infection.[12] Other studies, however, suggested the co-localization of the two viruses.[67,153] Recently, Dolei *et al.* have demonstrated that HIV infection increases HPV activity in an HIV-transmissive, HPV-positive cell line.[35]

A recent epidemiological study showed that persistence of anal HPV was associated in HIV-infected men with the presence of HIV DNA in the anal canal but not with CD4+ lymphocyte count, a measure of immune competence.[26] Another study demonstrated that the presence of oncogenic HPV DNA in the cervix and abnormal Pap smears are highly associated with plasma levels of HIV-1 RNA.[91] Also, regression of SILs occurred in patients treated with anti-retroviral therapy despite the persistence of high-risk HPV infection.[63] Moreover, there was no significant difference in either the decrease in plasma HIV load or the increase in CD4+ cell count between patients with regressing and non-regressing lesions. Whatever the explanation for these findings, they demonstrate that the *relationship between HPV-associated lesions and HIV infections cannot be explained simply by systemic immune dysfunction.*

Recently, Dolei *et al.* hypothesized that the increase of HPV shedding and of HPV-associated diseases in HIV-infected individuals could be due in part to a direct cytokine-mediated action of HIV, in addition to the HIV-induced systemic immunodeficiency.[35] Indeed, HIV infection substantially changes the cytokine expression of lymphocytes and macrophages.[16] The paradigm of the switch from Thl to Th2 cytokine patterns during HIV infection is well known.[102,122] Accordingly, HPV-infected cells are exposed to viral and cellular factors released within the tissue both by resident and by HIV-infected infiltrating cells.[2,4,41,42,102,120,142] At an early stage, the expression of interferon-alpha (IFN-α), IFN-γ, and transforming growth-factor-β (TGF-β), was found to be the most prevalent.[120] Peak expression of interleukin-4 (IL-4), IL-5, IL-6, and IL-10 was seen during the intermediate stage, and peak expression of tumor necrosis factor-α (TNF-α) and IL-Iβ was found in AIDS patients.[120] IL-10 expression is significant in the genital mucosa and in cervical mucus during HIV infection.[107,131] Moreover, this IL-10 expression was independent of peripheral or local CD4 counts.[107] Also, cytokine expression correlates with the level of HIV transcripts in HIV-infected cells.[88]

Pre-malignant progression seems to be accompanied by an increase in viral oncogene expression, which continues in the course of cancer progression. Only very weak transcription of early genes takes place in the replication-competent basal layers of low-grade SILs.[37] In contrast, transcription of the E6/E7 region is de-repressed in high-grade SILs and cancers, as demonstrated by evenly distributed signals throughout undifferentiated epithelium or cancer cells following RNA *in situ* hybridization.[37,70]

HPV gene transcription is regulated through the upper regulatory region (URR) of the HPV genome,[12,48] by cellular regulatory proteins such as AP-l, NFl, TEF1, YY1, NF-IL6, etc., which bind to the transcriptional enhancer. Cytokines are important regulators of HPV transcription,[80,83] and inflammatory cytokines, such as IFN-α, IFN-γ, IL-l, TNF-α and IL-6, inhibit mRNA levels of HPV genes through mostly unknown mechanisms.[9,31,83,105,162] Interestingly, IL-6 has also been found to increase the expression of HPV,[35] an observation in contrast to that found by others.[9,83]

Inflammatory cytokines probably exert their effects on HPV transcription through transcription factors that bind and affect the activity of the HPV promoter(s). For instance, repression of the URR activity has been demonstrated via NF-IL6 binding after IL-1 or TNF-α treatment.[84] However, the effects of anti-inflammatory (Th2-type) cytokines on HPV transcription are basically unknown. Altered cytokine profiles by HIV might enhance the activity of the HPV promoter.

Upon engagement with their receptors, various cytokines such as IFNs, ILs, TNFs, as well as epidermal growth factor (EGF) induce phosphorylation of specific transcription factors (STATs), which assemble to form transcription factor complexes (ISGF3 and STAT homodimers).[30,64,123,139,141] After translocation to the nucleus, these factors bind to specific DNA sites in the promoters of various responsive genes.[32,90] An imbalance between the available STAT factors might result in altered responses to cytokines.[124,156] Co-expression of various cytokines might lead to conflicting signals and, thus, to cross-inhibition of cytokine signaling.[10] This may be the case in the HIV-infected cervix in which pro-inflammatory and anti-inflammatory cytokines as well as various growth factors are present.

Inhibition of cytokine signaling could be achieved through a variety of negative regulators that curtail the biological response of cytokines. The families SOCS (suppressor of cytokine signaling) and PIAS (protein inhibitor of activated STAT) proteins are activated via various cytokines and suppress the JAK/STAT pathway at the level of tyrosine phosphorylation or by preventing STAT binding, respectively.[3,140] IL-10 is known to activate SOCS expression, leading to inhibition of inflammatory responses in monocytes.[36] Similarly, during HIV infection, the persisting IL-10 might represent a negative constraint for inflammatory cytokine signaling through regulation of SOCS/PIAS levels and result in a lack of HPV inhibition.

Thus, further investigations into the relationships between HIV, HPV, Th2 cytokines, and transcription factors may lead to better understanding and control of HPV oncogenesis in immunocompromised individuals.

13.4 DEVELOPMENT OF BETTER ANTIVIRAL AGENTS, IMMUNOMODULATORY DRUGS, AND HPV VACCINES

Only one antiviral agent, IFN-α, is approved for the therapy of HPV-associated lesions. Due to the need for multiple injections, cost, and the frequency of systemic side-effects, IFN-α never became a widely accepted therapy for HPV infections.

Imiquimod is an immunomodulatory drug, available in a topical formulation that acts, at least partially, via the induction of such antiviral proteins as IFN-α.[149] It is highly effective for the treatment of anogenital warts,[38] and is currently being evaluated for non-anogenital warts as well as for cervical dysplasia.

Another antiviral drug, cidofovir, appears promising for the therapy of HPV-associated benign lesions in case reports of small series of patients. Large controlled trials of cidofovir for HPV have not been reported, nor is it available in a topical formulation. *In vitro* studies of antisense oligonucleotides appeared very promising, but clinical trials did not support their efficacy.

In general, vaccines have been the most effective intervention for the control of viral diseases. Vaccines are also the most cost-effective intervention. Basic studies of HPV proteins and the immune response to these antigens are at the center of vaccine research. All existing viral vaccines are used only for prophylaxis. However, some HPV vaccines are being evaluated for therapy, while other HPV vaccines are being studied for prophylaxis. Thus far, clinical trials for HPV vaccines have only reached the phase I/II stage. Laboratory studies of the immune responses are ongoing regarding the induction of humoral immunity (especially mucosal immunity) and cell-mediated immunity. Questions to be answered include:

- Which antigens are most immunogenic?
- What type of immunity is important for protection against HPV and/or to clear infection?
- What are the immunologic laboratory correlates of successful vaccination?

An effective surrogate system for testing neuralizing antibody *in vitro* would markedly speed HPV vaccine development.[46]

13.5 CONCLUSION

In conclusion, many questions remain to be answered in the basic research laboratory, but data generated during the past decade have markedly increased our understanding of the molecular biology of HPV as well as of the immune response to HPV-associated antigens. Enhanced knowledge of the necessary components of an effective immune response to HPV can be gained from studies of people with significant defects in their immune systems. Another approach is to study the immune parameters of women who have undergone spontaneous remission of oncogenic HPV infection in their cervices.[155] There appears to be a range of genetic susceptibilities to HPV as well as to certain cofactors that may promote HPV oncogenesis. Thus, genetic analyses will lead to greater understanding of virus/host interactions. Such studies have the potential to result in better antiviral agents and immune modulators as well as to effective HPV vaccines, both prophylactic and therapeutic.

REFERENCES

1. Abercrombie PD, Korn AP. (1998) Lower genital tract neoplasia in women with HIV infection. *Oncology (Huntingt)* **12**: 1735–9; discussion 1742, 1745, 1747.
2. Akridge RE, Oyafuso LK, Reed SG. (1994) IL-10 is induced during HIV-1 infection and is capable of decreasing viral replication in human macrophages. *J Immunol* **153**: 5782–9.
3. Alexander WS, Starr R, Metcalf D, *et al.* (1999) Suppressors of cytokine signaling (SOCS): negative regulators of signal transduction. *J Leukoc Biol* **66**: 588–92.
4. Ameglio F, Cordiali Fei P, Solmone M, *et al.* (1994) Serum IL-10 levels in HIV-positive subjects: correlation with CDC stages. *J Biol Regul Homeost Agents* **8**: 48–52.
5. Anderson MC, Brown CL, Buckley CH, *et al.* (1991) Current views on cervical intraepithelial neoplasia [see comments]. *J Clin Pathol* **44**: 969–78.
6. Anwar WA, Abdel-Rahman SZ, El-Zein RA, Mostafa HM, Au WW. (1996) Genetic polymorphism of GSTM1, CYP2E1 and CYP2D6 in Egyptian bladder cancer patients. *Carcinogenesis* **17**: 1923–9.
7. Arany I, Tyring SK. (1998) Systemic immunosuppression by HIV infection influences HPV transcription and thus local immune responses in condylomas. *Int J AIDS STD* **9**: 268–71.
8. Arends MJ, Buckley CH, Wells M. (1998) Aetiology, pathogenesis, and pathology of cervical neoplasia. *J Clin Pathol* **51**: 96–103.
9. Bauknecht T, Randelzhofer B, Schmitt B, Ban Z, Hernando JJ. (1999) Response to IL-6 of HPV-18 cervical carcinoma cell lines. *Virology* **258**: 344–54.
10. Begley CG, Nicola NA. (1999) Resolving conflicting signals: cross inhibition of cytokine signaling pathways. *Blood* **93**: 1443–7.
11. Bell DA, Taylor JA, Paulson DF, Robertson CN, Mohler JL, Lucier GW. (1993) Genetic risk and carcinogen exposure: a common inherited defect of the carcinogen-metabolism gene glutathione S-transferase M1 (GSTM1) that increases susceptibility to bladder cancer. *J Natl Cancer Inst* **85**: 1159–64.
12. Bernard H-U, Apt D. (1994) Transcriptional control and cell type specificity of HPV gene expression. *Arch Dermatol* **130**: 210–15.
13. Board PG. (1981) Biochemical genetics of glutathione-S-transferase in man. *Am J Hum Genet* **33**: 36–43.
14. Boccalon M, Tirelli U, Sopracordevole F, Vaccher E. (1996) Intra-epithelial and invasive cervical neoplasia during HIV infection. *Eur J Cancer* **32A**: 2212–17.
15. Bond JA, Csanady GA, Leavens T, Medinsky MA. (1993) Research strategy for assessing target tissue dosimetry of 1,3-butadiene in laboratory animals and humans. Cleveland, OH, IARC Sci Publishers, 45–55.
16. Bornemann CMA, Verhoef J, Paterson PK. (1997) Macrophages, cytokines and HIV. *J Lab Clin Med* **129**: 10–16.
17. Bornstein J, Rahat MA, Abramovici H. (1995) Etiology of cervical cancer: current concepts. *Obstet Gynecol Surv* **50**: 146–54.
18. Bosch FX, Cardis E. (1990) Cancer incidence correlations: genital, urinary and some tobacco- related cancers. *Int J Cancer* **46**: 178–84.
19. Cappiello G, Garbuglia AR, Salvi R, *et al.* (1997) HIV infection increases the risk of squamous intra-epithelial lesions in women with HPV infection: an analysis of HPV genotypes. DIANAIDS Collaborative Study Group. *Int J Cancer* **72**: 982–6.
20. Carr AM. (2000) Cell cycle. Piecing together the p53 puzzle. *Science* **287**: 1765–6.
21. Carriere V, Berthou F, Baird S, Belloc C, Beaune P, de Groot IW. (1996) Human cytochrome P450 2E1 (CYP2E1): from genotype to phenotype. *Pharmacogenetics* **6**: 203–11.
22. Cavalcanti SM, Zardo LG, Passos MR, Oliveira LH. (2000) Epidemiological aspects of human papillomavirus infection and cervical cancer in Brazil. *J Infect* **40**: 80–7.

23. Charrier J, Maugard CM, Le Mevel B, Bignon YJ. (1999) Allelotype influence at glutathione S-transferase M1 locus on breast cancer susceptibility. *Br J Cancer* **79**: 346–53.

24. Chen C, Nirunsuksiri W. (1999) Decreased expression of glutathione S-transferase M1 in HPV16-transfected human cervical keratinocytes in culture. *Carcinogenesis* **20**: 699–703.

25. Coursen JD, Bennett WP, Gollahon L, Shay JW, Harris CC. (1997) Genomic instability and telomerase activity in human bronchial epithelial cells during immortalization by human papillomavirus-16 E6 and E7 genes. *Exp Cell Res* **235**: 245–53.

26. Critchlow CW, Hawes SE, Kuypers JM, *et al.* (1998) Effect of HIV infection on the natural history of anal human papillomavirus infection. *AIDS* **12**: 1177–84.

27. Crook T, Fisher C, Masterson PJ, Vousden KH. (1994) Modulation of transcriptional regulatory properties of p53 by HPV E6. *Oncogene* **9**: 1225–30.

28. Crook T, Wrede D, Tidy JA, Mason WP, Evans DJ, Vousden KH. (1992) Clonal p53 mutation in primary cervical cancer: association with human-papillomavirus-negative tumours. *Lancet* **339**: 1070–3.

29. Daly AK, Thomas DJ, Cooper J, Pearson WR, Neal DE, Idle JR. (1993) Homozygous deletion of gene for glutathione S-transferase M1 in bladder cancer. *BMJ* **307**: 481–2.

30. Darnell JE Jr. (1996) The JAK-STAT pathway: summary of initial studies and recent advances. *Recent Prog Horm Res* **51**: 391–403; discussion 403–4.

31. De Marco F, Di Lonardo A, Venuti A, Marcante ML. (1991) Interferon inhibition of neoplastic phenotype in cell lines harbouring human papillomavirus sequences. *J Biol Regulat Homeostat Agents* **5**: 65–70.

32. Decker T, Kovarik P, Meinke A. (1997) GAS elements: a few nucleotides with a major impact on cytokine-induced gene expression. *J Interferon Cytokine Res* **17**: 121–34.

33. Denissenko MF, Pao A, Tang M, Pfeifer GP. (1996) Preferential formation of benzo[a]pyrene adducts at lung cancer mutational hotspots in P53. *Science* **274**: 430–2.

34. Dimitrakakis C, Kymionis G, Diakomanolis E, *et al.* (2000) The possible role of p53 and bcl-2 expression in cervical carcinomas and their premalignant lesions. *Gynecol Oncol* **77**: 129–36.

35. Dolei A, Curreli S, Marongiu P, *et al.* (1999) Human immunodeficiency virus infection in vitro activates naturally integrated human papillomavirus type 18 and induces synthesis of the L1 capsid protein. *J Gen Virol* **80**: 2937–44.

36. Donnelly RP, Dickensheets H, Finbloom DS. (1999) The interleukin-10 signal transduction pathway and regulation of gene expression in mononuclear phagocytes. *J Interferon Cytokine Res* **19**: 563–73.

37. Durst M, Glitz D, Schneider A, zur Hausen H. (1992) Human papillomavirus type 16 (HPV 16) gene expression and DNA replication in cervical neoplasia: analysis by *in situ* hybridization. *Virology* **189**: 132–40.

38. Edwards L, Ferenczy A, Eron L, *et al.* (1998) Self-administered topical 5% imiquimod cream for external anogenital warts. *Arch Dermatol* **134**: 25–30.

39. El-Zein R, Zwischenberger JB, Wood TG, bdel-Rahman SZ, Brekelbaum C, Au WW. (1997) Combined genetic polymorphism and risk for development of lung cancer. *Mutat Res* **381**: 189–200.

40. El-Zein RA, Zwischenberger JB, Abdel-Rahman SZ, Sankar AB, Au WW. (1997) Polymorphism of metabolizing genes and lung cancer histology: prevalence of CYP2E1 in adenocarcinoma. *Cancer Lett* **112**: 71–8.

41. Emilie D, Fior R, Jarrousse B, *et al.* (1994) Cytokines in HIV infection. *Int J Immunopharmacol* **16**: 391–6.

42. Fan J, Bass HZ, Fahey JL. (1993) Elevated IFN-gamma and decreased IL-2 gene expression are associated with HIV infection. *J Immunol* **151**: 5031–40.

43. Farin FM, Bigler LG, Oda D, McDougall JK, Omiecinski CJ. (1995) Expression of cytochrome P450 and microsomal epoxide hydrolase in cervical and oral epithelial cells immortalized by human papillomavirus type 16 E6/E7 genes. *Carcinogenesis* **16**: 1391–401.

44. Farker K, Lehmann MH, Kastner R, *et al.* (1998) CYP2E1 genotyping in renal cell/urothelial cancer patients in comparison with control populations. *Int J Clin Pharmacol Ther* **36**: 463–8.

45. Franco EL. (1997) Understanding the epidemiology of genital infection with oncogenic and nononcogenic human papillomaviruses: a promising lead for primary prevention of cervical cancer. *Cancer Epidemiol Biomarkers Prev* **6**: 759–61.

46. Frazer IH. (1996) The role of vaccine in the control of STDs: HPV vaccines. *Genitourin Med* **72**: 398–403.

47. Frazer IH, Tindle RW. (1996) Cell mediated immunity to papillomaviruses. In *Papillomavirus reviews: Current research on papillomaviruses*, ed. C. Lacey. Leeds, Leeds University Press, 151–63.

48. Fuchs PG, Pfister H. (1994) Transcription of papillomavirus genomes. *Intervirology* **37**: 159–67.

49. Gadberry MG, DeNicola DB, Carlson GP. (1996) Pneumotoxicity and hepatotoxicity of styrene and styrene oxide. *J Toxicol Environ Health* **48**: 273–94.

50. Gaedigk A, Spielberg SP, Grant DM. (1994) Characterization of the microsomal epoxide hydrolase gene in patients with anticonvulsant adverse drug reactions. *Pharmacogenetics* **4**: 142–53.

51. Gelboin HV. (1980) Benzo[alpha]pyrene metabolism, activation and carcinogenesis: role and regulation of mixed-function oxidases and related enzymes. *Physiol Rev* **60**: 1107–66.

52. Giuliano AR, Papenfuss M, Schneider A, Nour M, Hatch K. (1999) Risk factors for high-risk type human papillomavirus infection among Mexican-American women. *Cancer Epidemiol Biomark Prev* **8**: 615–20.

53. Gu Z, Pim D, Labrecque S, Banks L, Matlashewski G. (1994) DNA damage induced p53 mediated transcription is inhibited by human papillomavirus type 18 E6. *Oncogene* **9**: 629–33.

54. Gut I, Nedelcheva V, Soucek P, Stopka P, Tichavska B. (1996) Cytochromes P450 in benzene metabolism and involvement of their metabolites and reactive oxygen species in toxicity. *Environ Health Perspect* **104**(Suppl. 6): 1211–18.

55. Hall PA, Lane DP. (1994) Genetics of growth arrest and cell death: key determinants of tissue homeostasis. *Eur J Cancer* **30A**: 2001–12.

56. Hand PA, Inskip A, Gilford J, *et al.* (1996) Allelism at the glutathione S-transferase GSTM3 locus: interactions with GSTM1 and GSTT1 as risk factors for astrocytoma. *Carcinogenesis* **17**: 1919–22.

57. Harada S, Abei M, Tanaka N, Agarwal DP, Goedde HW. (1987) Liver glutathione S-transferase polymorphism in Japanese and its pharmacogenetic importance. *Hum Genet* **75**: 322–5.

58. Hassett C, Aicher L, Sidhu JS, Omiecinski CJ. (1994) Human microsomal epoxide hydrolase: genetic polymorphism and functional expression in vitro of amino acid variants [published erratum appears in *Hum Mol Genet* (1994) **3**: 1214]. *Hum Mol Genet* **3**: 421–8.

59. Hassett C, Lin J, Carty CL, Laurenzana EM, Omiecinski CJ. (1997) Human hepatic microsomal epoxide hydrolase: comparative analysis of polymorphic expression. *Arch Biochem Biophys* **337**: 275–83.

60. Haverkos H, Rohrer M, Pickworth W. (2000) The cause of invasive cervical cancer could be multifactorial. *Biomed Pharmacother* **54**: 54–9.

61. Hayashi S, Watanabe J, Kawajiri K. (1991) Genetic polymorphisms in the 5′-flanking region change transcriptional regulation of the human cytochrome P450IIE1 gene. *J Biochem (Tokyo)* **110**: 559–65.

62. Heagerty AH, Fitzgerald D, Smith A, *et al.* (1994) Glutathione S-transferase GSTM1 phenotypes and protection against cutaneous tumours. *Lancet* **343**: 266–8.

63. Heard I, Schmitz V, Costagliola D, Orth G, Kazatchkine MD. (1998) Early regression of cervical lesions in HIV-seropositive women receiving highly active antiretroviral therapy. *AIDS* **12**: 1459–64.

64. Heim MH. (1999) The JAK-STAT pathway: cytokine signaling from the receptor to the nucleus. *J Recep Sig Trans Res* **19**: 75–120.

65. Helland A, Holm R, Kristensen G, *et al.* (1993) Genetic alterations of the TP53 gene, p53 protein expression and HPV infection in primary cervical carcinomas. *J Pathol* **171**: 105–14.

66. Hellberg D, Nilsson S, Haley NJ, Hoffman D, Wynder E. (1988) Smoking and cervical intraepithelial neoplasia: nicotine and cotinine in serum and cervical mucus in smokers and nonsmokers. *Am J Obstet Gynecol* **158**: 910–13.

67. Heng MC, Heng SY, Allen SG. (1994) Co-infection and synergy of human immunodeficiency virus-1 and herpes simplex virus-l. *Lancet* **343**: 255–8.

68. Hengstler JG, Arand M, Herrero ME, Oesch F. (1998) Polymorphisms of N-acetyltransferases, glutathione S-transferases, microsomal epoxide hydrolase and sulfotransferases: influence on cancer susceptibility. *Recent Results Cancer Res* **154**: 47–85.

69. Higgins GD, Davy M, Roder D, Uzelin DM, Phillips GE, Burrell CJ. (1991) Increased age and mortality associated with cervical carcinomas negative for human papillomavirus RNA. *Lancet* **338**: 910–13.

70. Higgins GD, Uzelin DM, Phillips GE, McEvoy P, Matin R, Burrell CJ. (1992) Transcription patterns of human papillomavirus type 16 in genital intraepithelial neoplasia: evidence for promoter usage within the E7 open reading frame during epithelial differentiation. *J Gen Virol* **73**: 2047–57.

71. Hildesheim A, Anderson LM, Chen CJ, *et al.* (1997) CYP2E1 genetic polymorphisms and risk of nasopharyngeal carcinoma in Taiwan. *J Natl Cancer Inst* **89**: 1207–12.

72. Hildesheim A, Chen CJ, Caporaso NE, *et al.* (1995) Cytochrome P4502E1 genetic polymorphisms and risk of nasopharyngeal carcinoma: results from a case-control study conducted in Taiwan. *Cancer Epidemiol Biomark Prev* **4**: 607–10.

73. Hirvonen A, Husgafvel-Pursiainen K, Anttila S, Vainio H. (1993) The GSTM1 null genotype as a potential risk modifier for squamous cell carcinoma of the lung. *Carcinogenesis* **14**: 1479–81.

74. Ho GY, Bierman R, Beardsley L, Chang CJ, Burk RD. (1998) Natural history of cervicovaginal papillomavirus infection in young women. *N Engl J Med* **338**: 423–8.

75. Ho GY, Kadish AS, Burk RD, *et al* (1998) HPV 16 and cigarette smoking as risk factors for high-grade cervical intra-epithelial neoplasia. *Int J Cancer* **78**: 281–5.

76. Holcomb K, Maiman M, Dimaio T, Gates J. (1998) Rapid progression to invasive cervix cancer in a woman infected with the human immunodeficiency virus. *Obstet Gynecol* **91**: 848–50.

77. Johnson JC, Bumett AF, Willet GD, Young MA, Doniger J. (1992) High frequency of latent and clinical human papillomavirus cervical infection in immuno-compromised human immunodeficiency virus-infected women. *Obstet Gynecol* **79**: 321–7.

78. Katoh T, Nagata N, Kuroda Y, *et al.* (1996) Glutathione S-transferase M1 (GSTM1) and T1 (GSTT1) genetic polymorphism and susceptibility to gastric and colorectal adenocarcinoma. *Carcinogenesis* **17**: 1855–9.

79. Ketterer B, Harris JM, Talaska G, *et al.* (1992) The human glutathione S-transferase supergene family, its polymorphism, and its effects on susceptibility to lung cancer. *Environ Health Perspect* **98**: 87–94.

80. Khare S, Pater MM, Pater A. (1995) Role of exogenous cofactors in HPV infection and oncogenesis. *Papillomavirus Rep* **6**: 89–93.

81. Kjellberg L, Hallmans G, Ahren AM, *et al.* (2000) Smoking, diet, pregnancy and oral contraceptive use as risk factors for cervical intra-epithelial neoplasia in relation to human papillomavirus infection. *Br J Cancer* **82**: 1332–8.

82. Kuhn L, Sun XW, Wright TC Jr. (1999) Human immunodeficiency virus infection and female lower genital tract malignancy. *Curr Opin Obstet Gynecol* **11**: 35–9.

83. Kyo S, Inoue M, Hayasaka N, *et al.* (1994) Regulation of early gene expression of human papillomavirus type 16 by inflammatory cytokines. *Virology* **200**: 130–9.

84. Kyo S, Inoue M, Nishio Y, Nakanishi K, *et al.* (1993) NF-IL6 represses early gene expression of human papillomavirus type 16 through binding to the noncoding region. *J Virol* **67**: 1058–66.

85. Lacey HB, Wilson GE, Tilston P, *et al.* (1999) A study of anal intraepithelial neoplasia in HIV positive homosexual men. *Sex Tran Inf* **75**: 172–7.

86. Landis SH, Murray T, Bolden S, Wingo PA. (1998) Cancer statistics, 1998 [published errata appear in *CA Cancer J Clin* (1998) **48**(3): 192; and (1998) **48**(6): 329]. *CA Cancer J Clin* **48**: 6–29.

87. Lang M, Pelkonen O. (1999) Metabolism of xenobiotics and chemical carcinogenesis. Cleveland, OH, IARC Science Publications, 13–22.

88. Lee B-N, Ordonez N, Popek EJ, *et al.* (1997) Inflammatory cytokine expression is correlated with the level of human immunodeficiency virus (HIV) transcripts in HIV-infected placental trophoblastic cells. *J Virol* **71**: 3628–35.

89. Lengauer C, Kinzler KW, Vogelstein B. (1998) Genetic instabilities in human cancers. *Nature* **396**: 643–9.

90. Levy DE. (1998) Analysis of interferon-regulated proteins binding the interferon-alpha-stimulated response element. *Methods* **15**: 167–74.

91. Luque AE, Demeter LM, Reichman RC. (1999) Association of human papillomavirus infection and disease with magnitude of human immunodeficiency virus type 1 (HIV-1) RNA plasma levels among women with HIV-1 infection. *J Infect Dis* **179**: 1405–9.

92. Magnusson PK, Sparen P, Gyllensten UB. (1999) Genetic link to cervical tumours. *Nature* **400**: 29–30.

93. Maiman M, Fruchter RG, Clark M, Arrastia CD, Matthews R, Gates EJ. (1997) Cervical cancer as an AIDS-defining illness. *Obstet Gynecol* **89**: 76–80.

94. Maiman M, Fruchter RG, Guy L, Cuthill S, Levine P, Serur E. (1993) Human immunodeficiency virus infection and invasive cervical carcinoma. *Cancer* **71**: 402–6.

95. Maiman M, Fruchter RG, Serur E, Remy JC, Feuer G, Boyce J. (1990) Human immunodeficiency virus infection and cervical neoplasia. *Gynecol Oncol* **38**: 377–82.

96. Majewski S, Jablonska S. (1998) Immunology of HPV infection and HPV-associated tumors. *Int J Dermatol* **37**: 81–95.

97. Mannervik B, Danielson UH. (1988) Glutathione transferases – structure and catalytic activity. *CRC Crit Rev Biochem* **23**: 283–337.

98. Martinez C, Agundez JA, Olivera M, *et al.* (1998) Influence of genetic admixture on polymorphisms of drug-metabolizing enzymes: analyses of mutations on NAT2 and C gamma P2E1 genes in a mixed Hispanic population. *Clin Pharmacol Ther* **63**: 623–8.

99. Maugard CM, Charrier J, Bignon YJ. (1998) Allelic deletion at glutathione S-transferase M1 locus and its association with breast cancer susceptibility. *Chem Biol Interact* **111–112**: 365–75.

100. McIndoe WA, McLean MR, Jones RW, Mullins PR. (1984) The invasive potential of carcinoma in situ of the cervix. *Obstet Gynecol* **64**: 451–8.

101. Memar O, Arany I, Tyring SK. (1995) Skin associated lymphoid tissue in HIV-1, HPV and HSV infections. *J Invest Dermatol* **105**: 99S–104S.

102. Meroni L, Trabattoni D, Balotta C, *et al.* (1996) Evidence for type 2 cytokine production and lymphocyte activation in the early phases of HIV-1 infection. *AIDS* **10**: 23–30.

103. Minkoff H, Feldman J, DeHovitz J, Landesman S, Burk R. (1998) A longitudinal study of human papillomavirus carriage in human immunodeficiency virus-infected and human immunodeficiency virus-uninfected women. *Am J Obstet Gynecol* **178**: 982–6.

104. Morrison EA. (1994) Natural history of cervical infection with human papillomaviruses. *Clin Infect Dis* **18**: 172–80.

105. Nawa A, Nishiyama Y, Yamamoto N, Maeno K, Goto S, Tomoda Y. (1990) Selective suppression of human papilloma virus type 18 mRNA level in HeLa cells by interferon. *Biochem Biophys Res Commun* **170**: 793–9.

106. Nuovo GJ, Forde A, MacConnell DD, Fahrenwald R. (1993) *In situ* detection of PCR-amplified HIV-1 nucleic acids and tumor necrosis factor cDNA in cervical tissues. *Am J Pathol* **143**: 40–8.

107. Olaitan A, Johnson MA, Reid WM, Poulter LW. (1998) Changes to the cytokine microenvironment in the genital tract mucosa of HIV+ women. *Clin Exp Immunol* **112**: 100–4.

108. Olsen AO, Dillner J, Skrondal A, Magnus P. (1998) Combined effect of smoking and human papillomavirus type 16 infection in cervical carcinogenesis. *Epidemiology* **9**: 346–9.

109. Omiecinski CJ, Aicher L, Swenson L. (1994) Developmental expression of human microsomal epoxide hydrolase. *J Pharmacol Exp Ther* **269**: 417–23.

110. Ozsaran AA, Ates T, Dikmen Y, *et al.* (1999) Evaluation of the risk of cervical intraepithelial neoplasia and human papilloma virus infection in renal transplant patients receiving immunosuppressive therapy. *Eur J Gynaecol Oncol* **20**: 127–30.

111. Palefsky JM, Holly EA, Hogeboom CJ, *et al.* (1998) Virologic, immunologic, and clinical parameters in the incidence and progression of anal squamous intraepithelial lesions in HIV-positive and HIV-negative homosexual men. *J AIDS Hum Retrovirol* **17**: 314–19.

112. Palefsky JM, Holly EA, Ralston ML, *et al.* (1998) Anal squamous intraepithelial lesions in HIV-positive and HIV-negative homosexual and bisexual men. *J AIDS Hum Retrovirol* **17**: 320–6.

113. Palefsky JM, Holly EA, Ralston ML, Jay N. (1998) Prevalence and risk factors for human papillomavirus infection of the anal canal in human immunodeficiency virus (HIV)-positive and HIV-negative homosexual men. *J Infect Dis* **177**: 361–7.

114. Parker SL, Davis KJ, Wingo PA, Ries LA, Heath CWJ. (1998) Cancer statistics by race and ethnicity. *CA Cancer J Clin* **48**: 31–48.

115. Persson I, Johansson I, Bergling H, *et al.* (1993) Genetic polymorphism of cytochrome P4502E1 in a Swedish population. Relationship to incidence of lung cancer. *FEBS Lett* **319**: 207–11.

116. Pim D, Storey A, Thomas M, Massimi P, Banks L. (1994) Mutational analysis of HPV-18 E6 identifies domains required for p53 degradation in vitro, abolition of p53 transactivation in vivo and immortalisation of primary BMK cells. *Oncogene* **9**: 1869–76.

117. Ponten J, Guo Z. (1998) Precancer of the human cervix. *Cancer Surv* **32**: 201–29.

118. Prokopczyk B, Cox JE, Hoffmann D, Waggoner SE. (1997) Identification of tobacco-specific carcinogen in the cervical mucus of smokers and nonsmokers. *J Natl Cancer Inst* **89**: 868–73.

119. Raunio H, Husgafvel-Pursiainen K, Anttila S, Hietanen E, Hirvonen A, Pelkonen O. (1995) Diagnosis of polymorphisms in carcinogen-activating and inactivating enzymes and cancer susceptibility – a review. *Gene* **159**: 113–21.

120. Reka S, Garro ML, Kotler DP. (1994) Variation in the expression of human immunodeficiency virus RNA and cytokine mRNA in rectal mucosa during the progression of infection. *Lymphokine Cytokine Res* **13**: 391–8.

121. Rezza G, Giuliani M, Serraino D, *et al.* (1998) Risk factors for cervical presence of human papillomavirus DNA among women at risk for HIV infection. DIANAIDS Collaborative Study Group. *Epidemiol Infect* **121**: 173–7.

122. Romagnani S, Maggi E. (1994) Th1 versus Th2 responses in AIDS. *Curr Opin Immunol* **6**: 616–22.

123. Sadowski HB, Shuai K, Damell JE Jr, Gilman MZ. (1993) A common nuclear signal transduction pathway activated by growth factor and cytokine receptors. *Science* **261**: 1739–44.

124. Sato T, Selleri C, Young NS, Maciejewski JP. (1997) Inhibition of interferon regulatory factor-1 expression results in predominance of cell growth stimulatory effects of interferon, due to phosphorylation of Stat 1 and Stat 3. *Blood* **90**: 4749–58.

125. Schafer A Friedmann W, Mielke M, Schwartlander B, Koch MA. (1991) The increased frequency of cervical dysplasia–neoplasia in women infected with the human immunodeficiency virus is related to the degree of immunosuppression. *Am J Obstet Gynecol* **164**: 593–9.

126. Schiffman MH, Brinton LA. (1995) The epidemiology of cervical carcinogenesis. *Cancer* **76**(10 Suppl.): 1888–901.

127. Schneider A. (1994) Natural history of genital papillomavirus infections. *Intervirology* **37**: 201–14.

128. Schneider A, Kirchhoff T, Meinhardt G, Gissmann L. (1992) Repeated evaluation of human papillomavirus 16 status in cervical swabs of young women with a history of normal Papanicolaou smears. *Obstet Gynecol* **79**: 683–8.

129. Seidegard J, DePierre JW. (1983) Microsomal epoxide hydrolase. Properties, regulation and function. *Biochim Biophys Acta* **695**: 251–70.

130. Serraino D, Carrieri P, Pradier C, *et al.* (1999) Risk of invasive cervical cancer among women with, or at risk for, HIV infection. *Int J Cancer* **82**: 334–7.

131. Sha BE, D'Amico RD, Landay AL, *et al.* (1997) Evaluation of immunologic markers in cervicovaginal fluid of HIV-infected and uninfected women: implications for the immunologic response to HIV in the female genital tract. *J Acquir Immune Defic Syndr Hum Retrovirol* **16**: 161–8.

132. Shamanin V, zur Hausen H, Lavergne D, *et al.* (1996) Human papillomavirus infections in nonmelanoma skin cancers from renal transplant recipients and nonimmunosuppressed patients. *J Natl Cancer Inst* **88**: 802–11.

133. Sillman FH, Sedlis A. (1991) Anogenital papillomavirus infection and neoplasia in immunodeficient women: an update. *Dermatol Clin* **9**: 353–69.

134. Simons AM, Phillips DH, Coleman DV. (1993) Damage to DNA in cervical epithelium related to smoking tobacco. *BMJ* **306**: 1444–8.

135. Sims P, Grover PL, Swaisland A, Pal K, Hewer A. (1974) Metabolic activation of benzo(a)pyrene proceeds by a diol-epoxide. *Nature* **252**: 326–8.

136. Six C, Heard I, Bergeron C, Orth G, *et al.* (1998) Comparative prevalence, incidence and short-term prognosis of cervical squamous intraepithelial lesions amongst HIV-positive and HIV-negative women. *AIDS* **12**: 1047–56.

137. Spinillo A, Tenti P, Zappatore R, *et al.* (1992) Prevalence, diagnosis and treatment of lower genital neoplasia in women with human immunodeficiency virus infection. *Eur J Obstet Gynecol Reprod Biol* **43**: 235–41.

138. Stanley MA, Chambers MA, Coleman N. (1995) Immunology of human papillomavirus infection, In *Genital warts. Human papillomavirus infection,* ed. A. Mindel. London, Edward Arnold, 252–70.

139. Stark GR, Kerr IM, Williams BRG, Silverman RH, Schreiber RD. (1998) How cells respond to interferons. *Ann Rev Biochem* **67**: 227–64.

140. Starr R, Hilton DJ. (1999) Negative regulation of the JAK/STAT pathway. *Bioessays* **21**: 47–52.

141. Starr R, Willson TA, Viney EM, *et al.* (1997) A family of cytokine-inducible inhibitors of signaling. *Nature* **387**: 917–21.

142. Stylianou E, Aukrust P, Kvale D, Muller, F, Froland SS. (1999) IL-10 in HIV infection: increasing serum IL-10 levels with disease progression – down-regulatory effect of potent anti-retroviral therapy. *Clin Exp Immunol* **116**: 115–20.

143. Sun XW, Kuhn L, Ellerbrock TV, Chiasson MA, Bush TJ, Wright TC Jr. (1997) Human papillomavirus infection in women infected with the human immunodeficiency virus. *N Engl J Med* **337**: 1343–9.

144. Svare EI, Kjaer SK, Smits HL, Poll P, Tjong AHS, ter Schegget J. (1998) Risk factors for HPV detection in archival Pap smears. A population-based study from Greenland and Denmark. *Eur J Cancer* **34**: 1230–4.

145. Szarewski A, Jarvis MJ, Sasieni P, *et al.* (1996) Effect of smoking cessation on cervical lesion size. *Lancet* **347**: 941–3.

146. Tornesello ML, Buonaguro FM, Beth-Giraldo E, Giraldo G. (1993) Human immunodeficiency virus type 1 *tat* gene enhances human papillomavirus early gene expression. *Intervirology* **36**: 57–64.

147. Tortolero-Luna G. (1999) Epidemiology of genital human papillomavirus. *Hematol Oncol Clin North Am* **13**: 245–57.

148. Tsutsumi M, Wang JS, Takase S, Takada A. (1994) Hepatic messenger RNA contents of cytochrome P4502E1 in patients with different P4502E1 genotypes. *Alcohol Alcohol* **29**(Suppl 1): 29–32.

149. Tyring SK, Arany I, Stanley MA, *et al.* (1998) A randomized, controlled, molecular study of condyloma acuminata clearance during treatment with imiquimod. *J Infect Dis* **178**: 551–5.

150. Uematsu F, Kikuchi H, Ohmachi T, *et al.* (1991) Two common RFLPs of the human CYP2E gene. *Nucleic Acids Res* **19**: 2803.

151. Unger ER, Vernon SD, Lee DR, *et al.* (1997) Human papillomavirus type in anal epithelial lesions is influenced by human immunodeficiency virus. *Arch Pathol Lab Med* **121**: 820–4.

152. Vernon SD, Hart CE, Reeves WC, Icenogle JP. (1993) The HIV-1 *tat* protein enhances E2-dependent human papillomavirus 16 transcription. *Virus Res* **27**: 133–45.

153. Vernon SD, Zaki SR, Reeves WC. (1994) Localization of HIV-1 to human papillomavirus associated cervical lesions [letter]. *Lancet* **344**: 954–5.

154. Vineis P, Malats N, Boffetta P. (1999) *Why study metabolic susceptibility to cancer?* Cleveland, OH, IARC Science Publishers, 1–3.

155. Wallin KL, Wiklund F, Angstrom T, *et al.* (1999) Type-specific persistence of human papillomavirus DNA before the development of invasive cervical cancer. *N Engl J Med* **341**: 1633–8.

156. Wang F, Sengupta TK, Zhong Z, Ivashkiv LB. (1995) Regulation of the balance of cytokine production and the signal transducer and activator of transcription (STAT) transcription factor activity by cytokines and inflammatory synovial fluids. *J Exp Med* **182**: 1825–31.

157. Warwick A, Sarhanis P, Redman C, *et al.* (1994) Theta class glutathione S-transferase GSTT1 genotypes and susceptibility to cervical neoplasia: interactions with GSTM1, CYP2D6 and smoking. *Carcinogenesis* **15**: 2841–5.

158. Watanabe J, Hayashi S, Kawajiri K. (1994) Different regulation and expression of the human CYP2E1 gene due to the RsaI polymorphism in the 5′-flanking region. *J Biochem (Tokyo)* **116**: 321–6.

159. Werness BA, Levine AJ, Howley PM. (1990) Association of human papillomavirus types 16 and 18 E6 proteins with p53. *Science* **248**: 76–9.

160. Wheeler CM, Parmenter CA, Hunt WC, *et al.* (1993) Determinants of genital human papillomavirus infection among cytologically normal women attending the University of New Mexico student health center. *Sex Transm Dis* **20**: 286–9.

161. Wiencke JK, Wrensch MR, Miike R, Zuo Z, Kelsey KT. (1997) Population-based study of glutathione S-transferase mu gene deletion in adult glioma cases and controls. *Carcinogenesis* **18**: 1431–3.

162. Woodworth CD, Chung J, McMullin E, Plowman GD, Simpson S, Iglesias M. (1996) Transforming growth factor β1 supports autonomous growth of human papillomavirus-immortalized cervical keratinocytes under conditions promoting cellular differentiation. *Cell Growth Diff* **7**: 811–20.

163. Wormhoudt LW, Commandeur JN, Vermeulen NP. (1999) Genetic polymorphisms of human N-acetyltransferase, cytochrome P450, glutathione-S-transferase, and epoxide hydrolase enzymes: relevance to xenobiotic metabolism and toxicity. *Crit Rev Toxicol* **29**: 59–124.

164. Wu X, Shi H, Jiang H, *et al.* (1997) Associations between cytochrome P4502E1 genotype, mutagen sensitivity, cigarette smoking and susceptibility to lung cancer. *Carcinogenesis* **18**: 967–73.

165. Zhong S, Wyllie AH, Barnes D, Wolf CR, Spurr NK. (1993) Relationship between the GSTM1 genetic polymorphism and susceptibility to bladder, breast and colon cancer. *Carcinogenesis* **14**: 1821–4.

166. zur Hausen H. (1996) Papillomavirus infections – a major cause of human cancers. *Biochem Biophys Acta* **1288**: F55–78.

Index

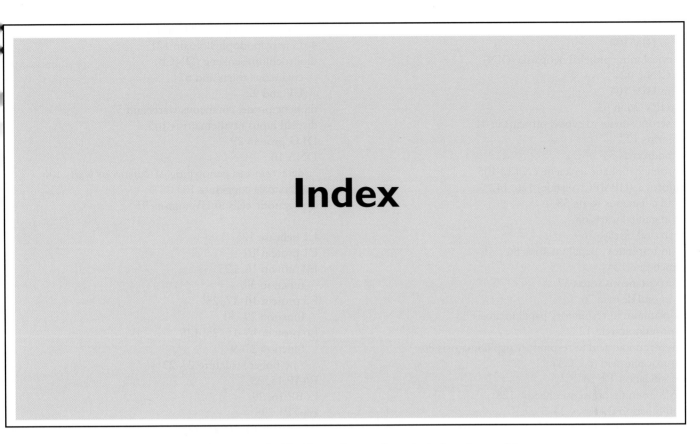

Page references in **bold** refer to figures; those in *italics* refer to tables